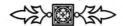

PRINCIPLES OF PUBLIC HEALTH PRACTICE

F. Douglas Scutchfield, M.D.
Graduate School of Public Health
College of Health & Human Services
San Diego State University
San Diego, California

C. William Keck, M.D., M.P.H.
Director of Health
Akron Health Department
Akron, Ohio

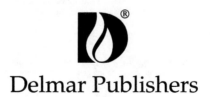

Delmar Publishers

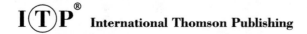 **International Thomson Publishing**

Albany • Bonn • Boston • Cincinnati • Detroit • London • Madrid
Melbourne • Mexico City • New York • Pacific Grove • Paris • San Francisco
Singapore • Tokyo • Toronto • Washington

Notice to the Reader

Publisher does not warrant or guarantee any of the products described herein or perform any independent analysis in connection with any of the product information contained herein. Publisher does not assume, and expressly disclaims, any obligation to obtain and include information other than that provided to it by the manufacturer.

The reader is expressly warned to consider and adopt all safety precautions that might be indicated by the activities herein and to avoid all potential hazards. By following the instructions contained herein, the reader willingly assumes all risks in connection with such instructions.

The publisher makes no representation or warranties of any kind, including but not limited to, the warranties of fitness for particular purpose or merchantability, nor are any such representations implied with respect to the material set forth herein, and the publisher takes no responsibility with respect to such material. The publisher shall not be liable for any special, consequential, or exemplary damages resulting, in whole or part, from the readers' use of, or reliance upon, this material.

Delmar Staff

Cover Design: *Carol D. Keohane*
Publisher: *William Brottmiller*
Editor: *Bill Burgower*
Assistant Editor: *Hilary Schrauf*
Project Editor: *Timothy Coleman*
Production Coordinator: *James Zayicek*
Art and Design Coordinator: *Carol D. Keohane*
Editorial Assistant: *Diane Biondi*

For more information, contact:

Delmar Publishers Inc.
3 Columbia Circle, Box 15015
Albany, New York 12212-5015

International Thomson Publishing
Berkshire House 168-173
168-173 High Holborn
London, WC1V7AA
England

Thomas Nelson Australia
102 Dodds Street
South Melbourne 3205
Victoria, Australia

Nelson Canada
1120 Birchmont Road
Scarborough, Ontario
Canada, M1K 5G4

International Thomson Editores
Campos Eliseos 385, Piso 7
Col Polanco
11560 Mexico D F Mexico

International Thomson Publishing GmbH
Konigswinterer Strasse. 418
53227 Bonn
Germany

International Thomson Publishing Asia
221 Henderson Road
#05-10 Henderson Building
Singapore 0315

International Thomson Publishing—Japan
Hirakawacho Kyowa Building, 3F
2-2-1 Hirakawacho
Chiyoda-ku, Tokyo 102
Japan

1 2 3 4 5 6 7 8 9 10 XXX 02 01 00 99 98 97 96

Library of Congress Cataloging-in-Publication Data

Scutchfield, F. Douglas.
    Principles of public health practice / F. Douglas Scutchfield, C.
  William Keck
        p.   cm.
    Includes bibliographical references and index.
    ISBN 0-8273-6271-4
    1. Public health administration—United States.   2. Public health.
  I. Keck, C. William.   II. Title.
  RA445.S44 1996
  362.1'0973—dc20   94-14785
                                                       CIP

This text is dedicated to two groups of individuals. The first is our wives, Phyllis and Ardith, for their patience and support during the preparation of this book. It was from them that we stole the nights and weekends to edit and write this text. Without their love and support, it would not be in your hands.

If we are able to see far, it is because we had mentors who allowed and encouraged us to stand on their shoulders. We also dedicate this book to them. They include Abram Benenson, Kurt Deutschel, William Foege, John Hanlon, Alex Langmuir, William McBeath, George Pickett, and William Willard.

Online Services

Delmar Online
To access a wide variety of Delmar products and services on the World Wide Web, point your browser to:
> **http://www.delmar.com/delmar.html**
> or email: info@delmar.com

thomson.com
To access International Thomson Publishing's home site for information on more than 34 publishers and 20,000 products, point your browser to:
> **http://www.thomson.com**
> or email: findit@kiosk.thomson.com

A service of I(T)P®

INTRODUCTION
TO THE SERIES

This Series in Health Services is now in its second decade of providing top quality teaching materials to the health administration/public health field. Each year has witnessed further strengthening of the market position of each of the principal books in the series, also reflecting the continued excellences of the products. Each author, book editor, and contributor to the series has helped build what is widely recognized as the top textbook and issues collection of books available in this field today.

But we have achieved only a beginning. Everyone involved in the series is committed to further expansion of the scope, technical excellence, and usability of the series. Our goal is to do more for you, the reader. We will add new books in important areas, seek out more excellent authors, and increase the physical attributes of the books to make them easier for you to use.

We thank everyone, the authors and users in particular, who have made this series so successful and so widely used. And we promise that this second decade will be dedicated to further expansion of the series and to enhancement of the books it contains to provide still greater value to you, our constituency.

Stephen J. Williams
Series Editor

DELMAR SERIES IN HEALTH SERVICES ADMINISTRATION

Stephen J. Williams, Sc.D., Series Editor

FOREWORD

◈

Public health has never received the recognition it deserves. The late nineteenth and the twentieth century have been referred to as the "Age of Modern Medical Miracles," yet it was not these miracles of high technology that brought this nation to the health status it now enjoys. Instead, it was public health advances that accomplished that: clean water, proper housing, immunization, eradication of smallpox, increased life expectancy, and the understanding of preventive medicine as exemplified by healthy lifestyle choices.

In recent years, when everyone seems to be an expert in the requirements for health care reform, public health measures still receive little recognition and even less money. Not quite three percent of the nation's total health care expenditure is allocated to public health and preventive medicine, despite the fact that 70 percent of the nation's premature mortality is related to issues amenable to public health preventive interventions.

The United States Public Health Service has articulated the goals for a healthy nation and outlined them well in *Healthy People: the Surgeon General's Report* as well as in *Health Promotion/Disease Prevention: Objectives for the Nation*. A few enlightened leaders have heard that message and acted upon it but not nearly to the extent this nation deserves. The Institute of Medicine also provided encouragement and direction for the revitalization of our nation's public health system in its report, *The Future of Public Health*.

The report from the Institute of Medicine defined the role of public health as assessing health status, defining health policy options, and assuring access to necessary services. In order for public health to be successful in these roles, it is imperative that there be a well–educated and competent public health workforce. There is no lack of tools with which to work. Indeed, there has been a knowledge explosion in the public health basic sciences, which provides contemporary practitioners with a list of options aimed at improving the health status of the public that was not available to their forebears.

There are nearly half a million individuals in the current public health workforce, but only a small proportion of these workers have received formal education in public health. Many of those without a formal educational background rely on informal, on the job learning experience and on continuing education activities to keep them up to speed. In the years I was Surgeon General, I was keenly aware of the need to keep current the knowledge of those charged with promoting and protecting the public's health. At least in the commissioned corps of the United States Public Health Service, we attempted to assure that our officers had the best public health professional education available.

There are 143 schools of medicine and osteopathic medicine in the United States training practitioners to treat injury and illness and return people to a previous status of health, without making much effort to take them beyond that. There are only 27 schools of public health, training practitioners to keep people well and teach them to prevent disease. Currently, about $35,000 in federal funds per year is spent on each physician's education, but only $35 on the education of a public health worker. This economic disparity illustrates the lack of balance in emphasizing treatment rather than prevention.

It is obvious, therefore, that there is an important role for a book that synthesizes state-of-the-art information about public health practice for the benefit of both students and current practitioners. I believe that Drs. Scutchfield and Keck have provided such a book. They have brought together the wisdom of many of the most knowledgeable health professionals in North America to provide the best information possible about current public health organizations and practice. For the new student, the book provides an introduction to the field of public health practice. For the current practitioner, it is a unique and vital reference. Those who make public health policy should not do so without understanding the content of this book. Only when there are enough knowledgeable and committed individuals will deplorable human suffering and unaffordable economic costs be prevented. This book is a step in that direction.

C. Everett Koop, M.D., Sc.D.
Surgeon General 1981 to 1989

PREFACE

Over the past 15 years an interesting dichotomy has developed in the field of public health. On the one hand, the contributions made by public health measures to the improvement of health status in the United States have been documented and increasingly appreciated, and the potential for future improvement has been recognized. On the other hand, those contributions have largely been taken for granted, and public health expenditures have been slashed as part of the effort to control governmental spending at the local, state, and federal levels. This has resulted in a growing awareness of the potential improvements that still can be made to the public's health, while, at the same time, the capacity of the "delivery system" in state and local health departments has been diminished.

Today's public health practitioner faces a changing and somewhat ambiguous environment. Possibilities are exciting, but resources are limited. Government's role is paramount, but there is public mistrust of government. Health reform is on the public's mind, but the focus is on illness care rather than health promotion and disease prevention. New public health crises call for effective responses, but the public is divided on priorities for action.

Successful management of health departments and other community health agencies will require enlightened and strong leadership. Public health leaders will need to understand the contributions that can be made by the application of public health principles to community health problems, to work with communities to involve them in understanding and addressing the problems that threaten them, and to engineer constructive evolution of their agencies to effectively perform in a changing and uncertain environment.

There are about 500,000 individuals employed as public health workers at all levels of government in the United States. Very few of these professionals have formal public health training or even share a common academic base. There are wide variations in the capacity of local health departments across the country, and there is uncertainty about the future place of public health departments in society. Nonetheless, improvement of the public's health will require that the core functions of public health be competently executed. A cadre of public health leaders must emerge, therefore, with a clear vision of public health's place in maintaining and improving health and with the skills required to make that vision a reality. This combination of problems and opportunities suggested to us the need for a modern text in public health practice and administration.

This book is designed to appeal principally to two audiences. The first is the public health professional who has come to work in the public health environment without having a formal exposure to course work in public health practice and administration or who wishes to have available a review of recent developments in the field. The second is students of the public health professions who would benefit from access to a broad text describing the organization, administration, and practice of public health.

The book is organized into five major sections. The first describes the current public health environment by introducing the reader to the concepts and development of public health practice, the factors that determine health status, and the legal concepts on which public health practice is based. The second tallies the contributions made to public health at the federal, state, and local levels and describes a number of our most prominent public health professional organizations. The third section contains chapters that describe and discuss the tools available to manage a typical health department well. The fourth section describes public health practice in a number of substantive areas. The topics are not all-inclusive, but an attempt has been made to include those that are serious problems nationally. The final section focuses on the role of the public health department in an evolving health system and suggests a vision of the ideal health department of the future.

ACKNOWLEDGMENTS

There are many people who have made important contributions to the successful completion of this book. The contributing authors merit the largest share of our gratitude, of course. The field of public health is broad and ever changing, and we felt the need to call widely on the expertise of many of our colleagues. Their willingness to participate with us in this endeavor is appreciated, as is their positive response to editing suggestions we made.

We especially thank Sue Phillips of the Akron Health Department for her skilled work in formatting chapter drafts received in a variety of styles and electronic word processing packages into a single, consistently typed document meeting our publisher's requirements. We also thank Neil Casey of the Akron Health Department for his assistance with several difficult computer program conversions and the Akron Health Commission for its understanding and support of this project.

The clerical staff of the Graduate School of Public Health at San Diego deserves our thanks for its yeomanly efforts to assure that this book reached the publication stage. In addition, we wish to thank faculty colleagues at many institutions for their review of and comments on our efforts. Our editors, Bill Burgower and Debra Flis, deserve special mention for their help and support in the preparation of this manuscript.

CONTENTS

CONTRIBUTORS

Myron Allukian, Jr., D.D.S., M.P.H.
Assistant Deputy Commissioner and Director
Bureau of Community Dental Programs
Boston Department of Health and Hospitals
Boston, Massachusetts

Trude Bennett, Dr.P.H.
Assistant Professor
Department of Maternal and Child Health
School of Public Health
University of North Carolina at Chapel Hill
Chapel Hill, North Carolina

Edward Brandt, M.D., Ph.D.
Professor, Health Administration and Policy
Director, Center for Health Policy
The University of Oklahoma Health Sciences Center
Oklahoma City, Oklahoma

Ronald L. Cada, Dr.P.H.
Director of Laboratories
Colorado Department of Health
Denver, Colorado

Terry L. Conway, Ph.D.
Research Director
San Diego State University
Graduate School of Public Health
San Diego, California

Alan Cross, M.D., M.P.H.
Professor of Social Medicine and Pediatrics
Director of the Center for Health Promotion
& Disease Prevention
University of North Carolina at Chapel Hill
Chapel Hill, North Carolina

Susan Dandoy, M.D., M.P.H.
Director
Virginia Beach Health Department
Virginia Beach, Virginia

Richard C. Dicker, M.D., M.Sc.
Chief, Epidemiology Training Activity
Division of Training
Epidemiology Program Office
Centers for Disease Control and Prevention
Atlanta, Georgia

Lori Dorfman, Dr.P.H.
Associate Director
Berkeley Media Studies Group
University of California, Berkeley
Berkeley, California

Christine C. Edwards, M.P.H.
Project Director
San Diego State University
Graduate School of Public Health
San Diego, California

John P. Elder, Ph.D., M.P.H.
Professor
Graduate School of Public Health
San Diego State University
San Diego, California

Gregory A. Ervin, M.P.H.
Deputy Director of Health
Akron Health Department
Akron, Ohio

Elizabeth Fee, Ph.D.
Professor of History and Health Policy
Johns Hopkins University School of Public Health
Baltimore, Maryland

Dominic Frissora, M.P.A.
Team Leader of Administrative Support
Rehabilitation Services Commission of Ohio
Columbus, Ohio

Larry J. Gordon, M.S., M.P.H.
Visiting Professor of Public Administration
University of New Mexico
Albuquerque, New Mexico

Robert G. Harmon, M.D., M.P.H.
Senior Vice President for Medical Services
Center for Corporate Health, Inc.
Oakton, Virginia

Jeffrey R. Harris, M.D., M.P.H.
Associate Director for Program Development
National Center for Chronic Disease Prevention
and Health Promotion
Centers for Disease Control and Prevention
Atlanta, Georgia

Alan R. Hinman, M.D.
Assistant Surgeon General
Director, Center for Prevention Services
Centers for Disease Control and Prevention
Atlanta, Georgia

Martha F. Katz, M.P.A.
Associate Director for Policy, Planning
and Evaluation
Centers for Disease Control and Prevention
Atlanta, Georgia

C. William Keck, M.D., M.P.H.
Director of Health
Akron Health Department
Akron, Ohio

Jeffrey P. Koplan, M.D., M.P.H.
Executive Vice President and Director
The Prudential Center for Health Care Research
Atlanta, Georgia

Marshall W. Kreuter, Ph.D.
Director
Health 2000
Atlanta, Georgia

John M. Last, M.D., D.P.H.
Emeritus Professor of Epidemiology
and Community Medicine
University of Ottawa
Ottawa, Canada

Deborah R. Maiese, M.P.A.
Senior Prevention Policy Advisor
United States Public Health Service
Washington, D.C.

J. Michael McGinnis, M.D.
Deputy Assistant Secretary for Health
Disease Prevention and Health Promotion
United States Public Health Service
Washington, D.C.

David V. McQueen, Sc.D.
Chief, Behavioral Surveillance Branch
Office of Surveillance and Analysis
National Center for Chronic Disease Prevention
and Health Promotion
Centers for Disease Control and Prevention
Atlanta, Georgia

James F. Mosher, J.D.
Research Fellow
The Marin Institute for the Prevention of Alcohol
and Other Drug Problems
San Rafael, California

K. Michael Peddecord, Dr.P.H.
Professor of Public Health and Director,
Laboratory Assurance Program
Graduate School of Public Health
San Diego State University
San Diego, California

Dennis D. Pointer, Ph.D.
Hanlon Professor of Health Services
Research and Policy
Graduate School of Public Health
San Diego State University
San Diego, California

Katharine C. Rathbun, M.D., M.P.H.
Associate Professor
Community and Family Medicine
University of Missouri at
Kansas City School of Medicine
Kansas City, Missouri

Nancy Rawding, M.P.H.
Executive Director
National Association of County and City Health
Officials
Washington, D.C.

Edward P. Richards, III, J.D., M.P.H.
Professor of Law
University of Missouri at Kansas City School of Law
Kansas City, Missouri

Mark L. Rosenberg, M.D., M.P.A.
Director, National Center for Injury Prevention and
Control
Centers for Disease Control and Prevention
Atlanta, Georgia

Julianne P. Sanchez, M.S.
Doctoral Candidate
Department of Sociology
University of Washington
Seattle, Washington

F. Douglas Scutchfield, M.D.
Graduate School of Public Health
San Diego State University
San Diego, California

David A. Sleet, Ph.D.
Acting Director, Division of Unintentional
Injury Prevention
National Center for Injury Prevention and Control
Centers for Disease Control and Prevention
Atlanta, Georgia

Carl W. Tyler, Jr., M.D.
Assistant Director for Academic Programs
Public Health Practice Program Office
Centers for Disease Control and Prevention
Atlanta, Georgia

Lawrence Wallack, Dr.P.H.
Professor of Public Health
Director, Berkeley Media Studies Group
University of California, Berkeley
Berkeley, California

Martin Wasserman, M.D., J.D.
Secretary
Maryland Department of Health and Mental Hygiene
Baltimore, Maryland

Katie Woodruff, M.P.H.
Program Assistant
Berkeley Media Studies Group
University of California, Berkeley
Berkeley, California

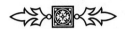

PART ONE

THE BASIS OF PUBLIC HEALTH

CHAPTER

Concepts and Definitions of Public Health Practice

F. Douglas Scutchfield, M.D.
C. William Keck, M.D., M.P.H.

The World Health Organization has defined health as ". . . a complete state of physical, mental, and social well-being and not merely the absence of disease or infirmity."[1] Societies that approach this ideal state will do so by appropriately balancing services for the diagnosis and treatment of illness with services that promote health and prevent disease.

Unfortunately, our current *system* of providing health services in the United States is unbalanced: it is tilted strongly toward interacting with people who are ill. This system, focused as it is on illness care, is not prepared to deal with the social issues that affect health. It is likely, for example, that health status is more closely linked to socioeconomic status and its attendant problems than to any other factor. Thus, improvement in our nation's health status will depend more on the ef-

fective application of public health techniques than on taking care of people who are ill.

This text is about public health. Public health is defined by John Last as:

> . . . one of the efforts organized by society to protect, promote, and restore the people's health. It is a combination of sciences, skills, and beliefs that are directed to the maintenance and improvement of the health of all the people through collective or social actions. The programs, services and institutions involved emphasize the prevention of disease and the health needs of the population as a whole. Public health activities change with changing technology and social values, but the goals remain the same: to reduce the amount of disease, premature death, and disease-produced discomfort and disability in the population. Public health is thus a social institution, a discipline and a practice.[2]

This chapter describes the discipline of public health and introduces concepts, problem areas, and approaches to problem solving that are part of public health practice. These issues, and others, will be referenced repeatedly and/or discussed in greater detail in subsequent chapters.

SCIENCE, SKILLS, AND BELIEFS

The scientific basis for public health rests on the study of risks to the health of populations (including risks related to the environment) and on the systems designed to deliver required services. Epidemiology and biostatistics are the scientific disciplines that underpin inquiry in all of public health. They provide the methods necessary for understanding the risks to the health of populations and individuals and for developing effective risk reduction and health promotion activities.

The skills required for effective public health practice begin with proficiency in applying the techniques required for a particular public health specialization. The most important skill, however, is the capacity to create a vision of the potential for health that exists within a community. With a clear vision come a sense of direction and a feeling of enthusiasm that are essential if one hopes to engage a population in a process of understanding and reducing risks to its health.

Health departments are the only entities statutorily responsible for the health of their constituent populations. As a result, an underlying belief and responsibility of public health departments is that all members of the community should have access to the health promotion, disease prevention, and illness care services they need for good health. Public health is firmly grounded in the concepts of social justice, and its practitioners should be strong proponents of the ethical distribution of resources.

ASSOCIATED DISCIPLINES

The public often has difficulty distinguishing between the practice of medicine and the practice of public health. It is important that public health practitioners are clear about the differences among them.

As with medicine, the practice of public health is rooted in science and the scientific method. Medicine applies what we learn from science to the benefit of the individual patient, usually in the pursuit of the diagnosis and treatment of illness. Public health applies the knowledge gained from science to the improvement of the health status of groups of people, usually through health promotion and disease prevention activities.

Preventive medicine and **community medicine** are medical disciplines that function, to some degree, as bridges between the practice of medicine and the practice of public health. Preventive medicine physicians work to assure the primacy and excellence of both individual and community health promotion and disease prevention efforts. Although they may interact primarily with individuals, they also deal with groups seeking to maintain and preserve their health.

Community medicine has developed as a discipline during the past 40 years, and its practitioners concentrate on the preservation of health status in communities rather than individuals. John Last defines community medicine as:

> . . . the field concerned with the study of health and disease in the population of a defined community or group. Its goal is to identify the health problems and needs of defined populations, to identify means by which these needs should be met and to evaluate the extent to which health services effectively meet these needs.[2]

Public health clearly includes some elements of medical practice, preventive medicine, and community medicine. It is greater than the sum of these parts, however. It includes many other disciplines, such as nutrition, health education, and environmental health, that contribute to the improvement of the public's health status. It also concentrates on **health promotion** and **disease prevention**.

Health Promotion

Health promotion refers to:

> . . . a wide variety of individual and community efforts to encourage or support health behavior and environmental improvement where these goals and objectives have been

previously determined, usually on the basis of epidemiological data, to be important.[3]

We know that prerequisites for health include a variety of factors such as shelter, food, and education among others. Good health promotion activities may involve educational, organizational, economic, and environmental interventions targeted toward specific lifestyle behaviors and environmental conditions that are harmful to health, with the intention of making health-promoting changes in those conditions.

Disease Prevention

Disease prevention techniques are usually described in one of three categories—primary prevention, secondary prevention and tertiary prevention.

Primary Prevention

The first category, **primary prevention,** includes those activities that are intended to prevent the onset of disease in the first place. The classic example of primary prevention is immunization against infectious diseases, but the use of seat belts, the installation of air bags in automobiles, the avoidance of tobacco use, the minimal intake of alcoholic beverages, and the inspection and licensure of restaurants, are all examples of common public health activities that exemplify primary prevention.

Secondary Prevention

Secondary prevention refers to techniques that find health problems early in their course so that action can be taken to minimize the risk of progression of the disease in individuals or the risk that communicable illnesses will be transmitted to others. Examples of this principle include the early diagnosis of hypertension with follow-up treatment to minimize the risk of future vascular disease and the early diagnosis and treatment of sexually transmitted diseases to minimize the transmission potential of those conditions to others.

Tertiary Prevention

Tertiary prevention is focused on rehabilitation in an effort to prevent the worsening of an individual's health in the face of a chronic disease or injury. Learn-

ing to walk again after an orthopedic injury or cerebrovascular accident is an example.

Acute Sickness Services

Although public health focuses principally on health promotion and disease prevention, in many circumstances it has become a provider of acute sickness services to those who cannot obtain these services otherwise. Not surprisingly, sickness services are most often provided by health departments found in inner-city and rural areas of lower socioeconomic status, where access to medical care is limited. This assumption of responsibility for illness care has been controversial. Many insist it is outside the purview of traditional public health functions. Others insist that the assurance of medical services, when they can't be obtained in any other way, is a clear public health mission, consistent with the responsibility for maintaining the public's health.

EVOLUTION OF THE DISCIPLINE

Public health departments began to appear in the United States in the middle of the nineteenth century. Since that time, public health methods and programs have evolved to meet the changing needs of the community. Many changes have been driven by scientific contributions to knowledge about risks to health and by improvements in the technology available to respond to public health issues. For more than a century, public health has moved from a period of limited scientific understanding, when infectious diseases were the major cause of death, to a period of significant and growing scientific capacity, as chronic diseases became the major killers.

INFECTIOUS DISEASE CONTROL

Scientists came to realize that the major health problems of the day were caused by microorganisms. They also realized that understanding how the microorganisms moved from person to person could lead to strategies to prevent the transmission of disease. This realization was so revolutionary that Milton Terris has called this period the "First Epidemiological

Revolution."[4] This allowed communities to develop policies and laws that would protect the public's health and to hire people to enforce them. These governmental *sanitarians* in the nation's first health departments used laws providing for quarantine, safe water, and sewage disposal to significantly reduce the toll taken by communicable disease. The later addition of vaccines and antibiotics increased the effectiveness of infectious disease control efforts. It became increasingly obvious, however, that improved socioeconomic status, decreased crowding, good nutrition, and better education had as much to do with this success story as did the newer medical interventions.[5] This reinforced the lesson that there are *determinants of health* that deserve as much attention as medical interventions when it comes to improving health status.

CHRONIC DISEASE CONTROL

Our struggles with infectious diseases continue in the present day. New organisms appear, such as the human immunodeficiency virus, or HIV, and *older* organisms, such as the tubercle bacillus that causes tuberculosis, return to fill new niches in our changing environment. The major causes of death and disability in the United States today, however, are chronic illnesses. Our efforts to understand and control them have led to what Terris calls the "Second Epidemiological Revolution."[4] We are in an era of rapidly increasing understanding of the causes of chronic disease. We have learned that heart disease, cancer, stroke, and many other chronic diseases are multifactorial in causation. A variety of genetic, environmental, and lifestyle factors interact to predispose individuals to chronic illness. In fact, up to 70 percent of premature mortality in the United States is directly related to environmental and lifestyle factors that are potentially controllable by individuals or society.[6] We describe these causes as **risk factors,** and we realize that such behaviors as the use of tobacco, the excessive use of alcohol, unhealthful nutritional practices, and sedentary lifestyles cannot be altered without the direct, willing participation of the individuals affected in an environment that is supportive of healthful choices.

We are moving beyond an era of professionals doing things *for* others to one of professionals doing things *with* others to help them minimize risks to their health. It is a time of trying to understand the motivations of human behavior and developing constructive and ethical mechanisms to support healthful behavioral choices. It is also a time of working with governments and communities to create the most healthful living environments possible.

SOCIAL ISSUES

New problems have emerged that have public health implications and will require a new level of understanding if effective intervention methods are to be devised. They include epidemics of violence, drug abuse, teenage pregnancy, and sexually transmitted disease, problems that are not clearly understood but probably due in part to racial and ethnic prejudice, increasing numbers of single-parent families, changing cultural values, and poverty as a social norm.

It appears that having a positive impact on these problems will require not only an expansion of our understanding of human behavior but also an increased understanding of community and family structures and their interaction. Unfortunately, we are only beginning to understand the epidemiology of these problems and do not yet have robust interventions for most of them.

NEW TOOLS FOR PUBLIC HEALTH PRACTICE

A number of new tools are available to public health professionals to help them carry out public health's core functions. Frequent reference will be made to these tools throughout this textbook because of the important roles they play in the conceptualization, organization, and delivery of public health services. They are just briefly introduced here.

Report on the Future of Public Health

The contributions made by public health over the past 100 years have largely been taken for granted. In fact, public health had languished, through inattention, for many decades. Fortunately, the 1988 report on *The Future of Public Health* by the Institute of Medicine (IOM) has focused attention on the discipline.[7] This study details the contributions made by public health while chronicling its current difficulties, and it makes very clear recommendations about how the nation's public health system should be improved to assure that every citizen in the country has access to needed public health services.

The report defines the mission of public health as "fulfilling society's interest in assuring conditions in which people can be healthy."[7] The Study Committee of the IOM that produced the report recognized that many components of a community must work together for that mission to be successfully accomplished, but they emphasized the unique responsibility of government, at all levels, to assure success. These governmental responsibilities are usually carried out by health departments, which are the jurisdiction's action arm to accomplish the mission articulated by the IOM. The committee suggested three core public health functions for local and state health departments: **assessment, policy development,** and **assurance.**

By assessment, the committee meant that each public health agency should:

. . . regularly and systematically collect, assemble, analyze, and make available information on the health of the community, including statistics on health status, community health needs, and epidemiologic and other studies of health problems.[7(p7)]

The committee noted that not every agency is large enough to conduct these activities in their entirety, but that each agency bears the responsibility for seeing that the assessment function is fulfilled. In essence, the committee recognized the public health department as the epidemiologic intelligence center for health in the community, providing the information necessary for effective health planning.

By policy development, the committee meant that each public health agency should:

. . . serve the public interest in the development of comprehensive public health policies by promoting use of

the scientific knowledge base in decision-making about public health and by leading in developing public health policy.[7(p8)]

Policy development links science with political, organizational, and community values. It includes information sharing, citizen participation, compromise, and consensus building in a process that nurtures shared ownership of the policy decisions.

By assurance, the committee meant that each public health agency should:

. . . assure their constituents that services necessary to achieve agreed upon goals are provided, either by encouraging actions by other entities (private or public sector), by requiring such action through regulation, or by providing services directly.[7(p8)]

The committee also felt that each public health agency should work with its community to guarantee access to a basic set of health services for each citizen.[7(p8)] This is the social justice element of public health. The effective health department will work with other service providers to be sure that good quality, basic services are available to all, even if the services are provided by someone other than the health department itself.

The areas of *assessment, policy development,* and *assurance* are now considered by most to define the core functions of public health. Unfortunately, most health departments will have to improve their capacity to carry out the functions and activities associated with these responsibilities. Many health departments are too small to perform them well. They might combine with others or form alliances that will allow the sharing of expertise. Strong liaisons with academic units, where available, may also provide access to analytical and other skills.

Healthy People 2000

The process of setting national goals and objectives for the nation began in 1979 with the publication of *Healthy People: The Surgeon General's Report on Health Promotion and Disease Prevention.*[6] It was the first such report to emphasize the importance of efforts to reduce premature mortality through health promotion and disease prevention programs, and it discussed a series of age-specific goals for the nation to accomplish by 1990. Following that report, the Centers for Disease Control and Prevention (CDC) convened a series of discussions that led to a publication entitled *Health Promotion/Disease Prevention: Objectives for the Nation.*[8] This document established 226 specific health objectives to be achieved by 1990. These objectives were measurable, specific, and tied to the various priority programs listed under the rubrics of health promotion, health protection, and preventive services.

In 1987, the Public Health Service's Office of Health Promotion and Disease Prevention began a new consultative process with the nation's public health professionals to develop a set of objectives for the year 2000. The resulting *Healthy People 2000: National Health Promotion and Disease Prevention Objectives*[9], which was published in 1990, articulated three major goals:

1. increase the span of healthy life for all Americans
2. reduce health disparities among Americans
3. achieve access to preventive services for all Americans

More than 300 objectives were listed within 22 priority areas and categorized as Health Status Objectives, Risk Reduction Objectives, and Service and Protection Objectives. *Healthy People 2000* has succeeded in establishing a national focus for attainable health status by the year 2000. It has been described by many as creating the *destination* for health promotion and disease prevention activities.

Healthy Communities 2000

While it is extremely worthwhile to have national objectives, in the final analysis, the achievement of national objectives is dependent upon activities within each local community. The American Public Health Association, together with the CDC and other public health professional associations, developed a *road map* for local communities to follow to help them do their part to reach the national objectives. *Healthy Communities 2000: Model Standards. Guidelines for Community Attainment of the Year 2000 National Health Objectives*[10] is intended to help communities organize and express their local public health needs in quantifiable objectives that are consistent with the national objectives.

Assessment Protocol for Excellence in Public Health

Before a community can translate its public health problems into objectives for action that are consistent, wherever possible, with national goals, those local public health problems must be identified and prioritized. We have moved beyond the time when significant progress in improved health status is possible by doing things for the community. We now realize that the community must be engaged in the process of identifying and understanding its health problems and determining the remedies to be applied. To this end, the National Association of County Health Officials, together with the CDC and other public health professional associations, developed the *Assessment Protocol for Excellence in Public Health (APEX).*[11] It guides public health agencies in the process of community assessment and public health program planning. APEX helps health departments assess their own internal strengths and weaknesses in terms of their capacity to carry out community needs assessment, to work with the community to understand its health problems and establish priorities for action, and to implement a community plan for reducing public health problems. Other, similar programs, such as the Planned Approach to Community Health (PATCH)[12] and the Healthy Cities Project[13] are discussed elsewhere in this text.

In the future, growing numbers of local and state health departments will be using APEX, PATCH, or Healthy Cities as guides to developing community-based plans for identifying and addressing community health problems. Inherent in that process will be accurate assessment of risks to health and a growing capacity to communicate those risks to the public at large. Increasingly, these tools will link communities with national efforts to improve health status so that the mission of public health, "fulfilling society's interest in assuring conditions in which people can be healthy," will be realized.

REFERENCES

1. Osamnczk EJ. *Encyclopedia of the United Nations and International Agreements.* Philadelphia, Pa: Taylor and Francis; 1985.

2. Last JM. *A Dictionary of Epidemiology.* 2nd Ed. New York, NY: Oxford University Press; 1988.

3. American Public Health Association. Technical report: criteria for the development of health promotion and education programs. *Amer J Public Health.* 1987;77(1):89–91.

4. Terris M. The complex tasks of the second epidemiological revolution: the Joseph W. Mountain lecture. *J Public Health Policy.* March 1983;8–22.

5. McKinlay JB, McKinlay SM. The questionable contribution of medical measures to the decline of mortality in the United States in the twentieth century. *Milbank Q.* 1977;55(3): 405–428.

6. *Healthy People: The Surgeon General's Report on Health Promotion and Disease Prevention.* Washington, DC: US Dept of Health and Human Services, Public Health Service; 1979.

7. Institute of Medicine, Committee for the Study of the Future of Public Health. *The Future of Public Health.* Washington, DC: National Academy Press; 1988.

8. *Health Promotion/Disease Prevention: Objectives for the Nation.* Washington, DC: US Dept of Health and Human Services, Public Health Service; 1981.

9. *Healthy People 2000: National Health Promotion and Disease Prevention Objectives.* Washington, DC: US Dept of Health and Human Services, Public Health Service; 1990.

10. *Healthy Communities 2000: Model Standards. Guidelines for Community Attainment of the Year 2000 National Health Objectives.* 3rd ed. Washington, DC: American Public Health Association; 1991.

11. *APEX/PH, Assessment Protocol for Excellence in Public Health.* Washington, DC: National Association of County Health Officials; 1991.

12. *Planned Approach to Community Health (PATCH): Program Descriptions.* Washington, DC: US Dept of Health and Human Services; November 1993.

13. *World Health Organization, Five Year Planning Project.* Fadl, Copenhagen: World Health Organization, Healthy Cities Project; 1988. WHO Healthy Cities Paper, No. 2.

CHAPTER

History and Development of Public Health

Elizabeth Fee, Ph.D.

This chapter discusses the history and development of public health in the United States and the factors that influenced them. The first section gives an overview of public health in the United States in the eighteenth and nineteenth centuries.

PUBLIC HEALTH IN THE EIGHTEENTH AND NINETEENTH CENTURIES

In the United States, before the twentieth century, there were few formal requirements for public health positions, no established career structures, no job security for health officials, and no formalized ways of producing new knowledge. Public health positions were usually part-time appointments at nominal salary; those who devoted much effort to public health typically did so on a voluntary basis. Until the midnineteenth century, public health, like other governmental functions, was usually the responsibility of the social elite. The public health officer was expected to be a *statesman* acting in the public interest, not a *politician* answering to a class constituency. Men of property and wealth were believed to be independent of special interests and therefore capable of disinterested judgement.

Charles Rosenberg has eloquently described an earlier conception of both poverty and disease as consequences of moral failure at the individual and social level.[1] Disease attacked the dirty, the improvident, the intemperate, the ignorant; the clean, the pious, and the virtuous, on the other hand, tended to escape. Epidemic diseases were the consequence of a failure to obey the laws of nature and God: they were indicators of social and moral dissolution. As cleanliness was linked to godliness, virtue was an essential qualification for managing the state. The conscientious, the respectable, the educated, and the affluent were seen as naturally qualified for public office. Physicians were frequently chosen as public health officers, but lawyers or gentlemen of independent means could also be appointed.

Earliest Public Health Programs and Activities

The first public health organizations were those of the rapidly growing port cities of the eastern seaboard in the late eighteenth century. Here, the American republic intersected with the world of international trade. Local authorities tried to protect the population from the threat of potentially catastrophic epidemic diseases, such as the yellow fever epidemic that had crippled Philadelphia in 1793, while they also tried to maintain the conditions for successful economic activity.[2] Public health programs, when organized at all, were organized locally. As Robert Wiebe has argued, the United States in the nineteenth century was a society of *island communities* with considerable economic and political autonomy.[3]

Public health in this period was also largely a police function. Traditionally, port cities had dealt with epidemics by means of quarantine regulations, keeping ships suspected of carrying disease in harbor for up to 40 days. However, quarantine regulations clearly interfered with shipping, and they were energetically opposed by those whose economic interests were tied to trade.[4]

Opponents of quarantine argued that diseases were internally generated by the filthy conditions of the docks, streets, and alleys, which provided an ideal environment for *putrefactive fermentation*. City health departments attempted to regulate the worst offenders: graveyards, tallow chandleries, tanneries, sugar boilers, skin dressers, dyers, glue boilers, and slaughter houses. They also cleaned the privies and alleys and removed dead animals and decaying vegetable matter from the streets and public spaces.[5(p50)]

Influence of Disease

The causes of disease were much in dispute by the midnineteenth century. The evidence available was contradictory and suggested no clear resolution to the dispute between those who believed that diseases were brought in from overseas and thus should be fought by quarantine regulations and those who believed that diseases were internally generated and thus should be fought by cleaning up the cities. Health regulations were written and revised more in response to political influence or pressure from merchants than in response to shifts in scientific thinking.

Official health agencies were sporadically moved to action by the threat of great epidemics—the devastating waves of yellow fever and cholera that periodically threatened from Europe, the Caribbean, or Latin America or were detected on ships arriving in New Orleans, Boston, or Philadelphia. These sudden, catastrophic events compelled even politicians and business leaders to devote their attention to sanitary improvements, city cleanliness, quarantines, and hospital construction.

At other times, adults and children were killed continually but in less spectacular numbers by tuberculosis, smallpox, typhus, dysentery, diphtheria, typhoid fever, measles, influenza, tuberculosis, malaria, and scarlet fever. These diseases were met with a stolid indifference born of familiarity and a sense of helplessness. It seemed that little could be done beyond attempts to maintain general cleanliness, backed by prayer, fasting, and exhortations to virtue.[5(p87)] When free of the immediate threat of an impending epidemic, politicians tended to ignore the fate of the multitudes of immigrant poor, unless compelled to action by the insistent demands of reform groups or the fear of popular unrest.[6–8]

Early Public Health Reforms

A few cities did have active and energetic reform groups. In New York in 1864, members of the Council of Hygiene and Public Health of the Citizens' Association conducted street-by-street investigations of tenement housing congestion, slaughterhouse and stable conditions, sewage drainage, garbage heaps, and filthy habitations of many sections of the city, and correlated these with outbreaks of infectious disease and premature infant deaths.[9] Dr. Ezra R. Pulling, for example, detailed every case of typhus, typhoid fever, and smallpox found in the notorious Five Points section of Manhattan's Lower East Side. He also carefully mapped all the stables, privies (especially "privies in an extremely offensive condition"), and other *insalubrious locations* in the area, making obvious the close geographical relationship between disease and its causes.[10]

In other parts of the country, a few farsighted men and women argued for the need to collect vital statistics, register birth and death rates, and keep careful records on the health of the population. The most notable of these was Lemuel Shattuck, a school teacher, bookseller, and publisher, who was largely responsible for implementing a system of vital statistics in Massachusetts. Shattuck is especially remembered for his *Report of the Sanitary Commission of Massachusetts*, an extraordinarily comprehensive set of recommendations for public health organization.[11,12]

Shattuck's report advocated a decennial census and collection of data by age, sex, race, occupation, economic status, and locality. It discussed the need for environmental sanitation, regulation of food and drugs, and control of communicable disease. Shattuck also recommended attention to well-child care, mental health, health education, smallpox vaccination, alcoholism, town planning, and the teaching of preventive medicine in medical schools.

Shattuck's report was well received by medical reviewers but essentially ignored by the Massachusetts state legislature. Although having little direct impact at the time it was written, the report would become a central reference point for later generations of public health practitioners.

By 1860, public health activities were just beginning to move beyond the confines of local city politics. Between 1857 and 1860, quarantine and sanitary conventions were held in Philadelphia, Baltimore, New York, and Boston.[13] Although these conventions gave public health reformers an opportunity to debate the causes of disease and the most appropriate public health responses, the possibility of implementing their ideas was interrupted by the outbreak of the Civil War.

Impact of the Civil War

In its own way, the Civil War helped enforce a national consciousness of epidemic disease: two-thirds of the 360,000 Union soldiers who died were killed by in-

fectious diseases rather than by bullets.[14,15] The ravages of dysentery, spread by inadequate or nonexistent sanitary facilities, were appalling. The United States Sanitary Commission, a voluntary organization inspired by Florence Nightingale's work in the Crimean War, promoted the health of the Union army by inspecting army camps, distributing educational materials, and providing nursing care and supplies for the wounded.

Formation of the American Public Health Association

In 1872, 10 health reformers from various parts of the country met in New York City at the home of Stephen Smith and announced the creation of the American Public Health Association (APHA). Its purpose was to advance *sanitary science* and promote the "practical application of public hygiene."[16,17] After a slow start, the new organization grew rapidly. Its members devoted themselves to the reform activities of citizens' sanitary associations and encouraged the formation and development of local and state health agencies. They organized annual meetings and presented papers on infectious diseases and on many of the practical public health issues of the day—from sewage and garbage disposal to occupational injuries and proposals for the medical inspection of prostitutes. The APHA was notable in welcoming physicians, engineers, lawyers, municipal officials, other professional groups, and lay reformers to its membership, and in this respect, it helped mold the specific character of American public health.[18,19]

First State and Local Boards of Health

In the late nineteenth century, state and local boards of health were created in many parts of the country. The first state board of health, formed in Louisiana in 1855, had largely been a paper organization. In the 1870s and 1880s, however, most states instituted their own boards of health. The first working state health board was formed in Massachusetts in 1869, followed by California (1870), the District of Columbia (1871), Virginia and Minnesota (1872), Maryland (1874), and Alabama (1875).[20] The impact of these state boards of health should not be overemphasized. By 1900, only three states (Massachusetts, Rhode Island, and Florida) spent more than two cents per capita for public health services.[21]

The Marine Hospital Service

The origins of a federal organization of public health lie in the provision of medical and hospital care for merchant seamen and sailors. In 1798, the United States Congress had passed the Act for the Relief of Sick and Disabled Seamen to finance the construction and operation of public hospitals in port cities.[22] These hospitals were poorly run and badly managed until 1871, when John Maynard Woodward became Supervising Surgeon of what was now named the Marine Hospital Service.

Woodward and other public health reformers urged the formation of a national system of quarantines and a national health board. In 1879, a disastrous yellow fever epidemic swept up the Mississippi Valley from New Orleans, prompting the United States Congress to create the National Board of Health. This consisted of seven physicians and one representative each from the army, the navy, the Marine Hospital Service, and the Department of Justice.

Responsible for formulating quarantine regulations between states, the National Board of Health soon became embroiled in fierce battles over states' rights. Many cities and states had discovered that local quarantine laws could be an excellent source of income as well as a valuable source of political patronage; they were naturally reluctant to relinquish these powers to the federal government.[7(pp157–174)] In 1883, after various battles in Congress, the National Board of Health was disbanded, and its quarantine powers reverted to the Marine Hospital Service.

Gradually, the Marine Hospital Service expanded its public health activities into public health research. In 1887, it set aside a single room as a *hygienic laboratory,* which would later be expanded into an important center for the investigation of infectious diseases.[23] In 1912, the Marine Hospital Service became the United States Public Health Service, specifically authorized to investigate the causes and spread of disease and to provide health information to the public.

PUBLIC HEALTH AS SOCIAL REFORM

The belief that epidemic diseases posed only occasional threats to an otherwise healthy social order had been shaken by the industrial transformation of the late nineteenth century. The burgeoning health problems of the industrial cities could not be ignored; almost all families lost children to diphtheria, smallpox, or other infectious diseases. Poverty and disease could not be treated simply as individual failings but were understood to be consequences of industrialization, urbanization, immigration, and exploitation.

Public Health Responses

The early efforts of city health department officials to deal with health problems were attempts to mitigate the worst effects of unplanned and unregulated growth—a kind of rearguard action against the filth and congestion created by anarchic economic and urban development.[24–29] As cities grew in size, as the flow of immigrants continued, and as public health problems became ever more obvious, pressures mounted for more effective responses to the problems.[30] New York, the largest city and the one with some of the worst health conditions, produced some of the most energetic and progressive public health leaders; Boston and Providence were also noted for their active public health programs; Baltimore and Philadelphia, however, trailed far behind.[25,31–33]

Social Reform

America no longer fit its self-image as a country of independent farmers and craftsmen. Like the countries of Europe, it displayed extremes of wealth and privilege, social misery, and deprivation. Labor and social unrest pushed awareness of the need for social and health reforms. The perceived social anarchy of the large industrial cities mocked the pretensions to social control of the traditional forces of church and state and highlighted the need for new approaches to the multiplicity of problems.[34]

Reformers and Reform Groups

An increasing number of reform groups devoted themselves to social issues and improvements of every variety. Health reformers, physicians, and engineers urged improved sanitary conditions in the industrial cities. Medical men were prominent in reform organizations, but they were not alone.[35] Barbara Rosenkrantz has contrasted public health in the late nineteenth century with the internecine battles within general medicine: ". . . the field of public hygiene exemplified a happy marriage of engineers, physicians and public spirited citizens providing a model of complementary comportment under the banner of sanitary science."[36]

Middle- and upper-class women, seizing an opportunity to escape from the narrow bounds of domestic responsibilities, joined in campaigns for improved housing, the abolition of child labor, maternal and child health, and temperance. They were active in the settlement house movement, the organization of trade unions, the suffrage movement, and municipal sanitary reform. The latter, as *municipal housekeeping,* was viewed as a natural extension of women's training and experience as *the housekeepers of the world.*[37] By the early years of the twentieth century, dozens of such voluntary health organizations were established around specific issues, thus providing the impulse and energy behind many public health reforms.[38]

The progressive reform groups in the public health movement advocated immediate change tempered by scientific knowledge and humanitarian concern. Sharing the revolutionaries' perception of the plight of the poor and the injustices of the system, they nonetheless counseled less radical solutions.[39-42] They advocated public health reforms on political, economic, humanitarian, and scientific grounds. Politically, public health reform offered a middle ground between the cutthroat principles of entrepreneurial capitalism and the revolutionary ideas of the socialists, anarchists, and utopian visionaries. As William Henry Welch, a leader of American medicine and public health, expressed it to the Charity Organization Society, sanitary improvement offered the best way of improving the lot of the poor, short of the radical restructuring of society.[43(p598)]

Economic Rewards of Reform

Economically, progressive reformers argued that public health should be viewed as a paying investment, giving higher returns than the stock market. In Germany, Max von Pettenkofer had first calculated the financial returns on public health *investments* to prove the value of sanitary improvements in reducing deaths from typhoid.[44] His argument would be repeated many times by American public health leaders. As William Henry Welch explained:

> . . . merely from a mercenary and commercial point of view it is for the interest of the community to take care of the health of the poor. Philanthropy assumes a totally different aspect in the eyes of the world when it is able to demonstrate that it pays to keep people healthy.[43(p596)]

Public health leaders argued that the demand for centralized planning and business efficiency required scientific knowledge rather than the undisciplined enthusiasms of voluntary groups.[45] Public health decisions should be made by an analysis of costs and benefits "as an up-to-date manufacturer would count the cost of a new process." The health officer, like the merchant, should learn "which line of work yields the most for the sum expended."[46]

NATIONAL AND INTERNATIONAL HEALTH

Public health was quickly becoming a national and even international issue. Although Congress was reluctant to enact federal health legislation, there were mounting pressures for United States attention to public health abroad. As American businessmen were seeking enlarged foreign markets, a vocal group of intellectuals and politicians argued for an assertive foreign policy. The United States began to challenge European dominance in the Far East and Latin America, seeking trade and political influence more than territory but taking territory where it could. National defense goals included broadening control of trade routes, building a Central American canal, and establishing strategic bases in the Caribbean and Western Pacific.

Cuba and the Panama Canal

In 1898, the United States entered the Spanish-American War, expanded the army from 25,000 to

250,000 men, and sent troops to Cuba. The war showed that the United States could not afford military adventures overseas unless more attention was paid to sanitation and public health: 968 men died in battle, but 5,438 died of infectious diseases.[47,48] Nonetheless, the United States defeated Spain and installed an army of occupation in Cuba. When yellow fever threatened the troops in 1900, the response was efficient and effective. An army commission under Walter Reed was sent to Cuba to study the disease and, in a dramatic series of human experiments, it confirmed the hypothesis that yellow fever was spread by mosquitoes. Surgeon Major William Gorgas then eliminated yellow fever from Havana.[49]

This experience confirmed the importance of public health for successful United States efforts overseas. Earlier attempts to dig the Panama Canal had been attended by enormous mortality rates from disease.[50] But in 1904, Gorgas, now promoted to General, took control of a campaign against the malaria and yellow fever that were threatening canal operations. He was finally able to persuade the Canal Commission to institute an intensive campaign against mosquitoes. In one of the great triumphs of practical public health, yellow fever and malaria were brought under control, and the canal was successfully completed in 1914.

Bringing the Lessons Home

United States industrialists brought some of the lessons of Cuba and the Panama Canal home to the southern United States. The South at that time resembled an underdeveloped country within the United States, characterized by poor economic and social conditions. Northern industrialists were already investing heavily in southern education as well as in cotton mills and railroads. John D. Rockefeller had created the General Education Board to support "the general organization of rural communities for economic, social and educational purposes."[51] Charles Wardell Stiles managed to convince the secretary of the General Education Board that the real cause of misery and lack of productivity in the South was hookworm, the *germ of laziness*. In 1909, Rockefeller agreed to provide $1 million to create the Rockefeller Sanitary Commission for the

Eradication of Hookworm Disease, with Wickliffe Rose as director.[52] This was to be the first installment in Rockefeller's massive national and international investment in public health.

Rose went beyond the task of attempting to control a single disease and worked to establish an effective and permanent public health organization in the southern states.[53] At the end of five years of intensive effort, the campaign had failed to eradicate hookworm but had greatly expanded the role of public health agencies. Between 1910 and 1914, county appropriations for local public health work increased from a total of $240 to $110,000.[52(pp220–221)]

Public Health at the National Level

In Washington, the Committee of One Hundred on National Health campaigned for the federal regulation of public health.[54,55] The committee was composed of such notables as Jane Addams, Andrew Carnegie, William H. Welch, and Booker T. Washington. Its president, the economist Irving Fisher, argued that a public health service would be good policy and good economics, in conserving *national vitality*.[56]

In 1912, the federal government made its first real commitment to public health when it expanded the responsibilities of the Public Health Service, empowering it to investigate the causes and spread of diseases and the pollution and sanitation of navigable streams and lakes.[57] The responsibilities of the Public Health Service included the medical inspection of immigrants arriving at Ellis Island, field investigations of endemic rural diseases such as trachoma, and groundbreaking research on diseases such as pellagra and Rocky Mountain spotted fever. By 1915, the Public Health Service, the United States Army, and the Rockefeller Foundation were the major agencies involved in public health activities, supplemented on a local level by a network of city and state health departments.

THE PROFESSIONALIZATION OF PUBLIC HEALTH

At the turn of the century existing health departments were often dominated more by patronage and political considerations than by economic or administrative efficiency. Progressives regretted *the evil of politics* and wanted to increase the pay and minimum qualifications for health officers to attract personnel on the basis of skill rather than influence. Their attempt to insulate boards of health from local political control was part of a broader movement to make all forms of public administration more *rational* and *efficient* by reducing the influence of political bosses and promoting a new group of professional administrators.[58] The goal was for a well-trained professional elite to conduct social reform on scientific lines.

These developments led to an increasing demand for people trained in public health to direct the new programs being created at the local, state, and national levels. Those attempting to develop such programs were increasingly critical of the lack of properly trained personnel; part-time public health officers were simply not adequate to staff the ambitious new programs. Public health reformers agreed that full-time practitioners, especially trained for the job, were needed. In 1913, the New York State legislature passed a law requiring public health officers to have specialized training, despite the fact that there was little agreement about what kind of specialized training was needed, much less where it could be obtained.[59,60]

Public health had been defined in terms of its aims and goals—to reduce disease and maintain the health of the population—rather than by any specific body of knowledge. Many different disciplines contributed to effective public health work: physicians diagnosed contagious diseases; sanitary engineers built water and sewage systems; epidemiologists traced the sources of disease outbreaks and their modes of transmission; vital statisticians provided quantitative measures of births and deaths; lawyers wrote sanitary codes and regulations; public health nurses provided care and advice to the sick in their homes; sanitary inspectors visited factories and markets to enforce compliance with public health ordinances; and administrators tried to organize everyone within the limits of health department budgets. Public health thus involved economics, sociology, psychology, politics, law, statistics, and engineering, as well as the biological and clinical sciences. However, in the period immediately following the brilliant experimental work of Louis Pasteur and Robert Koch, the bacteriological laboratory became the first and primary symbol of a new, scientific public health.

Bacteriology and Alternative Views of Health and Disease

The rise of bacteriology and other scientific advances in the understanding of disease contributed to the professionalization of public health.

The Rise of Bacteriology

The clarity and simplicity of bacteriological methods and discoveries gave them tremendous cultural importance: the agents of particular diseases had been made visible under the microscope. The identification of specific bacteria seemed to have cut through the misty miasmas of disease to define the enemy in unmistakable terms. Bacteriology thus became an ideological marker, sharply differentiating the *old* public health, the province of untrained amateurs, from the *new* public health, which would belong to scientifically trained professionals.

Young Americans who had studied in Germany brought back the new knowledge of laboratory methods in bacteriology and started to teach others. These young scientists were convinced that physicians should stop squabbling over medical ethics and politics and commit themselves to the purer values of laboratory research. Under their influence, the laboratory ideal soon spread throughout progressive public health circles. By the 1880s, Charles Chapin had established a public health laboratory in Providence, Rhode Island, and Victor C. Vaughan had created a state hygienic laboratory in Michigan.

In 1901, William Sedgwick reported on his bacteriological study of water supplies and sewage disposal at the Lawrence Experiment Station in Massachusetts.[61] Sedgwick demonstrated the transmission of typhoid fever by polluted water supplies, and he developed quantitative methods for measuring the presence of bacteria in the air, water, and milk. Describing the impact of bacteriological discoveries, he said, "Before

1880 we knew nothing; after 1890 we knew it all; it was a glorious ten years."[32(p57)]

The powerful new methods of identifying diseases through the microscope drew attention away from the larger and more diffuse problems of water supplies, street cleaning, housing reform, and the living conditions of the poor. The approach of locating, identifying, and isolating bacteria and their human hosts was a more elegant and efficient way of dealing with disease than environmental reform. The public health laboratory demonstrated the scientific and diagnostic power of the new public health. However, by focusing on the diagnosis of infectious diseases, it narrowed the distance between medicine and public health and brought public health into potential conflict with private medical practice. Physicians began increasingly to resent the public health officials' claim to diagnose, and often treat, infectious diseases.

Alternative Models

Although the narrow bacteriological view was dominant, there were several competing models for public health research and practice. It is worth noting the broad and comprehensive definition of public health offered by Charles-Edward A. Winslow, professor of public health at Yale University, in 1920:

> Public health is the science and art of preventing disease, prolonging life, and promoting physical health and efficiency through organized community efforts for the sanitation of the environment, the control of community infections, the education of the individual in principles of personal hygiene, the organization of medical and nursing service for the early diagnosis and preventive treatment of disease, and the development of the social machinery which will ensure to every individual in the community a standard of living adequate for the maintenance of health.[62,63]

Winslow's was not the only broad vision of public health. Alice Hamilton in Illinois conducted a survey of industrial lead poisoning and established the fact that thousands of American workers were being slowly killed by white lead.[64] Unaided by legislation, Hamilton argued, persuaded, shamed, and flattered individual employers into improving working conditions. Almost single-handedly, she created the foundations of industrial hygiene in America.

Joseph Goldberger's epidemiological studies of pellagra for the Public Health Service offer another example of a comprehensive approach to public health. In 1914, Goldberger announced that pellagra was due to dietary deficiencies and not to some unknown microorganism. He and his colleagues had cured endemic pellagra in a Mississippi orphanage by feeding the children milk, eggs, beans, and meat. He then teamed up with an economist, Edgar Sydenstricker, to survey the diets of southern wageworkers' families. They showed how the sharecropping system had impoverished tenant farmers, led to dietary deficiencies, and thus produced endemic pellagra.[65]

Alice Hamilton, Joseph Goldberger, and Edgar Sydenstricker were minority voices amid the growing majority focusing exclusively on bacteria. As most bacteriologists and epidemiologists concentrated on specific disease-causing organisms and the individuals who harbored them, only a minority continued to relate the problems of ill health and disease to the larger social environment.[66]

The Relationship Between Public Health and Medicine

While the broader conceptions of public health required an understanding of economics and politics, the dominant model of public health knowledge was based almost exclusively on the biological sciences. This redefinition of public health in bioscientific terms reinforced the medical profession's claim to preeminence in the field. Physicians felt that because they were the experts in infectious diseases, they were uniquely qualified to become the ultimate authorities in the new, scientific public health.

By the second decade of the twentieth century, non-medical public health officers were beginning to protest the dominance of public health by medical men. By this time, the sanitary engineers were the only professional group strong enough to challenge the physicians' assumption that the future of public health should be theirs. Civil and sanitary engineers had created clean city water supplies and adequate sewage systems, which were major factors in the declining death rates from infant diarrhea and other infectious diseases.[67-70]

Professional competition between the sanitary engineers and physicians became intense in the early years of the twentieth century as sanitary engineers vociferously complained about the increasing *medical monopoly* of public health. By 1912, 15 states required that all members of their boards of health be physicians, and 23 states required at least one physician member; only 10 states had no professional requirement for eligibility.[71]

With the increasing professionalization of public health, physicians came to hold a dominant but not exclusive role in the field. Leadership positions in public health departments and public health agencies were increasingly reserved for physicians. Other scientists, professionals, and nurses might be given subordinate positions. Physicians themselves were increasingly ambivalent about public health. The curious relationships between physicians and nonmedical public health practitioners would shape the subsequent development of public health practice.

PUBLIC HEALTH ORGANIZATION AND PRACTICE

The practical importance of public health was well recognized by the early decades of the twentieth century. The incidence of tuberculosis, diphtheria, and other infectious diseases was falling, apparently in response to energetic public health campaigns. School health clinics and maternal and child health centers were established in many cities with active public support. Registration for the draft in World War I revealed that a substantial proportion of young men were either physically or mentally unfit for combat, and this perception also led to increased political support for public health activities. The influenza epidemic that devastated families and communities in 1916 to 1918 underlined the continuing threat of infectious disease epidemics.

The Waning Influence of Bacteriology

After the first flush of enthusiasm for the achievements of bacteriology, many health departments were now paying more attention to community-based health activities and popular health education. In 1923, Charles-Edward A. Winslow went so far as to announce the ending of the bacteriological age and to describe popular health education as the keynote of the *new public health,* almost as far-reaching in its importance as the germ theory of disease had been some 30 years before.[63(pp53,55),72]

In the 1920s, state and municipal health departments developed new organizational units and increased their hiring of public health personnel, especially public health nurses. Although bacteriological laboratories continued to be important, divisions that were focused on tuberculosis, maternal and child health, venereal diseases, public health administration, and health education played a major role in most state and city health departments, as did divisions of sanitation and vital statistics.

Variation in Public Health Practice

Public health practice actually varied greatly throughout the states and cities across the country, as shown by an American Public Health Association survey of municipal public health department practice in 1923: although some cities had extensive, progressive, and imaginative programs, others did little beyond offering a few communicable disease clinics and public health inspections.[73]

Continuing Controversy with Medicine

The relationship between the emerging profession of public health and the well-established profession of medicine continued to be problematic and controversial. The increased activity of health departments in the identification and control of infectious diseases brought health officers into conflict with private practitioners. As soon as public health left the confines of sanitary engineering and took on the battle against specific diseases, it challenged the boundaries of medical autonomy. As John Duffy has argued, the medical profession moved from a position of strong support for public health activities to a cautious and sometimes suspicious ambivalence.[74]

Major battles would be fought over the Sheppard-Towner Maternity and Infancy Act of 1921, which provided grants to states to teach prenatal and infant care to mothers.[75] Conservatives denounced the measure as socialistic, and many physicians opposed it as interfering with the proper purview of medicine. These programs were allowed to expire in 1929, showing the difficulties faced by any innovative public health or social welfare legislation in a politically conservative period.

Federal Involvement

The most important federal organization in public health continued to be the United States Public Health Service, an arm of the Federal Security Agency. The Public Health Service aided the development of state health departments by giving grants-in-aid, loaning expert personnel, and providing advice and consultation on specific problems.[76] For example, if a state was facing an unexplained outbreak of typhoid fever or other epidemic disease, the Public Health Service would send epidemiologists to trace the source of the disease and suggest means of preventing its spread.

Influence of the Depression

A major stimulus to the development of public health practice came in response to the depression, with the New Deal and the Social Security Act of 1935. The Social Security Act represented America's first broad-based social welfare legislation, providing old-age benefits, unemployment insurance, and public health services. Unfortunately, the attempt to include basic medical insurance within the bill was abandoned because of the determined opposition of the medical profession, pharmaceutical companies, and the insurance industry.[77–79] From the public health point of view, however, the Social Security Act was a huge leap forward. Title V of the act established a program of grants to states for maternal and child health services, administered by the Children's Bureau, and provided funds for child welfare and crippled children's programs. Title VI of the act expanded financing of the Public Health Service and allotted federal grants to states to assist them in developing their public health services.

Federal and state expenditures for public health actually doubled in the decade of the depression, fueling the expansion of local health units. In most parts of the country, efficient provision of public health services to local communities depended on county health organizations, smaller and simpler units than the larger state health departments. In 1934, only 541 counties out of the 3,070 counties in the United States had any form of local public health service, but by June 1942, 1,828 counties could boast of health units directed by a full-time public health officer.[80] Much of this gain would be lost during the war; by the end of the war only 1,322 counties had an organized health service.[81(p125),82]

Federal Funding and Training

In 1935, for the first time, the federal government provided funds, administered through the states, for public health training. Federal regulations now required states to establish minimum qualifications for public health personnel employed through new federal grants. Thus, it was no longer sufficient for state programs to employ any willing physician; some form of professional public health training was expected.

As a result of the growing demand for public health education, several state universities began new schools or divisions of public health, and existing schools of public health expanded their enrollments. By 1936, 10 schools offered public health degrees or certificates requiring at least one year of attendance.[83] By 1938, more than 4,000 individuals, including about 1,000 doctors, had received some public health training with funds provided by the federal government through the states.

The economic difficulties of maintaining a private practice during the depression had pushed some physicians into public health; others were attracted by the new availability of fellowships or by increased social awareness of the plight of the poor. In 1939, the federal government allocated over $8 million for maternal and child health programs, more than $9 million for general public health work, and over $4 million for venereal disease control.

Several important trends were stimulated by these federal funds. The first was the development of programs to control specific diseases and of services targeted to specific population groups, the *categorical* approach to public health. Second was the expansion in the number of local health departments. Third was the increased training of personnel, and fourth, the assumption of responsibility for some phases of medical care on the part of health departments.[81(pxii)]

Categorical Approach to Public Health

The categorical approach to public health proved politically popular. Members of Congress were willing to allocate funds for specific diseases or for particular groups—health and welfare services for children were especially favored—but they showed less interest in general public health or administrative expenditures. Although state health officers often felt constrained by targeted programs, they rarely refused federal grants-in-aid and thus adapted their programs to the pattern of available funds. Federal grants came in turn for maternal and child health services and crippled children (1935), venereal disease control (1938), tuberculosis (1944), mental health (1947), industrial hygiene (1947), and dental health (1947). The pattern of funding started in the 1930s would thus shape the organization of public health departments through the postwar period. As institutionalized in the National Institutes of Health, it would also shape the future patterns of biomedical research.

PUBLIC HEALTH AND THE WAR

Mobilization for war acted as another major force in the expansion and development of public health in the United States.[84] Public health was declared a national priority for the armed forces and the civilian population engaged in military production. As James Stevens Simmons, brigadier general and director of the Preventive Medicine Division of the United States Army, announced:

> A civil population that is not healthy cannot be prosperous and will lag behind in the economic competition between nations. This is even more true of a military population, for any army that has its strength sapped by disease is in no condition to withstand the attack of a vir-

ile force that has conserved its strength and is enjoying the vigor and exhilaration of health.[85]

The Need for Personnel

Health departments again suffered from a critical shortage of personnel as physicians, nurses, engineers, and other trained and experienced professionals left to join the armed services.[86] In 1940, the United States Public Health Service expanded its program of grants to states and local communities, sending personnel to particularly needy areas. The Community Facilities Act, for instance, provided $300 million to fund health and sanitation facilities in communities with rapidly expanding populations because of military camps and war industries.[87,88]

The Selective Service Exams

The shock of the discovery that many of the young men being called into the army were physically unfit for military service provided a powerful impetus for increased national attention to public health. The Selective Service examinations represented the most massive health survey ever undertaken, with over 16 million young men examined. Fully 40 percent of the young men examined were declared physically or mentally unfit for service, with the leading causes of rejection being defective teeth, vision problems, orthopedic impairments (from polio, for example), diseases of the cardiovascular system, nervous and mental diseases, hernia, tuberculosis, and venereal diseases.[89,90]

Mosquitoes and the Centers for Disease Control

With the war mobilization, as hundreds of thousands of workers moved to areas with defense industry plants the troops moved to Army camps.[91] Army training camps often had been placed in areas with warm climates, where the *Anopheles* mosquito bred in profusion and malaria was endemic. In order to control malaria in the South, the Public Health Service established the Center for Controlling Malaria in the War Areas. After the war, when substantial funds were made available for malaria eradication efforts, this organization was gradually transformed into the Centers for Disease Control (now the Centers for Disease Control and Prevention), which would play a major national role in the effort to control both infectious and noninfectious diseases.[92]

POSTWAR REORGANIZATION

In the immediate postwar period, considerable optimism and energy were devoted to the possible reorganization of public health and medical care. Many of the discussions of a future national medical care system posited the potential unification of preventive and curative medicine. Some public health leaders were advocating the direct administration of tax-supported medical care by health departments. Others opposed such a development, feeling that if public health and medical care administration were combined, preventive and educational efforts would be submerged by the demand for costly therapeutic services.[93]

Hospital Construction

While public health officials were debating whether they wanted to take responsibility for medical care services, the Hospital Survey and Construction Act, more popularly known as the Hill-Burton Act, was passed in 1946. Hospital construction, especially in rural areas, promised to bring everyone the benefits of medical science, without disturbing the freedoms of the medical profession or the patterns of paying for their services. The federal government would pay one-third the costs of building hospitals, setting aside $75 million for each of the first five years. No health program had ever been so generous or so popular.

Hill-Burton addressed the national demand for access to medical care without challenging the private organization of medical practice. It thus answered the desire for acute-care services while essentially ignoring preventive care and public health. The United States could have been completely covered by local health departments for a fraction of the cost of Hill-Burton, but there was no strong political constituency for public health that could compete effectively for resources with curative medicine.

Local Health Services

In 1942, the American Public Health Association provided a plan for organizing local health services across the nation.[94] Haven Emerson's report, *Local Health Units for the Nation*, found that only two-thirds of the people of the United States were covered by local public health services. It also estimated the cost of providing a modest but adequate basic health service for each of the 1,197 additional local health units proposed. The committee noted that communities of over 50,000 should be able to provide a reasonably adequate local service at the cost of $1.00 per capita or a superior service for only $2.00 per capita.[94(p2)]

A survey of state health departments found that a multitude of agencies, state boards, and commissions were involved in public health activities, as many as 18 different agencies being involved in a single state.[95,96] The money spent for public health work also varied widely, ranging from $0.13 per capita in Ohio to $1.68 in Delaware. In most cases, the states spending the largest sums were spending most of these funds on hospital services rather than on prevention.

Changes in Disease

In the postwar years, the public health community clearly understood that the disease patterns of the country had changed: in 1900, the leading causes of death had been tuberculosis, pneumonia, diarrheal diseases, and enteritis; by 1946, the leading causes of death were heart disease, cancer, and accidents. Recognition of the importance of chronic diseases had been temporarily eclipsed by the more urgent demands of infectious disease control during the war. With the return to peace, health departments recognized that they must now come to terms with the problems and prevalence of the chronic diseases.

SOCIAL MEDICINE

In the late 1940s and early 1950s, some American public health officials welcomed the concept of social medicine as seeming to offer a fresh perspective on the problems of chronic illness. Iago Galdston, secretary of the New York Academy of Medicine, organized the Institute on Social Medicine in 1947, later publishing its papers as *Social Medicine: Its Derivations and Objectives.*[97] John A. Ryle, professor of social medicine at Oxford University, emphasized the distinctions between the new social medicine and the old public health. Public health, he said, was concerned with environmental improvement, while social medicine extended its view to "the whole of the economic, nutritional, occupational, educational, and psychological opportunity or experience of the individual or of the community."[98] Whereas public health was concerned with communicable diseases, social medicine would be concerned with all health problems—ulcers and rheumatism, heart disease and cancer, neuroses and injuries. Ryle stated that social medicine, in close alliance with clinical practice, posed the exciting challenge of the future.

The Role of Epidemiology

Ernest L. Stebbins, dean of the Johns Hopkins School of Public Health, argued that epidemiology was the essential discipline for dealing with both chronic and infectious diseases.[99] Margaret Merrell and Lowell J. Reed, statisticians from the Hopkins school, made a similar point in a brief paper that would become a classic statement on *the epidemiology of health.* They suggested a graded scale for measuring degrees of health, not simply the absence of illness:

> On such a scale people would be classified from those who are in top-notch condition with abundant energy, through the people who are well, to fairly well, down to people who are feeling rather poorly, and finally to the definitely ill.[100]

The ideas that health could be quantitatively measurable and that it could be advanced in the total absence of disease helped make connections between the new social medicine and the older public health. Epidemiology, broadening its scope to place more emphasis on the social environment, became newly fashionable as "medical ecology."[81] John E. Gordon, professor of preventive medicine and epidemiology at the Harvard School of Public Health and a prominent exponent of the "newer epidemiology," explained how the triad of "environment, host, and disease" could be applied to noncommunicable organic diseases such as pellagra, cancer, psychosomatic conditions, traumatic injuries, and accidents.[101,102] The notion of a single cause of disease (the agent) was now firmly rejected in favor of multiple causation.[99]

Troubles in Implementation

Social medicine brought considerable optimism about the possibilities for new approaches to the chronic diseases, for the integration of preventive and curative medicine, and for the extension of comprehensive health programs to the whole population.[103] In 1950, Eli Ginzberg introduced a tone of pessimism and caution, however, when he warned optimistic thinkers of an *anti-government attitude* in the United States and the prevalent assumption that health depended on medical care, with the ever increasing provision of doctors and hospital beds. He urged public health professionals to do a more effective job of persuading the public that advances in diet, housing, and public health nursing were more important to health than the construction of hospitals. He also noted that while hospitals were being built across the country, local health officer positions stood vacant because communities refused to provide reasonable salaries.[104]

Ginzberg's prognosis proved correct in the political climate of the 1950s. The theoretical innovations of social medicine were not translated into effective health programs; acute-care facilities and biomedical research expanded dramatically in the postwar period, while public health departments struggled to maintain their programs on inadequate budgets with little political support. The postwar construction meant massive expenditures for biomedical research and hospital construction, the partial payment for medical care by expanding private insurance coverage, but the relative neglect of public health services and a complete failure to implement the more radical ideas of social medicine through attention to the social determinants of health and disease.

POLITICAL PROBLEMS OF PUBLIC HEALTH

The Committee on Medicine and the Changing Order, supported by the Commonwealth Fund, the Milbank Memorial Fund, and the Josiah Macy Jr. Foundation, recommended the extension of public health services in 1947, but it argued that the quality of public health officers must be improved by better recruitment, training, assured tenure, and adequate salaries.[105] Harry Mustard, on the other hand, protested that the problems of public health were largely political. State health officers were of relatively low rank in the hierarchy of state officials and were limited in their freedom to introduce new proposals. Too often they accepted political constraints and bureaucratic barriers as natural and inevitable.[106] Too seldom were they willing to risk their positions by appealing to a larger constituency.

In retrospect, it also seems clear that public health failed to claim sufficient credit for controlling infectious diseases. The major scientific achievements of the war in relation to health, such as the discovery of penicillin and the use of DDT, were especially relevant to public health. In popular perception, however, scientific medicine took credit for both the specific wartime discoveries and the longer history of controlling epidemic disease. Medicine and biomedical research had essentially seized the public glory, the political interest, and the financial support given for further anticipated health improvements in the postwar world.

Public health departments needed to claim some share of the credit for declining infectious diseases and to move quickly to develop programs for the chronic diseases. Most health departments did neither of these things but simply continued running the same programs and clinics within already established bureaucratic structures. The political atmosphere of the 1950s did not support aggressive new programs, and health department budgets were stagnant, without the funding needed to develop broad new health programs.

The Fluoridation Fiasco

Health departments did implement, or try to implement, one important new and very cost-effective public health measure, the fluoridation of water supplies to protect children's teeth.[107] Despite virtually unanimous support from scientific authorities and professional organizations, however, fluoridation was denounced as a communist plot and effectively halted in many cities and towns through vocal local opposition. If such a simple and obviously effective measure could be so energetically opposed, health departments must have perceived the difficulty in instituting more adventurous or expensive interventions.

An Exception: Success with Polio

The one great triumph of the 1950s was the successful development of the polio vaccine and its implementation on a mass scale.[108–110] The success of the polio campaign was in large part due to private funding and a massive public relations campaign by the Foundation for Infantile Paralysis, which raised public awareness and developed public support, interest, and enthusiasm. The appeal for crippled children proved extremely popular, and the polio vaccination campaign, aside from some major setbacks, was a remarkable success.

DECLINE OF PUBLIC HEALTH IN THE 1950s

Despite such public success, in the 1950s the real expenditures of public health departments failed to keep pace with the increase in population.[111] Federal grants-in-aid to the states for public health programs steadily declined, falling from $45 million in 1950 to $33 million in 1959. Given inflation, the decline in purchasing power was even more dramatic. At a time when public health officials were facing a whole series of new, poorly understood health problems, they were also underbudgeted and understaffed.

Health officers were frequently limited to routine clinical responsibilities in child health stations, tuberculosis clinics, venereal disease clinics, and immunization programs, and to communicable disease diagnosis and treatment. They had little or no time for community health education, for studying new health problems, or for developing experimental programs. Indeed, in many areas health officer positions went unfilled, and local medical practitioners, working part-time, provided clinical services on an hourly basis.[112]

Some state legislatures were setting up new agencies to build nursing homes, abate water pollution, or promote mental health, and they simply bypassed health departments as not active or interested in these issues. Public health officials were expressing "frustrations, disappointments, dissatisfactions, and discontentments," said John W. Knutson in his Presidential Address to the American Public Health Association in 1957.[113] Public health professionals, he said, must develop more imagination, political skills, and knowledge of human motivation and behavior. Public health students needed a better understanding of social and political forces. Instead of simply learning soon-to-be-outdated factual information, they needed an in-depth knowledge of cultural anthropology, human ecology, epidemiology, and biostatistics.[113] Yet even with the best possible preparation, the bureaucratic controls of state health departments tended to assure conformity and discourage young professionals from initiating or taking responsibility for new programs or activities.[114]

In 1959, Milton Terris offered a forceful summary statement of the dilemma of public health. The communicable diseases were disappearing; their place had been taken by the noninfectious diseases that the public health profession was ill prepared to prevent or control. The public understood the fact that research was crucial, and federal expenditures for medical research had multiplied from $28 million in 1947 to $186 million 10 years later. Most of this money, however, was being spent for clinical and laboratory research; there was little understanding of the importance of epidemiological studies in addressing these problems. Schools of public health had been slow to deal with chronic illness, as had health departments, with a few notable exceptions as in the cases of New York and California. Yet even the small sums spent on epidemiological research had produced dramatic successes, including the discovery of the role of fluoride in preventing dental caries, the relation of cigarette smoking to lung cancer, and the suspected relation of serum cholesterol and physical exercise to coronary artery disease.[115]

In the late 1950s, public health leaders recognized and lamented the failure of their profession to assert a strong political presence or even to perceive the importance of politics to practical public health. The American Public Health Association devoted its annual meeting in 1958 to *The Politics of Public Health*.[116] The editor of the *American Journal of Public Health*, George Rosen, wrote that the education of public health workers should begin with teaching them to think politically and to understand the political process.[117] Raymond R. Tucker, mayor of St. Louis, the city hosting the APHA convention, insisted that public health officials must learn not to confuse the opposition of special interest groups with public opinion, for the general public solidly supported public health reform.[118]

THE 1960S AND THE WAR ON POVERTY

The 1960s saw the collapse of the conservative complacency of the 1950s, the growing power of the civil rights movement, riots in urban African-American ghettos, and federal support for the *war on poverty*. The antipoverty effort and other Great Society programs soon became deeply involved with medical care.[119] Growing concern over access to medical care and hospitalization, especially by the elderly population, culminated in Medicare and Medicaid legislation in 1965 to cover medical care costs for those on Social Security and for the poor. Both programs were built on the *politics of accommodation* with private providers of medical care, thus increasing the incomes of physicians and hospitals and leading to spiraling costs for medical services.[120] Other antipoverty programs, such as the neighborhood health centers that were intended to encourage community participation in providing comprehensive care to underserved populations, fared less well because they were seen as competing with the interests of private care providers.[121]

Most of the new health and social programs of the 1960s bypassed the structure of the public health agencies and set up new agencies to mediate between the federal government and local communities. Medicare and

Medicaid reflected the usual priorities of the medical care system in favoring highly technical interventions and hospital care, while failing to provide adequately for preventive services. Neighborhood health centers and community-based mental health services were established without reference to public health agencies.

When environmental issues attracted public concern and political attention in the 1960s and 1970s, separate agencies were also created to respond to these concerns. At the federal level, the Environmental Protection Agency was created to deal with such issues as solid wastes, pesticides, and radiation. At the state level, environmental agencies were often separate from public health departments and failed to reflect specific health concerns or public health expertise. Similarly, mental health agencies were often separate from public health agencies.

Thus, the broader functions of public health were again split between numerous different agencies. Losing a clear institutional base, public health had also lost visibility and clarity of definition. For a field that depends so heavily on public understanding and support, such a loss was disastrous.

PUBLIC HEALTH IN THE SEVENTIES AND EIGHTIES

In the 1970s, public health departments became providers of last resort for uninsured patients and for Medicaid patients rejected by private practitioners. By 1988, almost three-quarters of all state and local health department expenditures went for personal health services.[122] As Harry Mustard had predicted some 40 years earlier, direct provision of medical care absorbed much of the limited resources—in personnel, money, energy, time, and attention—of public health departments, leading to a slow starvation of public health and preventive activities.[122(p52)] The problem of caring for the uninsured and the indigent loomed so large that it eclipsed the need for a basic public health infrastructure in the minds of many legislators and the general public.

In the Reagan revolution of the 1980s, federal funding for public health programs was cut. Through the mechanism of the block grants, power was returned to state health agencies, but in the context of funding cuts, this was the unpopular power to cut existing programs.[123] In the context of general budget cuts, state health departments were often left the task of managing Medicaid programs and delivering personal health services to uninsured and indigent populations. State health departments also had to deal with the adverse health consequences of reductions in other social programs; with the problems of a growing poverty population, as evidenced in drug abuse, alcoholism, teenage pregnancy, infant mortality, family violence, and homelessness; and with the health and social needs of growing populations of illegal immigrants.

The AIDS epidemic and the resurgence of tuberculosis revealed the structural contradictions and weaknesses of national and federal health policy.[124] For state and local health agencies, AIDS and tuberculosis exacerbated their existing problems but gave a new visibility and urgency to their public health efforts.[125,126] The public health community urged a major national effort in AIDS education and prevention. Much of the new funding, when it did finally come, went into research and medical care; as usual, education and prevention received much less attention. But at the same time, the mobilization of public concern provided renewed attention to public health and increased political support. The report by the Institute of Medicine, titled *The Future of Public Health,* notes that:

> In a free society public activities ultimately rest on public understanding and support, not on the technical judgment of experts. Expertise is made effective only when it is combined with sufficient public support, a connection acted upon effectively by the early leaders of public health.[122(p130)]

PUBLIC HEALTH TODAY

Since the early 1990s, the whole country has been embroiled in debates over health care reform, welfare reform, drugs, violence, environmental health, and women's health issues. These are all issues of public health, yet public health as such is rarely mentioned. This is partly a failure of public health practice; we need a variety of model public health programs to demonstrate to the country what could be achieved with sufficient political will, expertise, and money. It is also in part a failure of communications. Public health professionals have not been very effective in presenting their views and accomplishments to the media, the politicians, and the public.

CONCLUSION

The growth in the technical knowledge of public health in the past 100 years has been extraordinary—and insufficiently addressed in this brief account—but our ability to implement this knowledge in health and social reform has advanced little. As we have noted, the issues of public health today include and intersect with the great social issues of modern America: health care reform and the coverage of the uninsured; environmental health and safety; welfare reform and child health; drugs and violence in the streets; women's health, reproductive freedom, abortion, and fertility control; family violence and child abuse; AIDS, tuberculosis, and emerging epidemics; the continuing problems of chronic disease; and the need for home health services and long-term care for an aging population.

Public health is a vitally important field for the future well-being of America, its citizens, and its communities. Public health professionals must learn to communicate better the vital importance of their activities, mobilize public support, build a more effective public health infrastructure, and demonstrate clearly the benefits of prevention to the public at large by finding innovative ways of responding to endemic social problems and new crises.

REFERENCES

1. Rosenberg C. *The Cholera Years: The United States in 1832, 1849 and 1866.* Chicago, Il: University of Chicago Press; 1962.

2. Powell JH. *Bring Out Your Dead: The Great Plague of Yellow Fever in Philadelphia in 1793.* Philadelphia, Pa: University of Pennsylvania Press; 1949.

3. Wiebe RH. *The Search for Order, 1877–1920.* New York, NY: Hill and Wang; 1967.

4. Ackerknecht EL. Anticontagionism between 1821 and 1867. *Bull Hist Med.* 1948;22:562–593.

5. Baltimore City Ordinance 11, approved April 7, 1797. In: Howard WT. *Public Health Administration and the Natural History of Disease in Baltimore, Maryland, 1797–1920.* Washington, DC: Carnegie Institution; 1924.

6. Rosen G. *A History of Public Health.* Expanded ed. Baltimore, Md: Johns Hopkins University Press; 1993.

7. Duffy J. *The Sanitarians: A History of American Public Health.* Urbana, Il: University of Illinois Press; 1990.

8. Rosner D, ed. *Epidemic! Public Health Crises in New York.* New Brunswick, NJ: Rutgers University Press; 1994.

9. Citizens' Association of New York. *Report of the Council of Hygiene and Public Health of the Citizens' Association of New York upon the Sanitary Condition of the City.* New York, NY: Arno Press; 1970:xxi–xxxv.

10. Hudson A. The mapping of property and environment in Manhattan since the 1600s. *Biblion.* Spring 1993;1:47–50.

11. Shattuck L. *Report of a General Plan for the Promotion of Public and Personal Health, Devised, Prepared, and Recommended by the Commissioners Appointed under a Resolve of the Legislature of the State.* Cambridge, Ma: Harvard University Press; 1948.

12. Rosen G. *A History of Public Health.* Baltimore, Md: Johns Hopkins University Press; 1993:216–219.

13. *Proceedings and Debates of the Third National Quarantine and Sanitary Conference.* New York, NY: Edward Jones; 1859:179–180.

14. Adams GW. *Doctors in Blue.* New York, NY: Henry Schuman; 1952.

15. Woodward JJ. *Chief Camp Diseases of the United States Armies.* Philadelphia, Pa: J.B. Lippencott; 1863.

16. Cavins HM. The national quarantine and sanitary conventions of 1857–1858 and the beginnings of the American Public Health Association. *Bull Hist Med.* 1943;13:419–425.

17. Kramer HD. Agitation for public health reform in the 1870s. *J Hist Med Allied Sci.* 1948;3:473–488.

18. Smith S. The history of public health, 1871–1921. In: Ravenel MP, ed. *A Half Century of Public Health.* New York, NY: American Public Health Association; 1921:1–12.

19. Ravenel MP. The American Public Health Association: past, present, future. In: Ravenel MP, ed. *A Half Century of Public Health.* New York, NY: American Public Health Association; 1921:13–55.

20. Patterson RG. *Historical Directory of State Health Departments in the United States of America.* Columbus, Oh: Ohio Public Health Association; 1939.

21. Abbott SW. *The Past and Present Conditions of Public Hygiene and State Medicine in the United States.* Boston, Ma: Wright and Potter; 1900.

22. Mullan F. *Plagues and Politics: The Story of the United States Marine Hospital Service.* New York, NY: Basic Books; 1989.

23. Harden VA. *Inventing the NIH: Federal Biomedical Research Policy, 1887–1937.* Baltimore, Md: Johns Hopkins University Press; 1986.

24. Blake J. *Public Health in the Town of Boston, 1630–1822.* Cambridge, Ma: Harvard University Press; 1959.

25. Rosenkrantz B. *Public Health and the State: Changing Views in Massachusetts, 1842–1936.* Cambridge, Ma: Harvard University Press; 1972.

26. Duffy J. *A History of Public Health in New York City, 1625–1826.* New York, NY: Russell Sage Foundation; 1968.

27. Duffy J. *A History of Public Health in New York City, 1866–1966.* New York, NY: Russell Sage Foundation; 1974.

28. Galishoff S. *Safeguarding the Public Health: Newark, 1895–1918.* Westport, Ct: Greenwood Press; 1975.

29. Leavitt JW. *The Healthiest City: Milwaukee and the Politics of Health Reform.* Princeton, NJ: Princeton University Press; 1982.

30. Kraut AM. *Silent Travelers: Germs, Genes, and the Immigrant Menace.* New York, NY: Basic Books; 1994.

31. Winslow CEA. *The Life of Hermann M. Biggs: Physician and Statesman of the Public Health.* Philadelphia, Pa: Lea and Febiger; 1929.

32. Jordan EO, Whipple GC, Winslow CEA. *A Pioneer of Public Health: William Thompson Sedgwick.* New Haven, Ct: Yale University Press; 1924.

33. Cassedy JH. *Charles V. Chapin and the Public Health Movement.* Cambridge, Ma: Harvard University Press; 1962.

34. Rosenberg CE, Rosenberg CS. Pietism and the origins of the American public health movement. *J Hist Med Allied Sci.* 1968;23:16–35.

35. Shroyck RH. The early American public health movement. *Am J Public Health.* 1937;27:965–971.

36. Rosenkrantz B. Cart before horse: theory, practice and professional image in American public health. *J Hist Med Allied Sci.* 1974;29:57.

37. Ryan MP. *Womanhood in America: From Colonial Times to the Present.* New York, NY: Franklin Watts; 1975:225–234.

38. Smillie W. *Public Health: Its Promise for the Future.* New York, NY: Macmillan; 1955:450–458.

39. Wiebe RH. *The Search for Order, 1877–1920.* New York, NY: Hill and Wang; 1967.

40. Hayes SP. The politics of reform in municipal government in the progressive era. In: Hayes SP, ed. *American Political History as Social Analysis.* Knoxville, Tn: University of Tennessee Press; 1980:205–232.

41. Hayes SP. *Conservation and the Gospel of Efficiency: The Progressive Conservation Movement, 1890–1918.* Boston, Ma: Beacon Press; 1968.

42. Rogers DT. In search of progressivism. *Rev Am Hist.* 1982;10:115–132.

43. Welch WH. Sanitation in relation to the poor. An address to the Charity Organization Society of Baltimore, November 1892. In: *Papers and Addresses by William Henry Welch, Vol. 3.* Baltimore, Md: The Johns Hopkins Press; 1920.

44. von Pettenkofer M. Sigerist HE, trans. *The Value of Health to a City.* Baltimore, Md: Johns Hopkins University Press; 1941:15–52.

45. Rotch TM. The position and work of the American Pediatric Society toward public questions. *Trans Am Pediatr Soc.* 1909;21:12.

46. Chapin C. How shall we spend the health appropriation? In: Chapin CV, Gorham FP, eds. *Papers of Charles V. Chapin, M.D.: A Review of Public Health Realities.* New York, NY: Commonwealth Fund; 1934:28–35.

47. Sternberg GM. Sanitary lessons of the war. In: Sternberg GM, ed. *Sanitary Lessons of the War and Other Papers.* Washington, DC: Byron S. Adams; 1912:2.

48. Cosmas GA. *An Army for Empire: The United States Army in the Spanish-American War.* Columbia, Mo: University of Missouri Press; 1971.

49. Kelley HA. *Walter Reed and Yellow Fever.* Baltimore, Md: Medical Standard Book Company; 1906.

50. Sternberg GM. Sanitary problems connected with the construction of the Isthmian Canal. In: Sternberg GM, ed. *Sanitary Lessons of the War and Other Papers.* Washington, D.C. Byron S. Adams; 1912:39–40.

51. Fosdick RB. *Adventure in Giving: The Story of the General Education Board.* New York, NY: Harper and Row; 1962:57–58.

52. Ettling J. *The Germ of Laziness: Rockefeller Philanthropy and Public Health in the New South.* Cambridge, Ma: Harvard University Press; 1981.

53. Rose W. First annual report of the administrative secretary of the Rockefeller Sanitary Commission; 1910:4. In: Fosdick RB,

ed. *The Story of the Rockefeller Foundation.* New York, NY: Harper and Brothers; 1952:33.

54. Rosen G. The committee of one hundred on national health and the campaign for a national health department, 1906–1912. *Am J Public Health.* 1972;62:261–263.

55. Marcus AI. Disease prevention in America: from a local to a national outlook, 1880–1910. *Bull Hist Med.* 1979;53:184–203.

56. Fisher I. *A Report on National Vitality, Its Wastes and Conservation.* Washington DC: Committee of One Hundred on National Health; 1909. US Govt Printing Office Bulletin 30.

57. Williams RC. *The United States Public Health Service, 1798–1950.* Washington, DC: US Govt Printing Office; 1951.

58. Schiesl MJ. *The Politics of Efficiency: Municipal Administration and Reform In America, 1880–1920.* Berkeley, Ca. University of California Press; 1980.

59. Fee E. *Disease and Discovery: A History of the Johns Hopkins School of Hygiene and Public Health, 1916–1939.* Baltimore, Md: Johns Hopkins University Press; 1987.

60. Fee E, Acheson RM, eds. *A History of Education in Public Health: Health That Mocks the Doctors' Rules.* New York, NY: Oxford University Press; 1991.

61. Sedgwick WT. The origin, scope and significance of bacteriology. *Science.* 1901;13:121–28.

62. Winslow CEA. The untilled fields of public health. *Science.* 1920;51:23.

63. Winslow CEA. *The Evolution and Significance of the Modern Public Health Campaign.* New Haven, Ct: Yale University Press; 1923.

64. Sicherman B. *Alice Hamilton: A Life in Letters.* Cambridge, Ma.: Harvard University Press; 1984:153–183.

65. Terris M, ed. *Goldberger on Pellagra.* Baton Rouge, La: Louisiana State University Press; 1964.

66. Kantor B. *The New Scientific Public Health Movement: A Case Study of Tuberculosis in Baltimore, Maryland, 1900–1910.* Baltimore, Md: Johns Hopkins University; 1985. Thesis.

67. Meeker E. The improving health of the United States, 1850–1915. *Explorations in Economic History.* 1972;9:353–373.

68. Haines RH. The use of model life tables to estimate mortality for the United States in the late nineteenth century. *Demography.* 1979;16:289–312.

69. Hoffman FL. The general death rate of large American cities, 1871–1904. *Publications of the American Statistical Association.* 1906–1907;10:1–75.

70. Duffy J. Social impact of disease in the late nineteenth century. *Bull NY Acad Med.* 1971;47:797–811.

71. Knowles M. Public health service not a medical monopoly. *Am J Public Health.* 1913;3:111–122.

72. Winslow CEA. Public health at the crossroads. *Am J Public Health.* 1926;16:1075–1085.

73. *Report of the Committee on Municipal Health Department Practice of the American Public Health Association, in cooperation with the United States Public Health Service.* Washington DC: US Govt Printing Office; 1923. Public Health Bulletin No. 136.

74. Duffy J. The American medical profession and public health: from support to ambivalence. *Bull Hist Med.* 1979; 53:1–22.

75. Meckel RA. *Save the Babies: American Public Health Reform and the Prevention of Infant Mortality, 1850–1920.* Baltimore, Md: Johns Hopkins University Press; 1990.

76. Mullan F. *Plagues and Politics: The Story of the United States Public Health Service.* New York, NY: Basic Books; 1989.

77. Committee on the Costs of Medical Care. *Medical Care for the American People.* Chicago, Il: University of Chicago Press; 1932. Final report.

78. Fee E. The pleasures and perils of prophetic advocacy: socialized medicine and the politics of medical reform. In: Fee E, Brown TM, eds. *Making Medical History: The Life and Work of Henry E. Sigerist.* Baltimore, Md: Johns Hopkins University Press; 1996. In press.

79. Berkowitz ED. *America's Welfare State: From Roosevelt to Reagan.* Baltimore, Md: Johns Hopkins University Press; 1991.

80. Kratz FK. Status of full-time local health organizations at the end of the fiscal year 1941–1942. *Public Health Rep.* 1943;58:345–351.

81. Corwin EHL, ed. *Ecology of Health.* New York, NY: The Commonwealth Fund; 1949.

82. Mustard HS. *Government in Public Health.* New York, NY: The Commonwealth Fund; 1945:190.

83. Leathers WS, et al. Committee on Professional Education of the American Public Health Association. Public health degrees and certificates granted in 1936. *Am J Public Health.* 1937;27:1267–1272.

84. Mustard HS, ed. Yesterday's school children are examined for the Army. *Am J Public Health.* 1941;31:1207.

85. Simmons JS. The preventive medicine program of the United States Army. *Am J Public Health.* 1943;33:931–940.

86. Mountain JW. Responsibility of local health authorities in the war effort. *Am J Public Health.* 1943;33:35–40.

87. Williams RC. *The United States Public Health Service, 1798– 1950.* Washington, DC: Commissioned Officers' Association of the United States Public Health Service; 1951: 612–768.

88. Furman B. *A Profile of the Public Health Service, 1798–1948.* Bethesda, Md: National Institutes of Health; 1973:418–458.

89. Perrott GStJ. Findings of selective service examinations. *Milbank Q.* 1944;22:358–366.

90. Perrott GStJ. Selective service rejection statistics and some of their implications. *Am J Public Health.* 1946;36:336–342.

91. Maxcy KF. Epidemiologic implications of wartime population shifts. *Am J Public Health.* 1942;32:1089–1096.

92. Ethridge EW. *Sentinel for Health: A History of the Centers for Disease Control.* Berkeley, Ca: University of California Press; 1992.

93. Stern BJ. *Medical Services by Government: Local, State, and Federal.* New York, NY: The Commonwealth Fund; 1946:31–32.

94. Emerson H. *Local Health Units for the Nation.* New York, NY: The Commonwealth Fund; 1945.

95. Mountain JW, Flook E. Distribution of health services in the structure of state government: the composite pattern of state health services. *Public Health Rep.* 1941;56:1676.

96. Mountain JW, Flook E. Distribution of health services in the structure of state government: state health department organization. *Public Health Rep.* 1943;58:568.

97. Galdston I, ed. *Social Medicine: Its Derivations and Objectives.* New York, NY: The Commonwealth Fund; 1949.

98. Ryle JA. Social pathology. In: Galdston I, ed. *Social Medicine: Its Derivations and Objectives.* New York, NY: The Commonwealth Fund; 1949:64.

99. Stebbins EL. Epidemiology and social medicine. In: Galdston I, ed. *Social Medicine: Its Derivations and Objectives.* New York, NY: The Commonwealth Fund; 1949:101–104.

100. Merrell M, Reed LJ. The epidemiology of health. In: Galdston I, ed. *Social Medicine: Its Derivations and Objectives.* New York, NY: The Commonwealth Fund; 1949:105–110.

101. Gordon JE. The newer epidemiology. In: *Tomorrow's Horizon in Public Health.* Transactions of the 1950 conference of the Public Health Association of New York City. New York, NY: Public Health Association; 1950:18–45.

102. Gordon JE. The world, the flesh and the devil as environment, host and agent of disease. In: Galdston I, ed. *The Epidemiology of Health.* New York, NY: Health Education Council; 1953: 60–73.

103. Smillie WG. The responsibility of the state. In: *Tomorrow's Horizon in Public Health.* Transactions of the 1950 conference of the Public Health Association of New York City. New York, NY: Public Health Association; 1950:95–102.

104. Ginzberg E. Public health and the public. In: *Tomorrow's Horizon in Public Health.* Transactions of the 1950 conference of the Public Health Association of New York City. New York, NY: Public Health Association; 1950: 101–109.

105. New York Academy of Medicine, Committee on Medicine in the Changing Order. *Medicine in the Changing Order.* New York, NY: The Commonwealth Fund; 1947:109.

106. Mustard HS. *Government in Public Health.* New York, NY: The Commonwealth Fund; 1945:112.

107. McNeil DR. *The Fight for Fluoridation.* New York, NY: Oxford University Press; 1957.

108. Benison S. *Tom Rivers: Reflections on a Life in Medicine and Science.* Cambridge, Ma: MIT Press; 1967.

109. Klein AE. *Trial by Fury: The Polio Vaccine Controversy.* New York, NY: Scribner's; 1972.

110. Paul JR. *A History of Poliomyelitis.* New Haven, Ct: Yale University Press; 1971.

111. Sanders BS. Local health departments: growth or illusion. *Public Health Rep.* 1959;74:13–20.

112. Aronson JB. The politics of public health—reactions and summary. *Am J Public Health.* 1959;49:311.

113. Knutson JW. Ferment in public health. *Am J Public Health.* 1957;47:1489–1491.

114. Woodcock L. Where are we going in public health? *Am J Public Health.* 1956;46:278–282.

115. Terris M. The changing face of public health. *Am J Public Health.* 1959;49:1113–1119.

116. American Public Health Association Symposium—1958. The politics of public health. *Am J Public Health.* 1959;49: 300–313.

117. Rosen G. The politics of public health. *Am J Public Health.* 1959;49:364–365.

118. Tucker RR. The politics of public health. *Am J Public Health.* 1959;49:300–305.

119. Davis K, Schoen C. *Health and the War on Poverty.* Washington, DC: Brookings Institution; 1978.

120. Starr P. *The Social Transformation of American Medicine.* New York, NY: Basic Books; 1982:374–378.

121. Sardell A. *The U.S. Experiment in Social Medicine: The Community Health Center Program, 1965–1986.* Pittsburgh, Pa; University of Pittsburgh Press; 1988.

122. Institute of Medicine, Committee for the Study of the Future of Public Health. *The Future of Public Health.* Washington, DC: National Academy Press; 1988.

123. Omenn GS. What's behind those block grants in health. *New Eng J Med.* 1982;306:1057–1060.

124. Fox DM. AIDS and the American health policy: the history and prospects of a crisis of authority. In: Fee E, Fox DM, eds. *AIDS: The Burdens of History.* Berkeley, Ca; University of California Press; 1988:316–343.

125. Fee E, Fox DM, eds. *AIDS: The Making of a Chronic Disease.* Berkeley, Ca: University of California Press; 1992.

126. Krieger N, Margo G, eds. *AIDS: The Politics of Survival.* New York, NY: Baywood; 1994.

CHAPTER

The Determinants of Health

John M. Last, M.D., D.P.H.

In this chapter, determinants of health are discussed in a conceptual framework based on definitions of health. Numerous examples are given to show that no single determinant of health is the most important; many are involved in promoting good health for individuals and communities. The examples also show that determinants often act synergistically rather than separately on the conditions that affect health. The chapter ends with a discussion of potential future challenges to public health practice.

DEFINITIONS OF HEALTH

The preamble to the constitution of the World Health Organization (WHO) describes health as "a state of complete physical, mental and social well-being, not merely the absence of disease or infirmity."[1] This is an ideal state. If this definition is taken literally, health is rarely attained by anyone for very long. The problems begin with the word *complete* and are compounded by the vague meaning of *social well-being*. Furthermore, this definition is operationally unsatisfac-

tory; one cannot measure or count any aspect of it. Therefore, it cannot be used to compare personal or community health status at different times, in different places, or among different kinds of persons.

In the early 1980s when WHO initiated its health promotion programs, new dimensions were added to its definition of health to convey the important idea that individuals and groups have some control over their own health:

> Health is . . . the extent to which an individual or a group is able, on the one hand, to realize aspirations and satisfy needs; and, on the other hand, to change or cope with the environment. Health is . . . a resource for everyday life, not the objective of living; it is a positive concept, emphasizing social and personal resources, as well as physical capacities.[2]

There are many other definitions of health. For those interested in measuring health status and calculating the rates or proportions of persons with good or poor health, a useful definition was given by Stokes et al.:

Health is a state characterized by anatomic integrity, ability to perform personally valued family, work and community roles; ability to deal with physical, biologic and social stress; a feeling of well-being; and freedom from the risk of disease and untimely death.[3]

There are valid instruments to measure all the components mentioned in this definition at both individual and population levels.

Humans do not live in a vacuum but interact with each other and with many other kinds of living creatures in local, regional, and global ecosystems. A definition that takes this into account describes health as "a state of equilibrium between humans and their physical, biologic, social and cultural environment that is compatible with full functional activity."[4] In personal communication to John M. Last, Maurice King called this definition deficient. In a provocative essay,[5] King argued that, for example, child survival strategies to improve community health in developing countries have led to exuberant population growth, overcultivation, and unsuitable agricultural practices in fragile environments. These, in turn, have caused the collapse of local ecosystems and subsistence agriculture, making the people in some developing countries dependent on food aid or forcing them to migrate out of the region as ecologic refugees, a phenomenon known as the demographic trap.[6] Another potential outcome is conflict.[7] Although King's views have been contested, there is no doubt that if present trends in population growth continue, the whole world will be caught in the demographic trap. If the environment is unable to sustain the population that inhabits it, then the population cannot be called healthy.[8] In response to this valid criticism, a modified definition of health might read:

Health is a sustainable state of equilibrium between humans and their physical, biologic, social and cultural environment, compatible with full functional activity of all interacting components in the ecosystem.

There are problems with this definition as well. If pathogens or their vectors are part of the ecosystem, for example, should they, too, be sustained? In other respects, however, this definition is useful. It cautions against taking a short-term view of health: if health is borrowed from the capital resources that future generations of humans will need for their survival, a present healthy state is an illusion.

DETERMINANTS OF HEALTH

All these definitions of health contain words or phrases that suggest or explicitly mention determinants of health. These determinants can be classified under headings such as **physical, biological, behavioral, social, cultural, and spiritual**. Another way to classify them is as **hereditary determinants,** which means those that are inborn or constitutional, or **acquired determinants**, which include everything from infections and trauma to cultural characteristics and spiritual values.

In medicine and human biology, however, nothing is simple. Few things can be categorized in neat, clearly circumscribed compartments, and fewer still in simple binary terms. Congenital conditions, for example, may be the result of factors in the physical environment, such as chemicals or radiation, or the result of invading microorganisms, such as the rubella virus. As another example, genetic makeup is determined by the mating patterns of one's ancestors, whose genetic makeup, in turn, was influenced by the inherent susceptibility or resistance of their ancestors to certain diseases (for example, measles, influenza, smallpox, plague, and malaria) that selectively attacked or spared particular genotypes.[9] Moreover, in virtually all settings, from primitive societies through rural agrarian states to modern industrial nations, mating tends to be more assortative than random, so patterns of gene frequency become a mosaic that is attributable to a combination of environmental, cultural, economic, social, and behavioral factors.

The *personal* qualities alluded to in the 1984 WHO definition include attributes routinely recorded in medical records and health statistics. We display health status in tables arranged according to the most important of these attributes, namely **age,** and **sex,** and sometimes according to others such as **race**.

Age and Sex

Age and sex are important determinants of health status. From conception through old age, mortality rates are higher for males than females, although health care utilization statistics nearly all show higher rates of utilization for females than males, even when reasons related to pregnancy and childbirth are excluded. However, females do not live longer on average than males because they use more health care services (perhaps in spite of it) but because of inherent, ill-defined biological characteristics.

Age is an obvious determinant of health. Infants, especially if they are underweight or prematurely born, are more vulnerable to many diseases than are older children. Indeed, recent record linkage studies have shown that premature infants are at increased risk of adult onset conditions, such as elevated serum cholesterol, hypertension, and coronary heart disease.[10] The peak of fitness and good health is reached after adolescence, and then health and physical vitality and efficiency slowly decline until the seventh or eighth decade. By the late 60s, most people are taking regular medication and can count their identified infirmities in double figures (failing eyesight and hearing, poor or no teeth, varicose veins, hernias, deteriorating genital tracts, and stiffening joints, among others). By the second half of the 80s, most people need personal care, often in a long-term care institution.[11]

Race

A race is defined as a group that is relatively homogeneous with respect to genetic inheritance. The most obvious marker of racial membership is skin color. Some conditions occur more commonly in certain racial groups than in others. For example, African-Americans have higher prevalence and mortality rates from hypertension and cancer of the prostate than Americans of European origin. Native Americans (Indians) have a higher prevalence of diabetes and, among some tribal groups, of arthritis when compared to Euro-Americans. Some Orthodox Jews carry the gene for Tay-Sachs disease.

These and other conditions that are described as racially determined are either of genetic origin (such as Tay-Sachs disease) or attributable to a combination of inherited, environmental, and socially and culturally determined factors. Both African-Americans and Native Americans include high proportions of persons

whose culture and values have been destroyed or gravely damaged. They often come from deprived socio-economic backgrounds, and the real "cause" of at least some of their high prevalence and mortality rates from the above conditions and others, such as alcohol and substance abuse, is confounded by these factors.

Physical Determinants

Physical determinants of health include first and foremost the radiant energy that reaches the earth from the sun. The sun is the giver of all life, the source of energy, the force that triggers the metabolism of carbon, nitrogen, and oxygen in plant and animal systems. However, too much sunshine is harmful: excess ultraviolet radiation impairs immune responses,[12] causes cancer,[13] and leads to cataracts.[14] Other forms of electromagnetic radiation, including some that have poorly understood effects on health, will be discussed later.

Another set of physical factors that determine health are elements essential for life, such as iron, iodine, and copper, among many others and those that may harm health, such as environmental lead,[15] mercury, cadmium, and organic compounds including PCBs. The air may be polluted with solid particulates, asbestos, or tobacco smoke. Drinking water may contain insufficient concentrations of fluoride for the manufacture of strong dental enamel, or it may contain toxic chemicals or any of innumerable pathogens.

Biological Determinants

The biological determinants of health include all the microorganisms that may cause harm, as well as biologic products such as sera and vaccines that help protect against disease. Some bacteria live in symbiosis with humans in the gastrointestinal tract, manufacturing vitamins that are needed for good health. There is an uneasy truce between humans and pathogenic microorganisms for much of the time, but this truce is in the interests of both parties. If invading pathogens are too harmful, they may die if they kill their human host; if humans are totally shielded from exposure to pathogens such as common cold viruses, they lose their immunities and can then be overwhelmed when they are eventually re-exposed. Many of the pathogenic microorganisms that cause ill health do so because of a combination of ecologic and behavioral factors.

Another class of biologic determinants of health are the essential dietary nutrients: the carbohydrates, proteins, fats, minerals, and vitamins that are derived from plant and animal sources. With these, as with many other determinants, health is optimal when the right balance is struck between deficit and excess.

Behavioral Determinants

Behavioral determinants of health are more difficult to describe, classify, and explain. Empirical observations dating from ancient times and Galen's system of medical beliefs[16] led to descriptions of personality types—phlegmatic, choleric, melancholic, sanguine—associated with predisposition or resistance to certain diseases. Such beliefs survive today in the names of some medical conditions and symptom complexes.

Emotions influence health and the sense of well-being in many ways. Health may be altered by a wide range of emotional states—the happiness of young lovers, the heartbreak of parents whose child is unexpectedly struck down by cancer or a fatal traffic crash, the grief of bereavement that sunders a long and happy marriage, the contentment of a secure and satisfying job, the anxiety that strikes when that job is lost. Interactions with family members, friends, and coworkers are fraught with emotional overtones that can influence and transform lives in innumerable ways. Each person is part of social networks that act as support systems[17] to sustain life and maintain health; health sometimes breaks down when support systems fail.

Peptic ulcer and hypertension are identified as *stress* diseases because there is abundant evidence for a relationship, which is probably at least indirectly causal, between these and other conditions and the occurrence of persistent emotional stress (although peptic ulcer may also be associated with *Helicobacter pylori* infection).

Psycho-neuro-immunologists identify and measure mind-body interactions using catecholamine or steroid levels. This field of science is leading to an increased understanding of psychological determinants of health, such as the impact life events have on the subsequent development of illness.

Social Determinants

Social determinants of health include many characteristics and phenomena. In 1911, the registrar-general of England and Wales, T. H. C. Stevenson, devised an occupational classification that grouped employed persons into five *social classes*. It was immediately observed that there were striking and consistent relationships between *social class*, now usually referred to as socioeconomic status (SES), and incidence of health and sickness.

There have been many refinements of Stevenson's classification with the recognition that educational level, occupation, income, and housing conditions are interrelated and all influence health. The relationship has held true at all times since the early twentieth century and in all nations and social contexts in which it has been examined. There have been many attempts to explain it, and to reduce the gap[18] between those who are endowed with wealth, education, and good health and those who are poor, uneducated, and sickly.

The relationship of SES to health has several underlying causes. It is not fully explained by the fact that well-educated people have higher incomes, live in better homes where they are less exposed to environmental risks to health, have better quality health care, and are more likely to avoid risk factors such as smoking, than the poorly educated. The relationship is not the same as the occupational association of health risks to dangerous trades such as underground mining. It is indirectly related, however, in that industrial and manual workers and their families tend to be financially worse off than clerical workers, to live in less salubrious housing conditions, and to more often have customs and habits, such as heavy use of alcohol and tobacco, that expose them to other risks.

Mind-body interactions and other intangible factors further complicate the relationship between SES and health. The subtle interaction between self-esteem, job satisfaction, and good health, for example, is influenced by levels of intelligence and insight, one's image of one's familial and social role, and many other factors.

Cultural Determinants

The cultural determinants of health, which are often confused with racial or ethnic characteristics, are striking and more complex than they appear. For example, variations in incidence rates of cancer of the reproductive organs (breast, cervix, and prostate) among people of different religious backgrounds seem sometimes to be related to differences in diet; sometimes to exposure, or lack of it, to sexually transmitted viruses that can cause cancer; and sometimes to culturally determined differences in reproductive behavior and breast-feeding practices.[19]

A nation's collective attitude towards human sexuality is culturally determined and can profoundly influence several aspects of reproductive health. Particularly notable are the risks of unwanted pregnancy and sexually transmitted diseases, including HIV infection, especially among sexually active teen-age children. Due to improved nutrition and probably other factors, children now become sexually mature at younger ages than they did 100 years ago, and they begin their sexual experiments and encounters earlier in life than they did in Victorian times. This reality is recognized in Sweden, the Netherlands, and, indeed, in virtually all western industrial nations except the United States, where a peculiar attitude of denial is widespread. Despite abundant evidence to the contrary, many responsible authorities in the United States seem to believe that provision of sex education and access to effective contraception will encourage promiscuous behavior. The consequence is much higher adolescent pregnancy rates in the United States than in any other industrial nation, as shown in Table 3.1.

In the United States, the pregnancy rate per thousand at ages 15 to 17 is 62, in Canada it is 28, in Sweden 20, and in the Netherlands 7. Indeed, the abortion rate among girls aged 17 and under is higher in the United States (45 per 1000) than the rate for *all* pregnancies in this age group in any of these other nations.[20] The impact of the HIV epidemic is also no doubt

TABLE 3.1 Pregnancy Rates at Ages for Females Under Age 19—Various Countries

	Total Pregnancy Rate	Abortion Rate
United States	96.0	43.3
Canada	44.3	17.9
Sweden	29.0	15.0
Netherlands	16.0	6.0

SOURCE: Jones EF, Forrest JD, Goldman N, et al. Teenage pregnancy in developed countries: Determinants and policy implications. *Fam Plann Perspect.* 1985; 17:53–63.

greater in the United States because of the timidity with which education about human sexuality has been approached and resistance to the suggestion that condoms be made more widely available to school children.

Spiritual Determinants

Spiritual determinants of health do not refer to religious beliefs but to more subtle phenomena, such as the view that individuals and communities hold of their place in nature. These views help to determine individual and community health. Reactions of individuals and families to the occurrence of life-threatening disease, for example, vary in ways that are best described as spiritual. The prevailing value system in the United States leads many people to believe that no expense or effort should be spared to prolong life to the maximum, even though the quality of life may be poor for many who survive for a few weeks or months more than they otherwise might, after the heroic interventions of modern, high-technology, tertiary medical care.[21] (Do we strive so officiously to keep alive the irretrievably ill because we do not believe in an afterlife, or because we do?)

Of greater importance than this are views of human relationships to the natural world. Judaism, Christianity, and Islam have in common an implicit belief that everything on earth was placed here by God for the benefit and use of humankind. This belief has led the species to the brink of ecological catastrophe.[22] So-called primitive or animist religions, and to some extent Hindu and Buddhist religious philosophies, by contrast, perceive humans as partners with other living creatures that share the planet. This perception is more compatible with the concept of health as a sustainable state than that of monotheist religions.

If a healthy human species is to live forever on a healthy planet, perhaps everyone should embrace primitive or animist religions. (Of course humanity will not live *forever.* On theoretical grounds, the total longevity of the human species has been calculated to be in the range of 0.2 to 8.0 million years, with a confidence interval of 95 percent.[23] This takes no account of the possibility of extermination in a nuclear holocaust or destruction of humans and many other life forms in a slower but equally relentless ecological catastrophe.)

Interactions and Multifactoral Causation

Tuberculosis is not caused by *Mycobacterium tuberculosis* alone, but by the combination of poverty, overcrowding, poor nutrition, ignorance, and often other environmental, social, and behavioral factors that together create circumstances in which *M. tuberculosis*, the seed, finds fertile human soil in which it can grow. *M. tuberculosis* is the essential precipitating factor. The other determinants—poverty, overcrowding, poor nutrition, and so on—are predisposing, enabling, and reinforcing factors.

Many infectious microorganisms behave similarly, although the reasons for susceptibility or resistance vary. The cholera vibrio, for example, strikes hardest at those who are poorly nourished and therefore often have little or no gastric acid to kill the cholera vibrio. Thus, cholera is to some extent a disease of the underprivileged. The cholera vibrio also thrives in the company of certain seasonally and climatically dependent algae,[24] which accounts for the occurrence of cholera in waves or pandemics that relate to climatic cycles, such as the natural fluctuations of the equatorial Pacific current, El Niño.

Malaria, too, behaves in ways that make it clear there are more than mosquitoes, plasmodia, and people involved in the mathematics that determines its incidence and prevalence. Rich people mostly live further from malarial swamps than poor people do. They also tend to live in houses that are better screened against mosquitoes and to have clothing that protects more of their skin surface. As a result, they are less often the source of the blood meal that the female mosquito requires to survive. Rich (educated) people also tend to know more about the habits of mosquitoes and can take steps to reduce the risks of being bitten by them.

The relationship between infection and poverty or deprivation is strong and consistent. Throughout history, scarlet fever, measles, whooping cough, typhoid, and diphtheria have all exacted a heavier toll from the poor than from the rich.[25] The mortality rates of all these diseases declined in the nineteenth century, well before effective preventive or therapeutic measures were available. Mortality rates varied inversely with the rising standards of living as the industrial revolution advanced.[26,27]

These mortality and morbidity differentials hold true for other environmentally determined conditions, such as industrial and domestic injuries. It is understandable that workers in dangerous trades such as mining, heavy transport, deep-sea fishing, and forestry should have higher rates of occupational causes of death and injury than white-collar workers. Their homes are often unsafe, too, so domestic accidents occur more frequently than in wealthy homes, and their children have higher rates of injury because they are less likely to have a safe place to play.

There are a few exceptions to the rule about affluence and good health. Until the recent past, poliomyelitis and hepatitis A have had higher attack rates among the affluent than the poor. The explanation is that higher proportions of the poor were exposed in infancy and early childhood, when subclinical infection is more common. Among well-off people, by contrast, first exposure to these fecal-oral infections more often occurred in later childhood or adolescence, when a more severe and clinically apparent manifestation of these diseases was likely to occur. Hodgkin's disease follows this pattern in some degree, raising the suspicion that an infectious organism may be implicated in its etiology as well. Breast cancer also tends to be a more common cause of death among wealthy than poor women, but this association is confounded by many other factors including breast-feeding practices and obesity, which is a risk factor for breast cancer.

PUTTING THE DETERMINANTS OF HEALTH IN CONTEXT

The necessary and sufficient causes of health and disease usually occur in specific environmental, social, occupational, and cultural contexts. In the urbanizing industrial world of the second half of the nineteenth century, horse-drawn transport was the rule. Horses had to be stabled, and they deposited large amounts of manure in these stables, which were often fairly close to the homes of even the most affluent citizens. Horse manure is an ideal breeding ground for flies, which, the social historians report, were ubiquitous in that era.

The invention of the internal combustion engine rapidly changed all this: motor cars replaced horses, stables (and streets) full of manure became a thing of the past, and with them went most of the flies, which had been the passive vector for a great many pathogens, notably the fecal-oral pathogens that cause diarrheal diseases. Increasing affluence that provided the wherewithal for screened windows and improved kitchen hygiene also helped reduce the contamination of food by the *filthy feet of fecal-feeding flies.* However, the principal determinant of reduced infant and child morbidity and mortality from diarrheal diseases in the first half of the twentieth century in the industrial world was probably the invention of the internal combustion engine, which led to this important transformation of urban ecosystems.

Ecological interactions are involved in modern public health problems in a similar manner. However, the critical links that must be broken in the causal chain have yet to be identified, even for the most common cause of premature cardiovascular death, coronary heart disease. Unsolved questions persist regarding the interaction of diet, exercise, addiction to cigarette smoking, hereditary factors, and relationships to family members and coworkers. For example, it is not yet completely understood why coronary heart disease mortality rates in men declined by about 40 percent in the United States, Australia, and Canada between the late 1960s and the early 1990s, while the rates did not decline in the same way or at the same pace among women or decline at all (indeed, they increased for a time) in Scotland, Sweden, and Switzerland. The relationship to changes in known risk factors, such as diet, exercise, and cigarette smoking, does not follow a consistent pattern. Clearly, some links are still missing.

Even when the critical links have been identified, society may lack the political will to do what is required to break them. This applies to the public health problems associated with addiction to tobacco. The fact that tobacco is addictive has consistently been denied by the tobacco industry and its supporters; to admit that tobacco is addictive would place the industry in a morally untenable position. Efforts to prevent the industry from recruiting new child smokers, to replace those in older cohorts who have been killed by their addiction, are frustrated by political and ethical restraints on censorship of tobacco advertising and by a failure to find convincing ways to convey the negative message, "Don't smoke," to a target population that is often inherently rebellious against parental and other adult authorities. The worldwide public health problem of tobacco addiction is more difficult to deal with because of the heavy investment of the tobacco industry in advertising and political lobbying in virtually every nation and increasingly in the developing nations.

Another prominent public health problem in the United States is intentional violence, especially homicide and particularly homicide caused by firearms among young, urban, male African-Americans, many of whom belong to an alienated underclass. Most of the links in this chain of causation probably have been identified. This is a culturally determined problem. Other western industrial nations have an urban underclass, often one that is racially distinct from the majority, but none have experienced intentional violence or homicide due to guns on a comparable scale.

The problem is usually attributed to the easy availability of handguns in the United States, which is facilitated by the constitutional *right* to bear arms and the highly successful lobbying efforts of the National Rifle Association. There is no doubt about the link between availability of handguns and homicide (as well as suicide and accidental death) caused by handguns; but it is too facile to suggest that this alone accounts for the very high mortality rates from firearm injuries experienced by young African-American males in the

TABLE 3.2 Homicide
Rates per 100,000—Various
Countries

Switzerland	0.1
Canada	2.2
United States	10.5

United States. Other cultures in which firearms are present in virtually every household, such as Switzerland, have orders of magnitude fewer deaths due to firearms,[28] as shown in Table 3.2.

The difference in mortality rates due to firearm injuries between the United States and other nations is probably due to a difference in value systems. Resort to firearms as a way of settling disputes seems to be an almost uniquely American value. It appears to have become firmly established and further enhanced over time since early in the twentieth century. It is reinforced by the presentation in movies and on television of fictional dramas in which the heroes and villains resolve their disputes with guns. Life then imitates art.

There is consistent and persuasive evidence for an association, probably causal, between the portrayal of violence on television and the occurrence of violence in real life.[29] The mind-set begins early in life, when toddlers and kindergarten children watch cartoons in which the road-runner blows up the coyote and the canary successfully thwarts the cat, always with great displays of violence that are presented as though they were hilariously funny. The process continues throughout childhood and into adult life, with entertainment (now no longer necessarily funny) incessantly emphasizing violent means of settling disputes. The preferred sports of many Americans also involve displays of brute force.

Contrast this with European nations, where the television programs and cartoons that children see are generally free of violence, the most popular films and television programs are mostly about aspects of civilized behavior and variations of normal adult interactions, and the preferred sports often emphasize elegance and skill rather than brute force. These culturally determined differences are striking, and changing them will not be easy.

CONTROVERSIES AND CONUNDRUMS

There are plenty of unsolved public health problems. Health may be linked to seemingly simple determinants that are anything but simple to deal with or to factors that remain altogether mysterious. Consider these examples.

Electromagnetic Field Exposure

Electromagnetic fields are generated by electric currents. When Wertheimer and Leeper[30] published the first report of an association between childhood malignant disease and residence close to high-voltage power lines, their paper was greeted with disbelief. Many studies later,[31] the association seems to be firm, although not all published reports have demonstrated it.[32] Some studies have yielded inconsistent findings, showing, for instance, an association of electromagnetic fields with leukemia but not brain cancer, or vice versa. Other studies have shown a relationship between exposure to electromagnetic fields from microwave radiation and emotional and intellectual dysfunction.[33]

There is no sound biological basis for these epidemiologically demonstrated associations, and even if there were, the implications for health and public policy remain unclear. The role of electricity in modern civilization is so pervasive and dominant that an ill-defined, weak association with possible adverse effects on a small proportion of humans will not alter the economic and social fabric through which electric power is inextricably woven. Nonetheless, if the association of electromagnetic radiation to human health can be clarified, the knowledge may be used to enhance health. More research on the biological basis of this phenomenon is needed.

Repetition Strain Illness (RSI)

Repetition strain illness is another contemporary disorder of uncertain provenance. This condition sometimes makes headlines or is the topic of learned discussions among experts on television talk shows. No textbook aimed at readers at the end of the millennium can afford to ignore it. There have been epidemics, notably in Australia,[34] following the recognition there of RSI as an industrially related disorder, so workers affected by it were able to claim compensation. The epidemic in Australia subsided after the conditions for claims under workers' compensation legislation were made more rigorous. In the United Kingdom, a recent court decision declared that the condition did not exist, apparently in an effort to forestall an epidemic similar to the one in Australia.

There seems no doubt that RSI exists and is related to ergonomically unsound positioning of hands and arms in repetitive motion exercise, such as the use of computer keyboards for prolonged periods. The best way to ameliorate the condition seems to be to avoid prolonged repetitive muscular activity by taking breaks from work and to assure that working conditions are ergonomically efficient. However, there may be more to RSI than this. The relationship, if any, of the condition to job satisfaction and harmony in the workplace requires further study.

Multiple Chemical Sensitivity

Multiple chemical sensitivity (MCS), also known as twentieth-century disease, environmental hypersensitivity, and generalized allergy, is an ill-defined condition whose very existence is debated, although it is well enough known to have developed its own cadre of specialists, called clinical ecologists, and to have become the subject of many articles in medical journals[35] and chapters in textbooks.[36] The clinical manifestations of MCS are poorly defined. It may be associated with sick-building syndrome.

These terms suggest environmental determinants but also hint at behavioral causes. The real cause may be the power of suggestion—although the condition does not necessarily occur in outbreaks resembling behavioral epidemics, which are generally acknowledged to be psychological in origin. The poorly defined clinical picture and obscure pathogenesis raise the possibility that MCS has suggestibility as at least one underlying cause. Clarifying the picture require first, precise clinical description, second, descriptive and analytic epidemiological study, and third, application and evaluation of

interventions based on testable hypotheses about causal factors. This sequence is unlikely to be implemented for some time, so MCS will no doubt remain a topic of debate and controversy in the years to come.

FUTURE CHALLENGES

By the early 1950s, many of the great infectious diseases that had scourged humans since prehistoric times were yielding to the combined onslaught of vaccines and antibiotics. Optimism was high about the ultimate conquest of all infectious diseases. All that was necessary, it was believed, was to discover more antibiotics and develop more vaccines.

The first inkling that the future would not be so rosy was the development of antibiotic resistant strains of common pathogens, including *Staphylococcus aureus*, *Proteus* and *Pseudomonas* organisms that menaced postoperative patients in hospitals. Optimism faded further in 1957 when a worldwide influenza pandemic took many lives. Meanwhile, malaria control was proving troublesome, as mosquitoes and parasites began to develop resistance. More recently, new varieties of infections, some highly lethal, have appeared in the United States and elsewhere: Lassa fever, Ebola virus disease, legionellosis, Hantavirus diseases, Lyme disease, and others. By 1981, when the first cases of AIDS were identified, the optimism had evaporated.

As we approach the millennium, we face the prospect of 40 million HIV infections worldwide. Tuberculosis has returned with new, often resistant, strains, both as a complication of HIV infection and as a public health problem in its own right among the growing numbers of homeless people in large cities in the United States and other countries. Tuberculosis remains, as it has always been, a prominent world health problem.

Compounding these problems is the fact that many people today live in parts of the world racked by low-intensity warfare, with deteriorating environments that cause them to be perpetually on the edge of famine. Undernutrition reduces further their resistance to infections of all kinds. Unprecedented numbers of people, great masses of humanity, are moving restlessly from one continent to another. Many are drawn to the seemingly affluent cities of the industrial world. Huge numbers come to the United States each year—a million or so legally, an unknown number, perhaps more than a million, illegally. The latter enter without any surveillance of their health. Increasing proportions belong to what has been called a *fourth world* of squalor and deprivation amidst the affluence all around them.

Migrants of all kinds, but especially environmental or ecological refugees, often carry pathogens that were common in their country of origin. They then acquire other pathogens at staging points on their migrations. Finally, they become exposed at their final destination to yet more pathogens. They may have little or no acquired resistance to these new pathogens, just as those who live around them may have little resistance to the pathogens that the new arrivals bring. Many of these immigrants are likely to be malnourished, some close to starvation, because they are escaping from droughts, or lands where the agricultural infrastructure has been destroyed by war. Malnutrition further decreases their resistance to new pathogens.

The situation worldwide is likely to get worse instead of better. The world is becoming increasingly crowded with people, with more than six billion projected by the year 2000. Many of these people will live—as many do today—in sprawling periurban slums in the developing world, lacking sanitation, clean water, safe food, and basic primary public health services. Add to this global warming, which is widening the range of vector-borne diseases such as arbovirus infections.[37] Also add increased ultraviolet radiation levels at the earth's surface (due to stratospheric ozone attenuation), which may impair human immunity.[12]

All these conditions set the stage for new epidemics and pandemics of infectious diseases, perhaps due to familiar pathogens, perhaps due to entirely new ones. Already in rich nations, such as the United States, essential public health services are strained by limited resources. The cost of new epidemics and pandemics will be overwhelming. It is clear that the most important determinant of good health in the next 50 years will be the successful control of infectious diseases, and that the most important handbook for public health practice will remain in the future, as it has been for the past half century, *Control of Communicable Diseases in Man.*[38]

REFERENCES

1. World Health Organization. *Preamble to the Constitution.* Geneva, Switzerland: WHO; 1948.

2. *Health Promotion: A Discussion Document on the Concepts and Principles.* Copenhagen, Denmark: WHO Regional Office for Europe; 1984.

3. Stokes J III, Noren JJ, Shindell S. Definition of terms and concepts applicable to clinical preventive medicine. *J Community Health.* 1982;8:33–41.

4. Last JM. *Public Health and Human Ecology.* Norwalk, Ct: Appleton and Lange; 1987:5.

5. King M. Health is a sustainable state. *Lancet.* 1990; 336: 664–667.

6. Population growth and ecological deterioration—the demographic trap. In: *From Alma Ata to the Year 2000; Reflections at the Midpoint.* Geneva, Switzerland: WHO; 1988:31–34.

7. Last JM. War and the demographic trap. *Lancet.* 1993; 342: 508–509.

8. Last JM. New pathways in an age of ecological and ethical concerns. *Int J Epidemiol.* 1994;23(1):1–4.

9. Khoury MJ, Beaty TH, Cohen BH. *Fundamentals of Genetic Epidemiology.* New York, NY: Oxford University Press; 1993.

10. Barker DJP, Martyn CN, Osmond C, Hales CN, Fall CHD. Growth in utero and serum cholesterol concentrations in adult life. *Br Med J.* 1993;307:1524–1527.

11. Suzman R, Riley MW, eds. The oldest old. *Milbank Q.* 1985;63:177–451.

12. Jeevan A, Kripke ML. Ozone depletion and the immune system. *Lancet.* 1993;342:1159–1160.

13. Tomatis, L, ed. *Monographs on the Evaluation of Carcinogenic Risks to Humans: Ultraviolet Radiation.* Lyon, France; 1992. IARC Monograph No. 55.

14. Taylor HR, West SK, Rosenthal FS, et al. Effect of ultraviolet radiation on cataract formation. *N Engl J Med.* 1988;319: 1429–1433.

15. McMichael AJ, Baghurst PA, Wigg NR, et al. Port Pirie cohort study: environmental exposure to lead and children's abilities at the age of four years. *N Engl J Med.* 1988;319:468–475.

16. Galen, Brock AJ, Trans. *Galen on the Natural Faculties.* London: Loeb Classical Library; 1916.

17. Cohen S, Syme SL, eds. *Social Support and Health.* Orlando, Fl: Academic Press; 1985.

18. Amler RW, Dull HB, eds. *Closing the Gap; The Burden of Unnecessary Illness.* New York, NY: Oxford University Press; 1987.

19. Tomatis L, Aitio A, Day NE, et al, eds. *Cancer—Causes, Occurrence and Control.* Lyon, France: WHO and IARC; 1990.

20. Jones EF, Forrest JD, Goldman N, et al. Teenage pregnancy in developed countries: determinants and policy implications. *Fam Plann Perspect.* 1985;17:53–63.

21. Callahan D. *Setting Limits.* New York, NY: Touchstone; 1988.

22. McMichael AJ. *Planetary Overload; Global Environmental Change and the Health of the Human Species.* Cambridge: Cambridge University Press; 1993.

23. Gott JR. Implications of the Copernican principle for our future prospects. *Nature.* 1993;363:315–319.

24. Epstein PR, Ford TE, Colwell RR. Marine ecosystems. *Lancet.* 1993;342:1216–1219.

25. McKeown T. *The Origins of Human Disease.* New York, NY: Blackwell; 1988;5:120–139.

26. McKeown T. *The Role of Medicine—Dream, Mirage or Nemesis?* London: Nuffield Provincial Hospitals Trust; 1976.

27. Black D, Morris JN, Smith C, Townsend P. *Inequalities in Health (The Black Report).* Harmondsworth, Middlesex, UK: Penguin; 1982.

28. Zwerling C, McMillan D. Firearm injuries; a public health approach. *Am J Prev Med.* 1993;9(suppl):3.

29. Reel violence. *Lancet.* 1994;343:127–128. Editorial.

30. Wertheimer N, Leeper E. Electrical wiring configurations and childhood cancer. *Am J Epidemiol.* 1979;109:273–284.

31. Feychting M, Ahlbom A. Magnetic fields and cancer in children residing near Swedish high-voltage power lines. *Am J Epidemiol.* 1993;138:467–481.

32. McDowall ME. Mortality of persons resident in the vicinity of electric transmission facilities. *Br J Cancer.* 1986;53:271–279.

33. Poole C, Kavet R, Funch DP, Donelan K, Charry JM, Dreyer NA. Depressive symptoms and headaches in relation to proximity to an alternating-current transmission line right-of-way. *Am J Epidemiol.* 1993;137:318–330.

34. Ferguson DA. "RSI"—putting the epidemic to rest. *Med J Aust.* 1987;147:213–214.

35. Ashford NA, Miller CS. Multiple chemical sensitivity. *Health & Environ Digest.* 1993(6);11:1–7.

36. Cullen MR. Multiple chemical sensitivities. In: Last JM, Wallace RB, eds. *Maxcy-Rosenau-Last Public Health and Preventive Medicine.* 13th ed. Norwalk, Ct: Appleton & Lange; 1992:459–462.

37. Rogers DJ, Packer MJ. Vector-borne diseases, models, and global change. *Lancet.* 1993;342:1282–1284.

38. Benenson AS, ed. *Control of Communicable Diseases in Man.* 16th ed. Washington, DC: American Public Health Association; 1995.

CHAPTER

The Legal Basis for Public Health

Edward P. Richards III, J.D., M.P.H.

Katharine C. Rathbun, M.D., M.P.H.

Public health is unique among medical specialties in being defined by law rather than physiology. While there are many public health practices that benefit affected individuals, the core of public health practice is coercive action under state authority, *the police power*. In the best of circumstances, this authority may be needed only to encourage educational efforts. At other times, however, public health authorities must seize property, close businesses, destroy animals, or involuntarily treat or even lock away individuals.

Such powers are rooted in earlier times, when the fear of pestilential disease was both powerful and well-founded. In a contemporary society dominated by concern with individual rights, such draconian powers may seem unnecessary or even unconstitutional. Many public health personnel believe that the rationale for such laws is past and that public health practitioners should restrict themselves to education and empowerment. Others, looking at the resurgence of tuberculosis and an increasing inability to treat other bacterial diseases, be-

lieve that the end of the antimicrobial era is near and that traditional public health restrictions will have to be employed, requiring the sacrifice of individual rights for the common good.

This chapter has three objectives: (1) to explain the history and constitutional basis for public health law; (2) to show how public health law fits into the general rules for administrative agency law; and (3) to outline basic public health law activities.

HISTORICAL PERSPECTIVE

Pestilence is one of the *Four Horsemen of the Apocalypse,* reflecting its position as a primal fear of society, yet it is difficult for individuals born after the ready availability of antimicrobial drugs and immunizations to appreciate the historic dread of deadly epidemics. In a society preoccupied with lifestyle diseases, we forget that civilizations have fallen because of communicable diseases and that pestilence has done more to eradicate indigenous cultures than has force of arms or religion.

Even in the United States, pestilence was once part of everyday life. Soon after the Constitution was ratified, for example, an epidemic of yellow fever raged in New York and Philadelphia. The flavor of that period was later captured in an argument before the Supreme Court:

> For ten years prior, the yellow-fever had raged almost annually in the city, and annual laws were passed to resist it. The wit of man was exhausted, but in vain. Never did the pestilence rage more violently than in the summer of 1798. The State was in despair. The rising hopes of the metropolis began to fade. The opinion was gaining ground, that the cause of this annual disease was indigenous, and that all precautions against its importation were useless. But the leading spirits of that day were unwilling to give up the city without a final desperate effort. The havoc in the summer of 1798 is represented as terrific. The whole country was roused. A cordon sanitaire was thrown around the city. Governor Mifflin of Pennsylvania proclaimed a non-intercourse between New York and Philadelphia.[1]

The extreme nature of the actions, including isolating the federal government, which was sitting in Philadelphia at the time, was considered an appropriate response to the threat of yellow fever. The terrifying nature of these early epidemics predisposed the courts to grant public health authorities a free hand in their attempts to prevent the spread of disease, as the following quote shows:

> Every state has acknowledged power to pass, and enforce quarantine, health, and inspection laws, to prevent the introduction of disease, pestilence, or unwholesome provisions; such laws interfere with no powers of Congress or treaty stipulations; they relate to internal police, and are subjects of domestic regulation within each state, over which no authority can be exercised by any power under the Constitution, save by requiring the consent of Congress to the imposition of duties on exports and imports, and their payment into the treasury of the United States.[2]

The American colonies adopted the English statutory and common law that recognized the right of the state to protect the health and safety of its citizens. This was called the police power, although police forces as we know them were not organized until much later. When the Constitution was written, public health power was left to the states:

> It is a well-recognized principle that it is one of the first duties of a state to take all necessary steps for the promotion and protection of the health and comfort of its inhabitants. The preservation of the public health is universally conceded to be one of the duties devolving upon the state as a sovereignty, and whatever reasonably tends to preserve the public health is a subject upon which the legislature, within its police power, may take action.[3]

The scope of the police power is broad. Defining the limits of the police power, and the rights of citizens to be protected from state actions taken pursuant to the police power, is the central legal issue in public health law.

PUBLIC HEALTH LAW AS ADMINISTRATIVE LAW

Governments act through laws passed by legislatures. These laws are of two types: criminal laws, which are intended to punish wrongdoing, and civil laws, which are intended to direct future behavior. Criminal laws are enforced by local prosecutors, state attorneys general, and the Justice Department. Civil laws are enforced by administrative agencies. These range in size and complexity from the Internal Revenue Service and the Department of Health and Human Services, which have bigger budgets than some states, to small, specialized agencies with no full-time staff. Public health departments are among the oldest of administrative agencies, with some dating from the colonial period.

As administrative agencies, public health departments have three advantages as compared to criminal law enforcement agencies: (1) they can act quickly; (2) they can write their own rules; and (3) they have experts on staff who can determine the agency's policies. Persons accused of violating agency rules have only a limited right to contest the agency's decisions or to have the courts overrule the agency.

In contrast, criminal laws and regulations must be passed by the legislature, they must be specific, and they cannot be modified by the law enforcement agency based on its expertise. In addition, persons accused of committing a crime have the right to remain silent, confront their accusers, and present witnesses, as well as the right to have counsel, a trial by jury, and certain other protections attendant on their criminal prosecution. These rights make criminal prosecutions slow and expensive, and they also limit the ability of law enforcement to respond to new problems.

The advantages of administrative agencies are so great that legislatures sometimes pass laws that impose punishments, while claiming they are administrative laws, in order to avoid giving individuals full criminal law protections. While the courts generally accept the legislature's determination that a law is not a criminal law, they do examine the law and its effects as it is applied.

A law that requires the permanent quarantine of persons accused of murder in order to protect the public's health, for example, would be a criminal law because it is based on past behavior rather than on proof of present danger to the community. Accused murderers are therefore entitled to full criminal law protections before being locked away. In contrast, if it can be assumed that a person who commits a violent sexual assault has a high probability of committing future assaults, then it would be acceptable to lock up the person as a threat to the public health without full criminal law protections. This is an administrative action, even though the person is locked up in a prison.[4] It is the purpose of the law that matters, not the conditions of confinement.

Public health restrictions frequently have been carried out in prisons and jails. In one case, disease carriers were quarantined in a prison. They petitioned the court for release, claiming that they were being punished by being put in prison and treated as prisoners. The court rejected their claim, concluding that:

> While it is true that physical facilities constituting part of the penitentiary equipment are utilized, interned persons are in no sense confined in the penitentiary, and are not subject to the peculiar obloquy which attends such confinement.[5]

The administrative rights of public health agencies are not without limit, however. Public health laws must be applied fairly. They cannot, for example, be a subterfuge for discrimination against racial or ethnic groups, who must be given equal protection under the United States Constitution. The courts have rejected laws that subjected the Chinese community to special health regulations without providing evidence that Chinese were at any greater risk of contracting or spreading disease.

Public health laws also must treat state residents the same as out-of-state residents. For example, courts have struck down several laws that imposed different sanitary restrictions on out-of-state milk processors. Even if the restrictions are the same for in-state and out-of-state businesses, the courts strike down laws that unnecessarily discriminate against out-of-state businesses. For example, a requirement that milk must be processed and delivered within 24 hours would put out-of-state dairies out of business. This law would be improper if there was no evidence that the 24-hour rule was necessary to protect the public's health.

If a public health law has a neutral purpose, it is constitutional even if it has a differential impact on different groups. Laws controlling the spread of gonorrhea, for example, are constitutional even if the disease is more prevalent in a specific racial or ethnic group. In the extreme case, abortion laws are constitutional even though they affect only women. As the court has pointed out in other cases involving pregnancy, the laws would also apply to pregnant men.

Most public health law cases were decided decades ago, and the Supreme Court gave individuals few rights. Some argue that these cases were superseded by the Supreme Court's civil liberties decisions in the 1960s and 1970s. In these rulings, the Supreme Court required criminal law protections in several cases where the legislature had said that the law was not intended to punish. In other cases, the Court recognized a right of privacy that might also apply to public health laws.

While the current Supreme Court has not directly affirmed traditional public health cases, it has upheld public health rationales in other contexts.[6] For example, it specifically rejected the Warren Court's consideration of the conditions of confinement in determining whether public safety detention is punishment. The Court rejected arguments that detainees should be held in the *least restrictive* manner necessary to assure their confinement. Instead, the Court allowed them to be kept with other prisoners and subjected to the same prison rules. Despite the detainees' apparent imprisonment, the Court ruled that their incarceration was not a punishment because the state's intent was merely to protect the public until the detainees could be tried.

Pretrial detention cases may prove more than is necessary to uphold public health restrictions. The difficult problem in the detention of criminally dangerous persons is determining the probability that they will endanger public safety by committing another crime. This probability is certainly less than 100 percent, perhaps substantially less. In contrast, communicable diseases can be objectively diagnosed and their risk assessed. Persons with diseases such as active tuberculosis are dangerous, irrespective of whether they intend to harm others.

INDIVIDUAL RIGHTS VERSUS PUBLIC SAFETY

There is pressure, even from some public health professionals, to give individuals more rights under public health laws than would be required by the Constitution. Indeed, this is the central legal issue in public health law, as stated above. Some states have amended their disease control laws to require court hearings before public health orders are issued against an individual. These hearings are modeled after the proceedings that are required before a mentally ill person is involuntarily committed to a psychiatric institution. Although such an expansion of individual rights seems desirable, it comes at a high price: potential paralysis of public health enforcement.

Court hearings are expensive and time consuming. No health department has a sufficiently large legal staff to have a court hearing before every enforcement action. Indeed, most health departments do not have *any* legal staff. They are at the mercy of city or county legal departments to provide attorneys when there is a hearing. Because most legal departments are understaffed, public health enforcement actions usually have low priority.

Another problem with hearings is that they take time. A hearing first must be scheduled with a judge,

and then the person subject to the order m... with notice of the hearing and given time to h... torney and present a defense. This prevents timely... strictions that are critical to effective disease control. Courts have recognized, in their rejection of requests for bail by persons under disease control orders, that disease carriers cannot be allowed to go free while restrictions are litigated, as the following argument shows:

> To grant release on bail to persons isolated and detained on a quarantine order because they have a contagious disease which makes them dangerous to others, or to the public in general, would render quarantine laws and regulations nugatory and of no avail.[7]

A final problem with hearings, and perhaps the most serious, is that they give the judge the opportunity to substitute her judgment for that of the public health officer. The proper role of the judge (or jury) was established in the original case ruling that involuntary immunizations are constitutionally permissible. The United States Supreme Court rejected the petitioner's claim that he was entitled to have a jury determine whether the state's actions were reasonable. The Court ruled that "It is no part of the function of a court or a jury to determine which of two modes was likely to be most effective for the protection of the public against disease."[8]

The courts are expected to defer to administrative agencies because agency personnel are experts in the subject matter being regulated and should be second-guessed only in limited circumstances. This view was recently reiterated in a case upholding the closing of a bathhouse as a disease control measure:

> It is not for the courts to determine which scientific view is correct in ruling upon whether the police power has been properly exercised. The judicial function is exhausted with the discovery that the relation between means and ends is not wholly vain and fanciful, an illusory pretense . . .[9]

Despite such clear judicial support for deference to agency decision makers, many judges are swayed by the emotional appeal of the case against restriction and reject the public health authority's recommendations. Such conflicts are most common in disputes over closing

oy friends of the local
e in disease control cases
are to not restrict individu-
a politically powerful group
not understand the danger to
cted person.

LIMITA. ON PUBLIC HEALTH POWER

There are three types of limitations on public health power: statutory limitations, the right of habeas corpus, and political limitations.

Statutory Limitations

An administrative agency may only exercise the powers given by the law that creates it, that is, its enabling legislation. Some enabling legislation, such as the tax code, is very detailed, running thousands of pages in length. This reflects the congressional desire to exercise close control over the agency.

The enabling legislation for health departments was traditionally a general grant of authority to protect the public health and safety, with little specific legislative guidance. The details were left to the public health officers because there was little disagreement in society over the goals and methods of public health practice. As public health departments were given broader responsibilities, however, their enabling legislation grew more complicated, and their freedom of action was increasingly constrained. In several states, legislatures have greatly limited the traditional constitutional powers of health departments.

The Right of Habeas Corpus

The second major restriction on public health power is the right of habeas corpus. While courts have been willing to allow persons to be restricted without a court hearing, they require that a restricted person have access to a court to review the public health order. This review is done through a habeas corpus proceeding, which the United States Constitution guarantees to every imprisoned or confined person. Habeas corpus, roughly trans-

lated, means *bring me the body*. It requires a judge to review the legality of a person's confinement, usually including a personal statement by the confined person.

Because a habeas corpus proceeding is held *after* the person has been confined, it does not interfere with the health department's ability to take quick action. Unlike routine court hearings, habeas corpus is only used when requested by the confined person. Many, perhaps most, people restricted by public health orders do not wish to contest the restriction. In the vast majority of cases, confinement is temporary—for a medical examination, initial treatment of a disease, or some other similarly minor inconvenience. By contrast, requiring hearings before enforcing routine or uncontested public health orders diverts limited resources from other public health agency functions.

Political Limitations

This is the most important restriction on public health authority. From the Surgeon General of the United States to the health officer in the smallest town, every public health official works for politicians. In some cases they work for independent boards, rather than directly for the elected officials, but the end results are the same. Public health officers who take actions that are politically unpopular in their community will be forced out of office. Public health officers also cannot do anything that elected officials will not pay for. For example, attempts to quarantine everyone with AIDS or other communicable diseases would be impossibly expensive as well as politically suicidal. Even with the resurgence of tuberculosis, it is politically difficult to get support and resources for confinement when it is necessary to treat an individual and prevent spread of the infection.

BASIC AREAS OF PUBLIC HEALTH LAW

Public health law falls into eight basic areas: environmental health, disease and injury reporting, vital statistics, disease control, involuntary testing, contact tracing, immunizations and mandated treatment, and personal restrictions. Each of these areas is considered in turn.

Environmental Health

Food sanitation, drinking-water treatment, and waste-water disposal have been mainstays of public health since the earliest times. As health departments were given the added responsibility of guarding against toxins in the broader environment, these regulatory functions were grouped into environmental health. Most public health orders are directed at environmental health problems. Because they affect property, not persons, they do not pose the difficult issues of personal freedom that arise with the rarer communicable disease control orders.

Environmental health regulations pose two central legal questions: whether the government owes compensation to the owners of regulated property, and under what circumstances health officers can enter private premises to look for public health law violations. Both questions arise from the United States Constitution, which requires that property owners be paid a fair price for property taken for public purposes and prohibits *unreasonable* searches and seizures. The difficult problem is deciding if the government has searched the property unreasonably or has taken the value of the property for which the owner must be compensated.

Regulation of Property

If a city condemns a house to widen a street, for example, the city has clearly taken the house and must pay its owner. In contrast, if property is destroyed because it poses a threat to the public health, the owner is not entitled to compensation because the property is not considered to have value. In the classic food sanitation case, public health officials ordered the destruction of frozen chicken stored in a cold storage plant that had lost its refrigeration. The owners of the plant demanded a hearing to determine whether the chicken was really spoiled and compensation for the chicken that was destroyed. The court ruled that there was no right to a hearing before the destruction of property and that property that endangered the public health had no value. Thus, the owners were entitled to no compensation.[10]

This decision echoed an earlier ruling involving a compensation claim for property that had been demolished to prevent the spread of a fire in San Francisco.[11] Unlike the rotten chicken, which arguably had no value, the property owners sued for their possessions, which they claimed could have been saved before the fire reached the building, had it not been destroyed. The court rejected their claims for compensation. It held that the police power included the right to destroy property if this was necessary to protect the public safety. This destruction was not taking the property for public purpose and thus no compensation need be paid. The court rejected the claim that the authorities should have allowed the owners time to remove their property because such a delay would have increased the danger to the public.

The most controversial modern cases involve regulatory actions that do not destroy property but limit the owner's use of the property. Examples include wetlands protection laws and endangered species acts. Such environmental laws are also based on the police power to protect the public health and safety, but the threat they address is much less direct and immediate than the threat posed by rotten chicken. The courts are increasingly reluctant to defer to the agency's expertise in these cases because the harm they seek to prevent is so difficult to measure. Although the courts still rule with the agencies in most cases, property owners are given extensive rights to court hearings to contest the actions before they are finalized.

Search and Seizure

The second legal issue in environmental health is the right of the health department to enter onto private property to assess environmental health risks. With certain exceptions, the police may not enter private property to search for evidence of criminal activity without a search warrant approved by a judge. Such warrants are difficult and expensive to get and will be granted only when there is evidence of wrongdoing.

In contrast, most environmental health inspections are done to assure that the owner is in compliance with the law, not because the inspector believes that the owner is violating the law. The courts do not require specific warrants for environmental health inspections, as long as there is no threat of criminal prosecution. Thus an inspection for rats does not require a search warrant based on probable cause, whereas one for toxic waste dumping in violation of criminal laws would. The courts do require that searches be related to a public health purpose. This can be satisfied by having a general plan for the inspections (called an area warrant) that describes which buildings will be searched and why.[12] Access by health inspectors can be made a condition of licensure, so that any establishment with a food handling or other public license has to admit inspectors without a warrant.

Disease and Injury Reporting

Basic to all public health is the reporting of communicable diseases, hazardous conditions, and injuries that are of public health significance. This information is used for tracking the course of epidemics and for intervening to protect the public health. Reporting duties transcend the patient's right to privacy and the health care provider's obligation to protect the patient's confidential information.

The constitutionality of reporting laws has been upheld in several recent United States Supreme Court decisions. In a case involving the reporting of controlled substances prescriptions, the Court addressed many of the concerns about public health reporting. The Court first noted that common law did not recognize the right to withhold medical information from the state. Such a right of physician-patient confidentiality arises from state or federal law and is subject to limitations such as public health reporting. The Court then held that:

Unquestionably, some individuals' concern for their own privacy may lead them to avoid or to postpone needed medical attention. Nevertheless, disclosures of private medical information to doctors, hospital personnel, insurance companies, and public health agencies are often an essential part of modern medical practice, even when the disclosure may reflect unfavorably on the character of the patient. Requiring such disclosures to representatives of the State having responsibility for the health of the community, does not automatically amount to an impermissible invasion of privacy.[13]

Every state has laws that require physicians to report certain diseases and injuries to a local or state health officer.[14] Many extend this requirement to nurses, dentists, veterinarians, laboratories, school officials, administrators of institutions, and police officials. For some diseases, health care providers are required to report only the number of cases they see. Other diseases and conditions require health care providers to provide identifying information, such as name, address, occupation, and birth date, as well as information on the disease and how it might have been acquired.

While states vary somewhat in which diseases must be reported, there are about 60 diseases that are commonly reportable in all jurisdictions. The state health department can provide information on which diseases to report and to whom the reports should be directed. Most health departments will accept reports for diseases that are not on the state list of reportable diseases, although they may choose not to act on them. Health care providers have no legal liability for making a report that is not required.

Legally required disease control reporting is not subject to informed consent. Health care providers do not need medical records releases for disease reporting because neither they nor their patients have the right to refuse the release of the information. Although patients have no right to be informed that they are being reported to the health department, it is good practice to do so for diseases such as syphilis or measles for which the health department will contact them for additional information.

Health care providers must never knowingly report false information to public health authorities, and they are liable for any injuries, such as transmission of HIV or tuberculosis, occasioned by false reports. Although health care providers are not required to personally investigate the information that patients provide, they must truthfully report what is known to them. In reality, very few health care providers do not know their patients' correct names and addresses, because few patients pay cash for medical care or never need a prescription or other order that requires a correct identity. Health care providers who provide information in good faith are not liable if the information is incorrect.

Disease registries are a special class of reporting laws. Most disease registries are statewide and involve either cancer or occupational illness. Some, such as the CDC registry of cases of toxic shock syndrome, are national. Reporting cases to the registry may be mandatory or voluntary. Because the objective is not to control a communicable disease, there is often no penalty for failing to report to a disease registry. However, it is always desirable to have a complete registry because registries are used to determine the extent of certain problems in the community and to try to determine causes. If they are inaccurate they may give false correlations and become useless for research and prevention.

Every jurisdiction requires health care providers to report certain types of injuries to law enforcement officials or protection agencies, generally including assaults, family violence, and criminal activity. Although the victim may have a plausible explanation of the injury and be anxious to avoid reporting for fear of reprisals or because he is under investigation already, proper reports should be made despite the victim's wishes. It is not up to the health care provider to investigate the incident before reporting it; that is the job of the law enforcement agency that receives the report.

Whenever a health care provider suspects that a child has been abused or neglected, that suspicion should be reported immediately to the child protective agency.[15] Child abuse is not a diagnosis, however, but a legal finding, and medical personnel who try to investigate this crime may confuse the evidence to the point that the law enforcement agency cannot protect the child.[16] Health care providers should defer to experts in child abuse and neglect rather than attempting to make an independent determination of abuse.[17] The experts will also act as consultants to the courts and protective services.

Generally, health care providers have a responsibility to report violent or suspicious injuries to the local law enforcement agency. These include all gunshot wounds, knifings, poisonings, serious motor vehicle injuries, and any other wounds that seem suspicious. The legal assumption is that anyone who has knowledge that a crime may have been committed has a duty to report it to the police. If the patient is brought to the hospital in the custody of the police or from the scene of a police investigation, then the health care provider may safely assume that the police have been notified. In all other cases, however, the health care provider should call the police and make the report.

Vital Statistics

Vital statistics, or birth and death records, are critical to public health and are required in all states. The keeping of good vital statistics is important to society for several reasons. For one, they are a good way to monitor a population's health. The infant mortality rate is generally considered to be the single best indicator of the health of a population. Accurate vital statistics also allow for allocation of health care funds to areas of greatest need. Vital statistics are of great historical value as well, documenting a population's health through time. On the individual level, the documentation of a birth certificate establishes a person's legal existence and her basic legal relationships, including citizenship and parentage.

Although there have been efforts to standardize state laws on keeping vital statistics, there are still significant differences among states. The registrar of vital statistics at the state health department is the best source of information about that state's laws. It is anticipated that vital statistics records will become a more useful resource as states centralize their records and begin to correlate them with other states and with federal social security records.

The quality of death records in the United States is generally poor because physicians are not well trained in filing these reports.[18] Death certificates are problematic for several reasons.[19] Unexpected deaths frequently occur outside the hospital. The cause of death may not be immediately obvious. There may be no one to provide information on the identity of the person who died. Occasionally, there may be a question of criminal activity having been involved in the death.

The cause of death is the most important information on a death certificate, but it is generally the most inadequate. Preferably, the causes of death that are listed are codable from the International Classification of Disease. For many certificates, however, the actual cause of the death is not clear, let alone codable. *Cardiac arrest*, for example, is a result of death, not a cause. A death certificate may list cardiac arrest as the cause of death and respiratory arrest following shock as the contributing cause, even though the patient actually died of a gunshot wound, terminal cancer, or heart disease. Ideally, the cause of death should reflect what killed the patient, not what the terminal events were.

Disease Control

Disease control is the prevention of disease in the community. While disease control specialists must be knowledgeable in the treatment of communicable diseases, the public health focus is different from that of the medical specialist who treats infectious diseases. Infectious disease specialists are concerned with the management and treatment of infected individuals. Effective public health disease control includes treatment, when indicated, but is much more comprehensive, attacking the roots of disease in the community.[20]

Disease control poses the most difficult legal questions because the rights and well-being of the individual patient are not paramount. Disease control measures frequently inconvenience a lot of people (smokers huddled in the freezing cold outside their office building are a classic example). Disease control measures also often pose a real, if small, risk of serious injury. In many cases, such as syphilis, the treatment (penicillin) that protects the public also benefits infected persons but not without some attendant risk (a possible allergic reaction to the penicillin). In some cases, such as erythromycin therapy for pertussis, the treatment makes the patient noninfectious but does not alter the course of the disease. The vaccine that prevents thousands of cases of paralytic polio may do so at the cost of an occasional case of vaccine-related polio.

Determining which disease control measures are indicated are scientific and political decisions more than legal decisions. As discussed earlier, courts generally defer to the expertise of the health officer, unless there is special legislation limiting the authority of the health officer. In most cases, however, health officers must temper good public health practice with the wishes of elected officials. Unfortunately, elected officials usually are loath to do anything that is opposed by a significant part of the community. For example, against the strenuous objections of most public health authorities, England stopped giving pertussis immunizations because of public outcries about the alleged dangers of the vaccine. Because pertussis had been under control for many years, most of the public had forgotten the terrible sequelae of the disease. As predicted, pertussis soon returned. Immunizations were resumed but only at the cost of many unnecessary childhood deaths and injuries.

Involuntary Testing

One of the least intrusive disease control measures is the involuntary testing of populations at risk for communicable disease. The most common example is testing for tuberculosis in high-risk populations. Involuntary testing has three benefits. First, it allows public health officials to learn the prevalence of a disease in the community, which is difficult to accomplish with voluntary testing because of statistical problems associated with self-selected data sets. Second, involuntary testing identifies infected individuals who may benefit from treatment, and third, it identifies individuals who may need to be restricted to protect the public health.

Involuntary testing for communicable diseases is legally different from testing for personal behaviors, such as drug use or the propensity to steal from an employer. For one thing, the presence or absence of a communicable disease may be objectively determined and the risk it poses easily quantified. Also, there are no criminal law consequences to the diagnosis of a communicable disease, so there is no need for protections against self-incrimination in disease screening. In many cases treatment will eradicate the condition. Even when treatment is not possible, only rare circumstances demand more than minimal workplace restrictions to prevent the spread of the disease. When these restrictions are required, their sole purpose is to protect others and not to punish the affected individual.

Contact Tracing

Contact tracing has been[21] used for decades to control endemic contagious diseases. It is done after disease reporting or involuntary testing identifies an individual as having a communicable disease. An investigator interviews the patient, family members, physicians, nurses, and anyone else who may have knowledge of the patient's contacts; anyone who might have been exposed; and anyone who might have been the source of the disease. Then the contacts are screened to see whether they have or ever have had the disease.

Many persons object to contact tracing as an invasion of privacy. It may be, but only in a very limited sense. Contact-tracing interviews are always voluntary; there is no legal coercion to divulge the names of contacts.[22] A more serious objection, especially with venereal diseases, is the risk of breaches of confidentiality. As a matter of law, the courts do not consider the risk of such breaches of confidentiality to be sufficient reason to restrict contact tracing. As a matter of public health practice, there have been no significant breaches of the confidentiality of public health records.[23] When suspected breaches of confidentiality have been investigated, they are usually traced back to the patient's own disclosures or to those of people whom the patient has told of the condition.

It has also been argued that contact tracing is not legally justified because it is too expensive or because it is ineffective. The courts have rejected these arguments because contact tracing is indeed highly efficient in finding infected persons.[24] This was best demonstrated in the campaign to eradicate smallpox, which was controlled not by universal immunization but by extensive contact tracing to find infected individuals.[25] Fellow villagers and tribesmen were encouraged in various ways to identify infected persons. When people with smallpox were identified, they were quarantined and everyone in the surrounding community or village vaccinated. In this way, smallpox was eventually reduced to isolated outbreaks and then eradicated.

Immunizations and Mandated Treatment

The police power to protect the public health and safety extends to involuntary treatment of persons who pose a threat to the community. The most common examples of involuntary treatment are state-mandated immunizations for childhood diseases. In the only immunization case ever decided by the United States Supreme Court, the Court held that it was constitutionally permissible to force an individual to be vaccinated for smallpox by arguing:

> We are not prepared to hold that a minority, residing or remaining in any city or town where smallpox is prevalent, and enjoying the general protection afforded by an organized local government, may thus defy the will of its constituted authorities, acting in good faith for all, under the legislative sanction of the state. If such be the privilege of a minority, then a like privilege would belong to each individual of the community, and the spectacle would be presented of the welfare and safety of an entire population being subordinated to the notions of a single individual who chooses to remain a part of that population.[8]

A patient who refuses to accept treatment for a contagious disease may be ordered to accept the treatment by a health officer or, depending on the jurisdiction, by a court. A common practice is to incarcerate a recalcitrant patient until the patient consents to the treatment. This coerced consent is not obtained as a sham of an informed consent but as a way to obviate the need for physically forcing the treatment on the patient. It also gives the patient an opportunity to contest the treatment through a habeas corpus proceeding.

Most mandatory immunization laws contain exemptions for individuals who have a high probability of being injured by the immunization. Many of these laws also exempt persons who have religious objections to immunization. Although the United States Constitution allows mandatory immunization of religious objectors, most states do not take advantage of this power. The effectiveness of immunization laws depends on compliance by health care providers and parents. If health care providers give medical exemptions to a large percentage of their patients, the level of immunity in their school system might drop low enough to support a disease epidemic. If a child is improperly exempted from immunization, the health care provider could be held liable should the child contract the disease and suffer any permanent sequelae.

The most difficult political problem in immunization law is the compensation of persons injured by vaccines. (This same issue arises when a person is injured by mandatory treatment for a communicable disease.) Just as persons inducted into the armed forces have no right to sue the government either for deprivation of liberty or for injuries suffered in the line of battle, so persons injured by disease control measures have no constitutional right to compensation. In many cases, however, such as injuries allegedly related to immunizations, the government has chosen to allow compensation.

Personal Restrictions

The most intrusive public health measures are ongoing restrictions of an individual's liberty. A classic example is the case of *Typhoid Mary*. Some people who are infected with typhoid become chronic carriers. If they work in food handling or preparation or in child care, they can spread the disease to others. If they work at other jobs, they pose no risk of disease transmission to their casual contacts. Typhoid Mary was a real person who was a typhoid carrier. She was a threat because she worked as a cook and refused to stop this work. Every time the health department located her, usually through a new outbreak of typhoid, she would move and change her name, but not her occupation. Typhoid Mary infected more than a hundred people, and several of them died of the disease. She was finally placed under house arrest to keep her from cooking and infecting others.

A 1941 case, also involving a typhoid carrier, is a good example of the court's view of the appropriateness of personal restrictions to control disease. The case concerned the issue of whether the identity of typhoid carriers could be disclosed if necessary to prevent them from handling food and thus exposing others to disease. It was argued that:

> The Sanitary Code which has the force of law . . . requires local health officers to keep the state department of health informed of the names, ages and addresses of known or suspected typhoid carriers, to furnish to the state health department necessary specimens for laboratory examination in such cases, to inform the carrier and members of his household of the situation and to exercise certain controls over the activities of the carriers, including a prohibition against any handling by the carrier of

food which is to be consumed by persons other than members of his own household. . . . Why should the record of compliance by the county health officer with these salutary requirements be kept confidential? Hidden in the files of the health offices, it serves no public purpose except a bare statistical one. Made available to those with a legitimate ground for inquiry, it is effective to check the spread of the dread disease. It would be worse than useless to keep secret an order by a public officer that a certain typhoid carrier must not handle foods which are to be served to the public.[26]

The most extreme public health restriction is quarantine, or isolation. The word **quarantine** derives from *quadraginta*, meaning 40. It was first used between 1377 and 1403 when Venice and the other chief maritime cities of the Mediterranean adopted and enforced a 40-day detention of all vessels entering their ports.[27] Quarantine was widely used until the 1950s. For self-limited diseases such as measles, the infected person was required to stay home without visitors. For chronic diseases, such as infectious tuberculosis before anti-tubercular agents were available, the infected person might be required to stay at a sanitarium with other infected patients.

With the advent of antibiotics and effective immunizations, quarantine was seldom necessary to prevent the spread of communicable disease. It was still used by tuberculosis control programs when dealing with recalcitrant tuberculosis carriers, but it was usually the homeless and alcoholics who were held because this was the only way to assure that they got their medicine.

When it was discovered that AIDS was a communicable disease, there was some discussion of using quarantine to prevent its spread. Although it was never considered seriously, the resulting hysteria made public health authorities reluctant to consider quarantine and isolation in any circumstances. Several states, bowing to public pressure, rewrote their disease control laws to make it very difficult to restrict disease carriers. These limitations on the use of restrictive measures are not mandated by the Constitution, and the United States Supreme Court has never ruled that public health restrictions of individuals are improper.

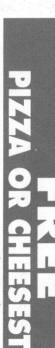

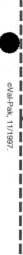

Jerry's
Subs · Pizza ®

PIZZA OR CHEESESTEAK

LANHAM
9001 ANNAPOLIS RD.
(301) 552-1157

FREE
WITH COUPON

PRINCESS GARDEN PKWY.
RT. 450
I-495
ANNAPOLIS RD
RT. 564
N →

FREE
MEDIUM PIZZA
WITH PURCHASE OF MEDIUM PIZZA OF EQUAL OR GREATER VALUE

Valid only at Jerry's of Lanham. Not valid with other coupons, promotions or value combo menu. Excludes tax.
Hurry! Expires: 12/14/97.

Jerry's Subs · Pizza

1.99
SMALL PIZZA & REG. COKE

Topping Extra. Valid only at Jerry's of Lanham. Excludes specialty pizzas. Not valid with other coupons, promotions or value combo menu. Excludes tax.
Hurry! Expires: 12/14/97

Jerry's Subs · Pizza

FREE
CHEESESTEAK
WITH PURCHASE OF CHEESESTEAK OF EQUAL OR GREATER VALUE

Excludes juniors and tax. Valid only at Jerry's of Lanham. Not valid with other coupons, promotions or value combo menu. Excludes tax.
Hurry! Expires 12/14/97

Jerry's Subs · Pizza

The repercussions of these policies are evident in the growing number of reports of the spread of tuberculosis and other diseases from known carriers to health care providers and members of the general population.[28] These are cases that could have been prevented but were not because of a reluctance to use effective isolation.[29] With the explosive growth of pandrug-resistant tuberculosis, public health authorities are facing a deadly, untreatable disease that is spread by casual contact. Isolation is the only way to protect the public from infection. Many public health officers are now facing the problem of persuading their legislatures and elected officials that quarantine and isolation are important measures that must not be limited by statutes that are overly biased toward individual liberties.

THE FUTURE OF PUBLIC HEALTH LAW

Public health faces several challenges: (1) an increasing threat of communicable diseases, both untreatable viral diseases, such as HIV, and bacterial illnesses, such as tuberculosis, that have become relatively resistant to antimicrobial drugs; (2) increasing public distrust of governmental programs, such as disease control measures, that interfere with private interests; and (3) increasing pressure to divert limited public health funds into acute medical care and lifestyle-related chronic diseases.

The key to understanding public health practice and policy is the realization that the mission of public health is to protect the population. Ideally, the interests of the population and the interests of affected individuals will be the same. When they are not, the United States Constitution allows individuals to be restricted for the public interest. This power should never be abused, and it should not be used unless necessary. Public health professionals must understand the law, however, and must defend their right to act in the public's interest. This is often politically unpopular, but it is critical to preserving public health authority. The greatest threats to the public's health are public health professionals who do not understand their legal duties and are guided instead by political expediency.

REFERENCES

1. *Smith v. Turner*, 48 U.S. (7 How.) 283, 340–341 (1849).

2. *Holmes v. Jennison*, 39 U.S. (14 Pet.) 540, 616 (1840).

3. In re Halko, 246 Cal. 2d 553, 556 (1966).

4. *Allen v. Illinois*, 478 U.S. 364 (1986).

5. *Ex Parte McGee*, 185 P. 14, 16 (Kan. 1919).

6. Richards EP, Rathbun KC. *Law and the Physician, A Practical Guide.* Boston: Little, Brown and Company; 1993.

7. *Varholy v. Sweat*, 15 So. 2d 267, 270 (Fla. 1943).

8. *Jacobson v. Massachusetts*, 197 U.S. 11 358, 363 (1905).

9. *City of New York v. New St. Mark's Baths*, 497 N.Y.S. 2d 979, 983 (1986).

10. *North Am. Cold Storage Co. v. City of Chicago*, 211 U.S. 306 (1908).

11. *Surocco v. Geary*, 3 Cal. 69 (1853).

12. *Camara v. Municipal Court of City and County of San Francisco*, 387 U.S. 523 (1967).

13. *Whalen v. Roe*, 429 U.S. 589, 602 (1977).

14. Chorba TL, Berkelman RL, Safford SK, Gibbs NP, Hull HF. Mandatory reporting of infectious diseases by clinicians. *JAMA.* 1989;262:3018–3026.

15. Gaus SM. Reporting child abuse. "Whistle blower protection" and physician responsibility. *Mich Med.* 1988;87(4): 191–193.

16. Johnson CF, Showers J. Injury variables in child abuse. *Child Abuse Negl.* 1985;9(2):207–215.

17. Morris JL, Johnson CF, Clasen M. To report or not to report. Physicians' attitudes toward discipline and child abuse. *Am J Dis Child.* February 1985;139(2):194–197.

18. Cole SK. Accuracy of death certificates in neonatal deaths. *Community Med.* February 1989;11(1):1–8.

19. Davis BR, Curb JD, Tung B, et al. Standardized physician preparation of death certificates. *Control Clin Trials.* June 1987;8(2):110–120.

20. Richards EP. The jurisprudence of prevention: society's right of self-defense against dangerous individuals. *Hastings Const Law Q.* 1989;329:16.

21. Hothcote HW, Yorke JA. *Gonorrhea Transmission Dynamics and Control.* New York: Springer-Verlag; 1984.

22. Woodhouse DE, Muth JB, Potterat JJ, Riffe LD. Restricting personal behaviour: case studies on legal measures to prevent the spread of HIV. *Int J STD AIDS.* March/April 1993;4(2): 114–117.

23. *Guide to Public Heath Practice: Principles to Protect HIV-Related Confidentiality and Prevent Discrimination.* Washington, DC: Association of State and Territorial Health Officers; 1988.

24. Potterat JJ, Spencer NE, Woodhouse DE, Muth JB. Partner notification in the control of human immunodeficiency virus infection. *Am J Public Health.* 1989;79(7):874(3).

25. Carrell S, Zoler ML. Defiant diseases: hard-won gains erode. *Med World News.* 1990;31(12):20(7).

26. *Thomas v. Morris*, 36 N.E.2d 141, 142 (N.Y. 1941).

27. Bolduan C, Bolduan N. *Public Health and Hygiene.* Philadelphia: W.B. Saunders; 1941.

28. Haley CE, McDonald RC, Rossi L, et al. Tuberculosis epidemic among hospital personnel. *Infect Control Hosp Epidemiol.* 1989;204:10.

29. Dooley SW, Villarino ME, Lawrence M, et al. Nosocomial transmission of tuberculosis in a hospital unit for HIV-infected patients. *JAMA.* 1992;267:2632.

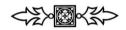

PART TWO

SETTINGS FOR PUBLIC HEALTH PRACTICE

CHAPTER

The Federal Contribution to Public Health

Edward Brandt, M.D., Ph.D.

The federal government is a major player in public health today, but that has not always been the case. Indeed, because the United States Constitution does not mention health and does not, therefore, list health as a responsibility of the government, little was done in the early days of our country. In fact, presidents during the 1800s were very reluctant for the federal government to be involved in health and welfare issues. They felt it violated the constitution. The advent of the *New Deal* of President Franklin Roosevelt ushered in the modern role of the federal government in social and health matters.

HISTORY OF FEDERAL INVOLVEMENT IN PUBLIC HEALTH

Despite such views, the federal government has a long history of involvement with public health. The first federal public health action was taken with the pas-

sage of An Act for the Relief of Sick and Disabled Seamen, which was signed into law by President John Adams on July 16, 1798 and defended as constitutional under the clause, *to promote the general welfare*. The act led to the creation of the Marine Hospital Service, the forerunner of the United States Public Health Service.

The Marine Hospital Service, as conceived by the United States Congress, had two major purposes. One, a public health purpose, was the protection of Americans from infectious diseases that might be imported from foreign countries by merchant seamen. The other, an economic purpose, was to provide a stimulus to foreign trade by giving some assurance to seamen that they would receive care for their illnesses and injuries. The act therefore was meant to provide incentives to people to become merchant seamen, which was a dangerous occupation at that time.

In the nineteenth century, the major public health threats were infectious diseases, such as malaria, typhus, and tuberculosis. The Marine Hospital Service, recognizing that a major problem was a lack of scientific understanding of these illnesses, created a laboratory at the Staten Island Marine Hospital to study methods for their treatment and prevention. This laboratory was the forerunner of the National Institutes of Health, which will be described later. In 1944, the Marine Hospital Service was renamed the Public Health Service and its structure and mission more clearly defined. In the 1950s, the Public Health Service became part of the Department of Health, Education, and Welfare.

POWERS AND ACTIONS OF THE FEDERAL GOVERNMENT

Today the federal government has numerous ways to influence public health and individual health behavior, including the enactment of laws, the imposition of taxes and tax exemptions, the provision of incentives, the execution of studies, and the issuance of regulations. In addition, the federal government may appoint advisory committees to define problems and propose solutions. It may also issue statements concerning public health, and it may set examples. Federal officials often use their offices as *bully pulpits,* adding visibility and credibility to health messages. Over the past 15 years, all of these mechanisms have supported a health promotion and disease prevention revolution.

Until the objectives-for-the-nation process began in the 1980s, the federal government lacked a method of setting priorities for its actions. Instead, the government funded important initiatives that required state and local governments to adapt their needs to the programs defined by federal policy makers. Nonetheless, the federal government was aggressively involved in public health policy development, as the following examples demonstrate.

Traffic Safety

A useful illustration of the federal government's involvement in health issues is provided by traffic safety. Federal action in this area has been directed primarily to occupant protection in crashes rather than to crash avoidance with some exceptions. For example, federal law now requires states to legislate mandatory seat belt and motorcycle helmet use or lose federal highway funds. In addition, the federal government requires interior padding and passive restraints in automobiles. The federal government also issues regulations on braking systems, mirrors, and other safety features of automobiles.

As the result of federal urging or regulation, automobile manufacturers have introduced much technology to assist drivers in maintaining control over automobiles, thereby preventing crashes. Antilock braking systems, improved steering and suspension, and better information displays and outside vision are examples.

Federal taxes have not played an important direct role in automobile safety. However, taxes on gasoline are used to improve roads and signage, which do contribute to safety. In addition, the development of the interstate highway system in the 1950s certainly led to greater traffic safety, with improved construction and maintenance of highways, more traffic lanes, limited access, wider shoulders, and better signage.

Smoking

Unfortunately, not all federal government involvement in public health has been positive. For example, the provision of free cigarettes to American troops in World War II made smokers—and tobacco addicts—out of many soldiers, with a subsequent cost in significant disease and death. In this instance, the military and several private organizations raised the money to purchase the cigarettes for free distribution to the troops.

Indeed, little was done at the federal level about smoking and health until the release of the first surgeon general's report on smoking in 1965. This report detailed the panoply of illnesses linked to smoking. Following this report, a number of events occurred, illustrating the bully pulpit actions of the federal government. First, thousands of Americans began to quit smoking; second, additional research was initiated to document other smoking-related illnesses; and third, state and local governments began to examine their policies with respect to tobacco.

The federal government has continued its effort to decrease tobacco use. For example, there have been a series of surgeon general's reports on tobacco. Reduction in tobacco use also has a very prominent place in the year 2000 health objectives. In addition, the CDC's Office on Tobacco and Health has provided important information on the nation's battle to decrease tobacco use.

Alcohol

Alcohol abuse and alcoholism are significant sources of morbidity and mortality. Nearly 50 percent of fatal automobile crashes involve a drinking driver,[1] and the list of diseases caused, or aggravated, by alcohol is quite long. The federal government has been involved with alcohol abuse, but to a lesser extent than it has been with tobacco. For example, the federal government taxes alcohol and has used the bully pulpit, especially to deter teenage drinking and drinking while driving, but it has little other direct involvement in the fight against alcohol abuse.

ORGANIZATION OF THE FEDERAL GOVERNMENT

The federal government is comprised of three separate but equal components—the legislative, judicial, and executive branches. The federal government was established by the Constitution so that each component would serve as a **check and balance** against the other two, thereby decreasing the possibility of tyranny.

The Judicial Branch

The judicial branch generally does not play a large part in the public's health, although the privacy rulings of the United States Supreme Court certainly contributed to the ability of public health departments to provide family planning services. Chapter 4, on the legal basis of public health, illustrates the nature of the judicial branch's impact on public health. As that chapter

suggests, the underlying basis for public health in the United States is the police power of the state, a well-defined constitutional, judicial, and legal concept.

The Legislative Branch

The legislative branch of the federal government is composed of the two houses of Congress: the Senate and the House of Representatives. Each is unique in its own way, with a style and nature of doing business that reflects its history and tradition and the nature of its processes. The legislative branch, because it is responsible for establishing law and providing funding, certainly influences public health status in the United States.

The Executive Branch

When there is discussion of the federal government's role in public health, however, it is usually the executive branch of government that is under discussion. This branch of government is headed by the president of the United States and consists of the employees of the federal government whose responsibility it is to carry out the mandates of the legislative branch.

Departments and Agencies

Most cabinet departments and independent agencies of the executive branch are involved in public health in some way. For example, the Department of the Treasury administers tax policy, which is important in determining tax exemptions that impact the public's health. The Department of State is involved in international public health activities, such as the participation of the United States in the World Health Organization (WHO). As one of the countries with a seat on the Security Council of the United Nations, the United States is assured a seat on the Executive Council of WHO for two out of every three years. The State Department also works with the United States Department of Health and Human Services to assure that international health policy is consistent with United States foreign policy.

The Labor Department administers the Occupational Safety and Health Administration (OSHA), which is concerned with workplace safety. OSHA accomplishes its work by inspections of workplaces and by the development of safety standards based on research performed by the National Institute of Occupational Safety and Health (NIOSH), an agency of the Public Health Service. The Department of Agriculture administers the Women, Infants, and Children (WIC) nutrition program (the largest public health program in terms of funding), the school lunch program, and the food stamp program.

The Environmental Protection Agency (EPA) is concerned with environmental threats to health. Of special importance to public health is the EPA's responsibility for protection against water and food contamination, especially by pesticides and herbicides. The Department of Energy examines the health effects of various forms of energy. It has also played a role in the development of therapeutic radiographic equipment.

The Department of Defense (DOD) provides health care to active-duty military personnel and their dependents. In addition, on all military bases it provides all of the traditional public health activities, including epidemiologic studies and assurance of food and water quality. DOD also has an extensive health research program. The Department of Veterans Affairs (DVA) is responsible for the provision of health care, including long-term care, for eligible military veterans. DVA carries out relevant health research as well.

Coordination of Activities

It is important to emphasize the overlapping responsibilities of these executive branch departments and agencies and to realize that their efforts must be coordinated if the federal government is to have consistent public health policies and programs. For example, nutrition efforts involve the Departments of Agriculture, Defense, Veterans Affairs, and Health and Human Services. Consider the case of food biotechnology that makes it possible, through gene transfer, to improve the nutritional content of vegetables and grains and to develop crops that are pest, drought, and freeze resistant. Responsibility for this technology is divided among the Department of Agriculture, the Environmental Protec-

tion Agency, and the Department of Health and Human Services.

THE DEPARTMENT OF HEALTH AND HUMAN SERVICES

The cabinet department most concerned with health is the Department of Health and Human Services. This department bears primary responsibility for the federal government's major efforts in welfare and health. Figure 5.1 outlines the organization of the department.

All four of the department's major operating divisions—the Health Care Financing Administration (HCFA), the Administration for Children and Families (ACF), the Administration on Aging (AOA), and the Public Health Service (PHS)—are involved in public health. The Health Care Financing Administration administers Medicaid policy and all aspects of Medicare. Through its research and data sources, it can also identify significant public health issues, especially those affecting the elderly and the poor. The Administration for Children and Families is concerned with developmental disabilities, family assistance, and community services. The Administration on Aging is concerned with the welfare and health needs of older Americans. However, the major component of the Department of Health and Human Services that is concerned with public health is the United States Public Health Service.

The United States Public Health Service

The Public Health Service is responsible for a variety of health functions, including research, health infrastructure, direct provision of health services, disease control, and health regulation. It is arguably the most important public health organization in the country, being an essential component of all federal efforts to promote health and prevent disease.

The PHS formerly was headed by an assistant secretary for health (ASH), who was appointed by the president and confirmed by the Senate. Recently, the Social Security Administration was removed from the DHHS. With this change, the position of ASH appeared superfluous and was merged into the secretary of DHHS's office to improve access of the PHS to the secretary.

Office of the Assistant Secretary for Health

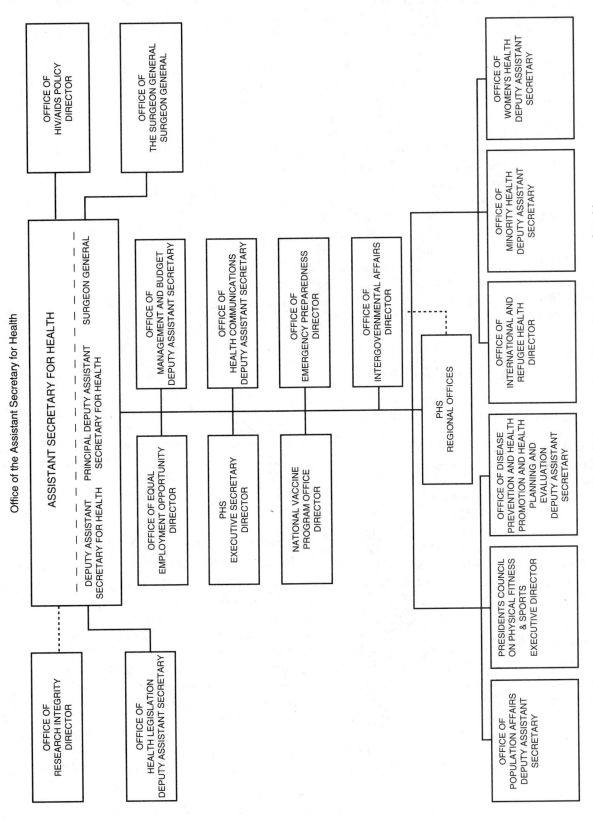

FIGURE 5.1 U.S. Department of Health and Human Services, Public Health Service, Office of the Assistant Secretary of Health

The PHS is undergoing substantial change as the result of both congressional pressure to downsize DHHS and efforts growing out of the *reinventing government* task force of the executive branch of federal government. The new administrative structure of the PHS has not yet been finalized, but it is likely that its operating agencies will remain the same—National Institutes of Health (NIH), Centers for Disease Control and Prevention (CDC), Indian Health Service (IHS), Health Resources and Service Administration (HRSA), Substance Abuse and Mental Health Services Administration (SAMHSA), Agency for Health Care Policy and Research (AHCPR), Food and Drug Administration (FDA), and Office of Health Promotion and Disease Prevention (ODPDP). The role of the PHS is best examined by looking briefly at each of these agencies that comprise it.

National Institutes of Health (NIH)

The largest PHS agency, in budgetary terms, is the NIH. The primary mission of the NIH is health-related research, conducted both intramurally (i.e., by full-time staff of the NIH) and extramurally (i.e., by grant programs to universities, research institutes, and private corporations worldwide). NIH consists of 24 institutes, centers, and divisions, the National Library of Medicine, and a number of multidisciplinary programs, such as the Fogarty International Center and the Offices of Disease Prevention, Women's Health, AIDS Research, and Minority Health. NIH is, unquestionably, the premier health research organization in the world.

Centers for Disease Control and Prevention (CDC)

The CDC is charged with disease surveillance and the epidemiology and control of infectious diseases, chronic diseases, and injuries. It includes eight centers and four program offices. The CDC accomplishes its missions by intramural disease prevention and health promotion activities and extramural grants and by providing personnel to state and local health departments. CDC also provides epidemiologic, laboratory, and other support to state health agencies. The CDC is the major agency responsible for protecting the American public against disease and injury.

Agency for Toxic Substances and Disease Registry (ATSDR)

The ATSDR, created in 1980, is one of the newer agencies of the PHS and is closely affiliated with CDC. Indeed, its administrator is the director of CDC. The ATSDR's mission is to conduct studies relevant to prevention of disease due to toxic substances.

Indian Health Service (IHS)

The IHS is charged with providing funding for, or direct health care services to, Alaskan natives and members of federally qualified Native American tribes. Most of its constituents receive services directly from IHS personnel, but many tribes are now organizing their own health care delivery systems, funded by the IHS under the Indian Self Improvement Act. Although primarily a health care delivery agency, the IHS also provides public health services to Native Americans, including sanitation, water quality, preventive services, disease surveillance, and health education.

Health Resources and Services Administration (HRSA)

The HRSA is arguably the most complex of the PHS agencies in that its mission is to provide infrastructure for a variety of public health activities. For example, it funds health professions education, community health centers, and related activities. It is the home of the National Health Service Corps and other programs that are aimed at providing service to underserved populations. HRSA operates through four bureaus—Health Resource Development, Primary Health Care, Maternal and Child Health, and Health Professions. HRSA also has four interdisciplinary offices—Rural Health Policy, AIDS Programs, Minority Health, and Public Health Practice.

Substance Abuse and Mental Health Services Administration (SAMHSA)

The mission of SAMHSA is to provide substance abuse and mental health services, primarily to the poor and medically underserved. It was created from an older agency, the Alcohol, Drug Abuse and Mental Health Administration (ADAMHA), by transfer to it of the mental health research components from the NIH. SAMHSA administers grant programs designed to establish substance abuse services and community mental health clinics.

Agency for Health Care Policy and Research (AHCPR)

The AHCPR's mission is to enhance health care service delivery through the design of clinical protocols and guidelines that lead to improved clinical outcomes. It also studies health care delivery systems to improve their efficiency, effectiveness, quality, and productivity. It accomplishes its mission through competitive grant programs, intramural research programs, and special advisory groups. AHCPR consists of four centers—Medical Effectiveness Research, General Health Services Intramural Research, General Health Services Extramural Research, and Research Dissemination and Liaison. It also has two offices, the Forum for Quality and Effectiveness in Health Care and Health Technology Effectiveness.

Food and Drug Administration (FDA)

The FDA is the largest regulatory body of the federal government, regulating over two-thirds of the nation's economy. The mission of the FDA is to promote public health by assuring that human and animal drugs and medical devices are both safe and effective and that food is safe. The latter mission includes assuring that animal feeds and drugs do not contaminate meat and other animal products.

As a result of its responsibilities, the FDA generates a great deal of controversy. For example, it is charged with causing suffering and deaths both for not approving new therapeutic modalities quickly enough as well as for approving them too quickly. One of the principal problems of the FDA is that it shares regulatory responsibilities with the Department of Agriculture and the Environmental Protection Agency.

Office of Disease Prevention and Health Promotion (ODPHP)

Prior to 1995, ODPHP was the staff office within PHS responsible for health promotion and disease prevention. It coordinated, both within PHS and between DHHS and other cabinet departments, the federal government's health promotion and disease prevention activities. ODPHP led the development of the 1990 and year 2000 objectives for the nation and monitored progress toward achieving those objectives.[2] With the recent reorganization of functions within DHHS, ODPHP's functions were transferred to the secretary's office, and ODPHP no longer exists as such.

OBJECTIVES FOR THE NATION

One of the more notable achievements of the federal government's public health activities in the past 20 years has been the definition of objectives for the nation. In the late 1970s, a large group of public health experts came together to define 15 major priority program categories with 226 specific, measurable objectives. The objectives were published[3,4] and formed a framework for public health workers, at all levels, to set priorities and allocate resources.

Groups of people from the various PHS agencies were assigned to monitor the objectives. One of the early problems that surfaced was a lack of well-developed data systems to track progress toward meeting a quarter of the objectives. However, using data from the National Center for Health Statistics,[5] success or failure in achieving most of the 1990 objectives has been tracked.[2] Of the 205 objectives for which data are available, 85, or 41 percent, were achieved by 1990, ranging from 6 percent of the objectives in the nutrition program to 78 percent of the objectives in the high blood pressure program.

Beginning in 1987, the PHS started developing objectives for the year 2000. Regional hearings were held, draft objectives widely circulated, and comments reviewed.[6] The final result was the publication of *Healthy People 2000: National Health Promotion and Disease Prevention Objectives*,[7] which includes 300 specific objectives grouped into 27 categories. Benefiting from the lessons learned from the 1990 objectives, there is more emphasis on minority and low-income populations as well as on the availability of data to monitor progress towards achievement of the objectives.[2]

The direct accomplishments of the objectives process are impressive. Equally important, however, have been the results of giving states and communities national objectives to use as a basis for developing objectives of their own. Also important have been improvements in data systems and the involvement of individuals, agencies, and groups critical to progress in public health and not usually considered in health planning.[2] Chapter 10 describes the objectives process in more detail.

CLINICAL PREVENTIVE SERVICES

An important aspect of improving the health status of Americans and achieving the objectives is the provision of personal preventive services. In the past, a major impediment to this effort was the lack of agreement about the scientific effectiveness of preventive services and, therefore, about which preventive services should be provided. In 1984, the ASH appointed the Preventive Services Task Force to identify preventive services that had documented scientific efficacy. Following careful study and consultation with numerous experts, the task force presented its findings in May 1989 in a publication entitled *Guide to Clinical Preventive Services*.[8] The report focused on 60 illnesses and 169 preventive interventions.

The process of developing clinical preventive service guidelines has continued with the establishment of the National Coordinating Committee on Clinical Preventive Services (NCCCPS). In 1993, this group published a report extending the work of the Task Force on Clinical Preventive Services and providing information about the costs of preventive services. According to the report, the cost of providing recommended services averaged $62 per year for children, $84 per year for

adult females, and $52 per year for adult males.[9] The NCCCPS also has responsibility for updating and expanding the *Guide to Clinical Preventive Services.*

LEGISLATION AND ITS EFFECTS

Since the beginning of this century, there have been numerous laws passed to improve the health of the public. During the Eisenhower administration, for example, the Department of Health, Education and Welfare (DHEW) was created by legislative action in an effort to bring most federal public health activities into one department. With the movement in 1979 of activities related to education to the newly created Department of Education, DHEW was renamed the Department of Health and Human Services.

Health Care for the Poor and Elderly

Since 1960, the pace of federal public health legislation has increased. For example, in 1960 there was major debate over the provision of health care to the poor and to the elderly. Senator John F. Kennedy advocated a federal system to provide such care, and this was at least partly the basis for his election to the office of president. This represented a change in public opinion. Although some form of national health insurance had been advocated by Presidents Roosevelt and Truman and by several members of Congress in the 1930s and 1940s, prior to 1960 the idea had been rejected by business, organized medicine, and Congress as a whole.

Legislation to accomplish President Kennedy's goals was not enacted until 1965, when his successor, President Lyndon Johnson, obtained passage of Titles XVIII and XIX of the Social Security Act. Medicare (Title XVIII) and Medicaid (Title XIX) have made health care available to many Americans who previously had been unable to obtain it.

The public health aspects of Medicare and Medicaid have been limited, but there are some important public health features of this legislation. For example, preventive procedures, such as immunizations against pneumococcal pneumonia and influenza, are now covered by Medicare, as are some early detection measures, such as mammography. Medicaid pays for prenatal care for poor and nearly poor women and for Early Periodic Screening, Diagnosis, and Treatment (EPSDT) services, which have led to improved infant health. In addition, many states include mammography screening, immunizations, and other preventive services as reimbursed Medicaid benefits.

Several pieces of legislation were enacted during the 1960s and 1970s that were intended to improve the provision of health services to medically underserved populations. These included funds to establish and operate community health centers, community mental health centers, and family planning services, and for the establishment of the National Health Service Corps, which was designed to provide health personnel to underserved areas. It did so by providing students in health professions with scholarship money in exchange for their service to underserved populations.

Categorical Grants Versus Block Grants

A major issue in the transfer of funds from federal to state and local governments has been the nature of the mandate and constraints associated with federal funding. In federal funding, the pendulum has consistently swung between categorical grants and block grants. The former are tied to a specific purpose, for example, rat control or sudden infant death syndrome. The latter are broad and intended to allow state and local agencies to use their discretion to allocate resources based on local need.

Traditionally, there has been a series of categorical programs funded by the federal government, frequently related to problems experienced by particular members of Congress who sponsor enabling legislation or by an important constituency. There is recognition that this categorical funding has placed too many constraints on those in positions to know best the health problems of the community and make resource allocations based on those community problems.

The Omnibus Budget Reconciliation Act of 1981 (Public Law 97-35) created a series of block grants, one of which was the Preventive Health and Health Services Block Grant. Originally proposed by the Reagan ad-

ministration as one major block grant to permit state governments to have total control over priority setting and allocation of federal funds, Congress actually set up four separate block grants. Although the grants impeded states' abilities to allocate funds, they did permit greater control over priorities than previous categorical programs did.[10] At the same time, allocated funds were cut by 20 percent, reflecting the administration's judgment of the cost of complying with federal requirements for administration of a large number of categorical programs rather than a single large block of funds.

The Preventive Health and Health Services Block Grants, coupled with the objectives for the nation, did give states the opportunity to institute a coordinated approach to health promotion and disease prevention that was aimed at their special problems. In response to this initiative, virtually all of the 57 states and territories have set up public health objectives and programs to achieve them.

Recent changes in Congress have again accelerated the pace of block grants. There are two unique block grants under development. The first would shift, on a block grant basis, all Medicaid revenues back to the states. Given the dependence of many local health departments on Medicaid funds to cross-subsidize other services, the implications of this for public health are significant.

The second block grant seeks to create *performance partnerships*. In this block grant, PHS funds would be put in large blocks and given to the states, which would be held accountable for achieving various health objectives. This *reinventing of public health* has become a major theme of the Clinton administration.[11]

NEW STATE INITIATIVES

The combination of federal agenda setting through objectives for the nation and the provision of relatively unencumbered federal funds has resulted in many new state public health initiatives.

Massachusetts

In Massachusetts seven of the fifteen major program priorities were selected as state priorities.[12] This priority setting was based on a model that used epidemiological findings and the availability of effective intervention strategies to establish program priorities. As Massachusetts has experienced success with these programs, the state legislature has provided additional funding to enhance them.

Minnesota

A second example is Minnesota, where the Department of Health selected nine of the fifteen program priorities to work on, including smoking cessation.[13] The Minnesota commissioner of health established the Center for Nonsmoking and Health. This subsequently led to the development and implementation of a statewide tobacco plan. The result has been a significant reduction in the Minnesota smoking rate.[14]

Summary

These steps taken by the states—setting of objectives based on the objectives for the nation, exercising control over priorities and resource allocation, and taking action to achieve the objectives—have put the entire country in a position to make significant public health gains. All of these steps were made possible by federal actions. Furthermore, continuation of federal policies to increase the capacity of state and local health departments, publishing the year 2000 objectives, and targeting minorities and others at high risk for health problems hold promise for further gains in the future.

THE FUTURE

There is little question that federal and state governments will remain active in health promotion and disease prevention. The fact that most states and territories have defined public health objectives based on those developed by the federal government is an indication of the commitment of state governments to improving health status. Governments at all levels are now approaching health problems and disease prevention in a more systematic, coordinated fashion. Public involvement in priority setting and resource allocation gives greater assurance of widespread commitment to achieving objectives and broadening available resources.

Arguably, the most significant public health step taken by the federal government in the past 20 years has been the development of the *1990 Objectives of the Nation* and *Healthy People 2000*. The progress made towards those objectives, the resultant implementation by the states, and the openness of the development process, which has involved numerous groups and the public, should lead to actions for the further achievement of health promotion and disease prevention goals.

In 1994, the federal government was involved in debate over reform of the health care system. Several goals were proposed, including decreasing the costs of health care to individuals; increasing access to health care for the poor and nearly poor and for those with *preexisting conditions;* making insurance coverage portable; and increasing the supply of primary care practitioners. Most of the proposals ignored public health issues. For a variety of reasons, Congress decided not to act on any of the legislation that was introduced, and responsibility has now shifted to the states. However, state governments have been faced with dramatic increases in the cost of Medicaid and as a result, funding for public health services has been cut, or at least not increased. History has shown clearly that reform of the health care system without significant enhancement of the public health system will not lead to improved health status.

CONCLUSION

Throughout the history of this country, the federal government has made significant contributions to the health of the public. It has been a participant in the development of the nation's public health system, although the major responsibility has been assumed by state and local governments. In recent years, there have been legitimate concerns raised as to the status of the public health system of the country.[15] Nonetheless, the public health system keeps growing stronger and the federal government continues playing a significant role.

REFERENCES

1. National Highway Traffic Safety Administration. Press release. August 26, 1991.

2. McGinnis MJ, Richmond JB, Brandt EN Jr, Windom RE, Mason JO. Health progress in the United States: results of the 1990 objectives for the nation. *JAMA.* 1992;268:254–255.

3. *Promoting Health/Preventing Disease: Objectives for the Nation.* Washington, DC: US Dept of Health and Human Services; 1990.

4. *Healthy People: The Surgeon General's Report on Health Promotion and Disease Prevention.* Washington, DC: US Dept of Health Education and Welfare; 1979. PHS publication 79-55071.

5. National Center for Health Statistics. *Health United States, 1991, and Prevention Profile.* Hyattsville, Md: US Dept of Health and Human Services; 1992. PHS publication 92-1232.

6. McGinnis JM. National priorities in disease prevention. *Issues in Sci Tech.* 1989;46.

7. *Healthy People 2000: National Health Promotion and Disease Prevention Objectives.* Washington, DC: US Dept of Health and Human Services; 1990. PHS publication 91-50212.

8. US Dept of Health and Human Services. *Guide to Clinical Preventive Services.* Baltimore, Md: Williams and Wilkins; 1989.

9. *Preventive Services in the Clinical Setting, What Works and What It Costs.* Washington, DC: US Dept of Human Services; 1993.

10. Brandt EN Jr. Block grants and the resurgence of federalism. *Public Health Rep.* 1981;96:495

11. Lee PR. Advancing America's Health. *JAMA.* 1995;273: 248–249.

12. Havas S, Blik C. The Preventive Health and Services Block Grant: the Massachusetts experience. *Public Health Rep.* 1987;102:284.

13. Dean AG, et al. The Minnesota Plan for nonsmoking and health: a multidisciplinary approach to risk factor control. *Public Health Rep.* 1986;101:270.

14. Perry CL, Kelder SH, Murray DM, Klepp KI. Community aide smoking prevention: long-term objectives of the Minnesota Heart Health Program and the Class of 1989 Study. *Am J Public Health.* 1992;82:1210.

15. Institute of Medicine, Committee for the Study of the Future of Public Health. *The Future of Public Health.* Washington DC: National Academy Press; 1988.

CHAPTER

The State Public Health Department

Susan Dandoy, M.D., M.P.H.

Massachusetts was the first state to take responsibility for the health of its people by creating a board of health in 1869. By 1909, all states had health departments whose tasks focused primarily on the recording of births and deaths and the control of communicable diseases. Today, state health departments have expanded their activities to include improving the health of children and pregnant women, controlling chronic diseases, preventing injuries, regulating health care facilities, developing emergency medical services and other health care resources, and protecting the environment.

In its 1988 report, the Institute of Medicine's Committee for the Study of the Future of Public Health (IOM Committee) noted that states are close enough to the people to maintain a sense of their needs and preferences, yet large enough, in most cases, to command the resources necessary to get the important jobs done.[1] In fact, because state health departments were created to meet the differing needs and preferences of the people in each state, their functions and activities show wide variation. Departments also vary in organizational structure, per capita expenditures, staffing patterns, re-

sponsibility for local health services, political influence, and relationships with other agencies.

Each of these topics is explored in this chapter, which focuses on trends over time and current issues. IOM Committee recommendations regarding specific topics are included as a yardstick for comparison with actual conditions.

FUNCTIONS OF STATE HEALTH DEPARTMENTS

Government responsibility in public health includes the *agenda setting function*.[2] Each state health department must identify goals and strategies to improve the health of its citizens. To set and implement this agenda, the state health department assesses the health status and needs of the population; plans strategies and health programs to address unmet needs; obtains financial assistance to support these plans; sets and enforces standards; provides technical assistance to local health departments and other governmental and nongovernmental agencies; and, in limited circumstances, delivers health services directly (in most states, local health departments are the primary government entity providing public health services directly to individuals).

Traditional Versus Newer Functions

Until the 1940s, state health departments focused almost solely on six basic public health services: collection of vital records and statistics; control of communicable diseases; environmental sanitation; laboratory services; public health education; and maternal and child health. Concern for the health of the labor force led states to add industrial hygiene services.[3]

As antibiotics and vaccines became available to control the spread of communicable diseases, citizens voiced their desire for government to give attention to other health problems. In the late 1950s, the United States Congress began offering states federal funds to support specific new services for certain groups of people or for particular diseases. These *categorical* programs addressed areas in which state health departments traditionally had not been involved, such as heart disease, diabetes, migrant labor, mental retardation, rheumatic fever, and the construction of new hospitals and clinics. This expansion of state health department activity has continued, stimulated by the availability of federal funds, the necessity of meeting federally enacted mandates, and the growth of state health laws.

Typical Responsibilities

Typical responsibilities of a state health department are presented in Table 6.1. Many of these activities are expansions and variations on the original six basic functions, particularly health information (vital records and statistics), disease and disability prevention (communicable disease control and laboratory services), health protection (environmental sanitation), health promotion (public health education), and maternal and child health services.

Health Information

The collection and preservation of vital records, and the analysis and use of information from such records,

TABLE 6.1   Responsibilities of a State Health Department

Health Information
- Recording and issuing certified copies of birth and death certificates
- Publishing health statistics
- Birth defects registry
- Cancer registry

Disease and Disability Prevention
- Screening newborns for inborn errors of metabolism
- Immunization programs
- AIDS screening, counseling, and partner notification
- Tuberculosis control
- Screening children for lead
- Investigating disease outbreaks
- Laboratory testing for infectious diseases
- Medical care for children with handicapping conditions
- Education on use of occupant restraints in vehicles

Health Protection
- Testing waters in which shellfish are grown
- Issuing permits for sewage disposal systems
- Monitoring drinking water systems
- Inspecting dairies
- License hospitals, nursing homes, and home health agencies
- Examining and certifying emergency medical personnel
- Inspecting clinical laboratories

Health Promotion
- Food vouchers for pregnant women, infants, and children (WIC)
- Prenatal care for low-income families
- Dental care for low-income children and adults
- School health education
- Family planning services
- Cholesterol and high blood pressure education programs

Improving the Health Care Delivery System
- Scholarships for medical and nursing students
- Certificates of need for construction of health facilities
- Development of rural health policies and services

are major functions of state health departments. Now states also gather and analyze data on the health of the population and the characteristics of the medical care delivery system. State health departments are the legal repositories for birth and death records in most states, and they may also keep records of marriages, divorces, and terminations of pregnancy.

Data from these vital records, along with data from disease registries, surveys of health care providers and facilities, disease case reports, screening programs, and laboratory analyses, are used for several purposes: to influence the creation, continuation, or modification of programs; to identify disease patterns or outbreaks; to determine priorities for resource allocation; and to assist in planning health care delivery sites and facilities.

Disease and Disability Prevention

Preventing disease and disability, particularly communicable disease, is a unique function of health departments in every state; no other state agency is given the lead responsibility for this function. As pertussis, measles, and other communicable diseases have been brought under control, state health department attention and resources have shifted to other health problems, such as AIDS, hepatitis, breast cancer, injuries, and cardiovascular disease. State activities in these areas include screening programs, laboratory testing, health education, technical advice, issuance of isolation and quarantine orders, immunizations, public information, and chemotherapy.

Health Protection

Citizens extended their concern with the general cleanliness of the environment to require state oversight of public drinking water, ambient air, food service facilities, sewage systems, and sources of radiation. State health departments have also been asked to regulate the medical care delivery system. Initially, this was to assure the hygiene, proper staffing, and safety of health facilities. However, anxiety over the increasing costs of health care led policy makers to give state health departments responsibility for regulating facility charges, bed capacity, and service enhancement; gathering data on health care costs; and, most recently, monitoring the availability of medical care to the population. To improve access to care, health departments recruit physicians for medically underserved areas and provide scholarships and loans for medical and nursing students. Thus, state health departments have been charged with protecting not only the public's health but also the public's access to quality medical care.

Health Promotion

Going beyond educating the population on how to avoid infectious diseases, health promotion efforts in state health departments now focus on lifestyle issues, maintenance of health, and prevention of injury. Health education programs at schools and workplaces address diet, exercise, tobacco use, and stress reduction, with emphasis on reducing risk factors for cancer and cardiovascular diseases.

Health Care Delivery

The involvement of state health departments in direct delivery of care began with clinics for pregnant women and children. As federal and state funds have become available, direct services have expanded to include family planning, cancer screening, dental health, treatment for tuberculosis and sexually transmitted diseases, and, most recently, primary medical care. In each of these undertakings, the state's role centers on program planning, setting and enforcing standards, developing procedures, and providing technical assistance and funding, while the clinical care is actually delivered at the local level.

ORGANIZATIONAL ISSUES

Before 1960, almost all public health functions provided by states were located in state health departments. As programs became more complex and as demands for new types of services increased, the newer functions as well as some traditional health department activities were assigned to other state agencies.[3] Table 6.2 shows this for Virginia. Lewis-Idema and Falik maintain that, although public needs are ever changing, public agencies tend to be static, with institutionalized perspectives and responsibilities.[4] Thus, new problems tend to generate new programs that are assigned to new agencies rather than to generate changes in existing agencies. Public health leaders may be perceived as having no in-

TABLE 6.2 Health Responsibilities in State Agencies Other than the State Health Department: Virginia

Department of Agriculture
• Inspects grocery stores
• Inspects food processing plants

Department of Education
• Supervises health teaching in schools
• Supervises delivery of health services in schools

Department of Environmental Quality
• Controls air pollution
• Controls water pollution
• Oversees solid and hazardous waste disposal

Department of Health Professions
• Licenses twelve categories of health professionals

Department of Labor and Industry
• Regulates occupational health and safety

Department of Medical Assistance Services (Medicaid)
• Finances medical care to the indigent and categorically needy
• Funds a health status screening program for children
• Provides case management services for newborns

Department of Mental Health, Mental Retardation, and Substance Abuse Services
• Operates mental hospitals
• Directs community mental health and substance abuse services

Department of Motor Vehicles
• Educates the public on occupant safety and seat belt use

Health Services Cost Review Council
• Collects, analyzes, and publishes data on health care costs

Joint Commission on Health Care
• Develops legislative proposals for improving access to medical care

terest in new ideas or as not having the political skills needed to lead and direct a particular program. Often, special interest groups want separate administration for their particular programs so they can exert more control over their operation.

Major governmental health functions that are assigned to other agencies include mental health, financing of medical care for the indigent, and environmental protection. The IOM Committee analyzed this frag-

mentation of public health functions and made specific recommendations regarding closer linkages between programs that now exist in separate agencies.[1]

Mental Health

In only four states are health departments also the state mental health authority, reflecting a long trend in segregating physical and mental health problems.[5] This division of leadership at the state level results in separate service delivery systems at the local level, with little coordinated planning around client needs. The IOM Committee recommended that public health and mental health leaders devote efforts to strengthening the linkages between the two fields, particularly to integrating these functions at the service delivery level.

Financing Medical Care

The state's participation in financing medical care usually resides outside the state health department. When the federal Medicaid program started in 1965, states had to select a single state agency to manage the program. Initially, some states assigned this role to health departments. As the Medicaid program grew, both in dollars and in numbers of people receiving care, responsibility for operating the program shifted either to a separate state agency or to the social services/welfare agency. According to unpublished data from the Public Health Foundation, in 1991 only five state and three territorial health departments managed their state's Medicaid program.

Coordination and Control of Services

When a state health department retains responsibility for the program, there is greater integration of Medicaid-financed services with other public health services, using the same delivery system. Thus, both federal Medicaid and state public health funds are coordinated to provide services to eligible clients. When public health and Medicaid are administered separately, on the other hand, the state health department loses some of its control, particularly over programs for pregnant women and children—the largest constituency served by Medicaid.

As Medicaid eligibility has been expanded by Congress to cover more pregnant women, children, and adolescents, every state's Medicaid budget far exceeds its public health budget. State funds allocated to Medicaid bring federal dollars to each state, on a matching basis, while state funds appropriated for public health stand alone. Therefore, Medicaid and public health compete for state funds, with public health usually losing the battle.

IOM Committee Recommendations

Although the IOM Committee report recommended that each state health agency include responsibility for Medicaid, most state health officers oppose any attempt to take back this function.[6] They believe it will detract from, rather than enhance, their public health activities, by linking them too closely to **welfare** programs.

Environmental Protection

Although mental health has never been a significant part of state health departments and medical care financing has moved to separate agencies without much protest from state health officials, the removal of environmental health programs from state health departments has been viewed as a significant loss to public health. Many environmental monitoring and control activities previously handled by state health departments, in areas such as air pollution, groundwater contamination, and solid and hazardous waste disposal, have been transferred to separate environmental protection agencies.

Background

These programs grew from the health department's original work in sanitation but became increasingly complex as technology advanced and more potential pollutants were identified. Citizens demanded more protection of and from the environment, businesses became concerned about the costs of compliance with environmental health standards, and regulatory decisions became more complicated. Directors of state health departments frequently had no expertise in new environmental issues. Governors and legislators, wanting to give greater visibility to environmental issues, created new environmental agencies, following the example of the federal Environmental Protection Agency.

IOM Committee Recommendations

The IOM Committee noted that this separation of environmental health functions has led to a lack of coordination of efforts and an inadequate analysis of the health effects of environmental problems. Environmental protection agencies are more likely to focus on regulatory requirements and engineering technology than on risk to human health. Therefore, the IOM Committee recommended that state and local health agencies strengthen their capacities for identifying, understanding, and controlling environmental problems as health hazards. In some states, even after environmental programs were transferred, expertise in environmental health risk assessment was retained within the state health department as a resource for the environmental agency.

Recent Trends

The number of state health agencies that are the lead environmental agencies has shown a steady decrease, from 19 in 1978 to 8 in 1991.[7] However, most state health departments have lead responsibility for at least one environmental health function, usually food sanitation, safe drinking water, radiation control, or consumer protection.[8] Only the state health departments of Guam, Maryland, and the District of Columbia have no environmental health responsibilities.

CURRENT ORGANIZATION OF STATE HEALTH DEPARTMENTS

In the United States there are 55 state health agencies (one in each of the 50 states, the District of Columbia, American Samoa, Guam, Puerto Rico, and the United States Virgin Islands), each of which may be a freestanding, independent department or a component of a larger state agency. Because some of these agencies are not truly "departments" of state government, the Association of State and Territorial Health Officials adopted the term *state health agency* to signify that agency of state government that is vested with primary responsibility for public health within the state.[9]

Superagencies and Umbrella Agencies

Beginning in the 1960s, state health departments were merged with other departments, usually social services or welfare departments, to form **superagencies,** or they were placed under a secretariat in an **umbrella agency,** following the pattern of the federal Department of Health, Education, and Welfare (now the Department of Health and Human Services). The main difference between these two types of consolidation is that a state health agency usually retains more autonomy under the umbrella arrangement.

In 1952, only Maine and Missouri had state public health functions in a superagency. By 1969, there were 8 states with such arrangements, by 1972, 16 states, and by 1980, 22 states.[3,10,11] State health agencies in 19 states plus the District of Columbia were part of superagencies in 1990, indicating that some states had reversed this consolidation.[5] A typical organization chart of such a superagency is presented in Figure 6.1.

Rationale

The stated purpose of bringing together several separate departments under one roof was to increase coordination between programs serving the same population groups and to provide more political control over policy decisions. These superagencies most often bring together health and social services for the aged, children and adolescents, families, the developmentally disabled, those needing income assistance, and those with substance abuse problems. In the example shown in Figure 6.1, the Department for Health Services, which is the state public health agency, is part of the Cabinet for Human Resources, which also includes Departments for Employment Services, Social Services, Medicaid, Social Insurance, and Mental Health and Mental

Retardation Services. The director or secretary of such an agency is usually a political appointee, frequently with little or no health expertise.

Public Health Opposition

Public health leaders have generally opposed such mergers because the superagencies focus more on services for the poor or families with problems, rather than on protecting or improving the health of the total population.[1] Unless service delivery at the local level has also been merged or colocated, there may be little benefit to clients from such mergers of agencies at the state level.

Name of the State Health Agency

If it is an independent entity or part of an umbrella agency, or secretariat, the state health agency is titled the Department of Health, Department of Public Health, or Department of Health Services.[12] If it is combined with another agency, the public health unit is usually called a Division of Health or Public Health.

When public health functions have been combined with environmental functions, *health* is more likely to appear in the agency title, for example, Department of Health and Environment, than when public health is combined with social services agencies. The latter are frequently named the Department of Human Resources or Human Services, supporting the assertion that public health's visibility is lost when such a merger occurs. The IOM Committee recommended that each state have a department of health that groups all primarily health-related functions under professional direction and separate from income maintenance functions of state government.[1]

STATE BOARDS OF HEALTH

State governments created boards of health even before state departments of health to make rules to prevent the spread of diseases and improve general sanitary conditions in the states. As these boards hired employees to enforce the rules, departments of health were organized. In 1972, all but four states had a state board of health in some form.[11]

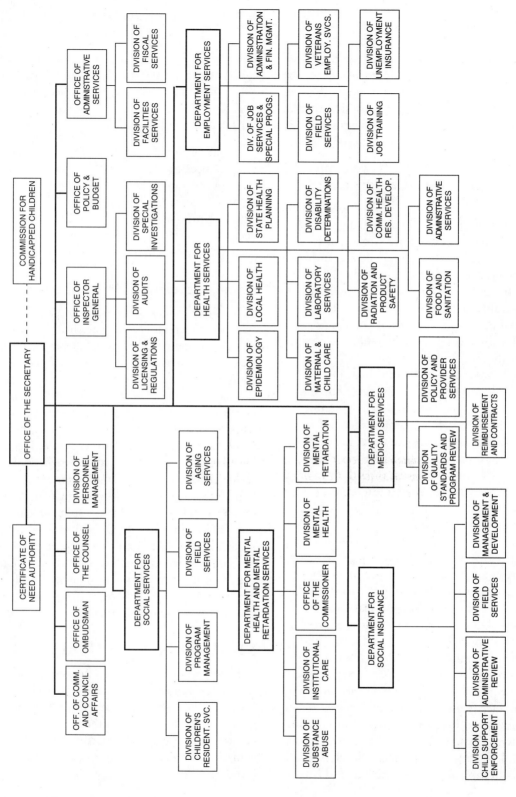

FIGURE 6.1 Cabinet for Human Resources. Source: Public Health Foundation. *State Health Agency Organization Charts*. Washington DC: Public Health Foundation; 1992.

Role of Boards of Health

Thirty-seven (80 percent) of the 46 boards in 1972 were policy making, that is, responsible for making, adopting, promulgating, and enforcing rules and regulations pursuant to state health codes.[11] The remaining nine boards were advisory only and usually located in states where public health functions had been consolidated into a superagency or an umbrella agency.

From 1971 to 1980, major structural changes took place in state health departments. In addition to those that were consolidated with other departments of state government, 13 state boards of health were disestablished in this time period.[13] By 1990, only 23 states had boards still making policy, and 17 others just had advisory boards or committees at the department level.[5] Two-thirds of states with freestanding departments of health retained a board of health, whereas only half the states in which public health was located in a superagency or an umbrella agency had a board.[14] From 1972 to 1981, the number of boards of health responsible for hiring the state health director also decreased—from fifteen to eight. By 1992, only four state health directors were appointed by a board.[13,15]

Gilbert and Miller concluded that the potential for boards of health to influence public health policy, rules and regulations, and budgeting, as they had in the past, was declining rapidly.[13] Their functions were being taken over by the executive branches of state governments, with policy decisions being made by political appointees instead of citizens' groups. As governors sought more control over health policy, they needed the ability to select health directors who would carry out political platforms.

Composition of Boards of Health

Even when state boards of health had a stronger role, they were never representative of the state's population. Governors appoint 91 percent of the 427 positions on state boards of health.[13] The remaining 9 percent of board members are appointed by professional associations or the state health director. Consumers have held only 11 to 12 percent of seats on state boards of health, because state laws generally delineate the categories from which board appointments are to be made.[11,13]

About 70 percent of board members are medical care providers and, among these, the majority are physicians.[1,13] Indeed, physicians are the majority of board members in 12 states and hold at least one-third of the seats in two-thirds of the states. Undoubtedly, this special interest focus of boards contributed to their demise, as state legislators viewed the boards as unable or unwilling to tackle the broad range of issues facing state health agencies.

Specialized Boards and Committees

Replacing or supplementing the board of health in many states are specialized boards or committees established by state statute to oversee particular programs. Many of these boards are technical, bringing to the state health agency particular expertise not found in the staff, for example, in genetics or rural health. Other special boards are established to make decisions on a particular function in the state health department, such as rules regarding physician loan repayment, certification of emergency medical technicians, licensure of hearing aid dispensers, or expansion of health facilities. Special interest groups have lobbied state legislatures to establish these boards, with defined membership representing the regulated community and the public, in preference to having policies made by a board of health or the state health director.

IOM Committee Recommendation

The IOM Committee recommended that each state have a health council that reports regularly on the health of the state's residents, makes health policy recommendations to the governor and legislature, promulgates public health regulations, reviews the work of the state health department, and recommends candidates for director of the department.[1] The committee proposed that the purpose of the council should not be the control of health matters by health professionals but the making of policy judgments on public health by lay citizens. In reality, however, most states appear headed in a different direction, with less power given to such a representative group and more control residing in the elected and appointed officials of the executive branch of state government.

STATE HEALTH DIRECTORS

The title of the chief executive of the state health agency is usually director or commissioner; in a few states the position is called state health officer or secretary. The important factor is not the title but who makes the appointment. Whether the director of the department is appointed by the governor, a board, or the head of an umbrella agency or superagency is crucial in determining the health director's level of authority, access to state policy makers, and participation in health policy decisions.

The director of the state health agency is appointed by the governor to a cabinet level position in 36 states and the territories, by the head of a superagency in 14 states, by the state board of health in 4 states, and by the mayor in the District of Columbia.[5] Where there is direct access to the governor, the health director has a greater opportunity to influence health policy in both the executive and legislative branches.

Qualifications of State Health Directors

Traditionally, a physician held the position of state health officer, with medical requirements being part of state law. At first, most of these physicians had no training in public health. As schools of public health were created, however, physicians trained specifically for positions in public health administration directed most state health departments. In 1977, all but six states had physician health directors.[15] Twenty-three of the 44 physicians were specialists in public health and preventive medicine, and 30 had a public health degree.

Changes with Reorganization

Concomitant with the consolidation of some state health departments into superagencies or umbrella agencies in the 1970s, states began removing the medical criteria for appointment. Even after the trend to merge health departments with other state agencies declined, states continued to repeal the requirements for physician directors. By 1992, only 28 states required a medical degree for their state health official, and the number of state health officials who were physicians

was down to 30.[16] Public health training or experience was required in just 15 states.

These changes in qualifications of state health directors related to the transition occurring in the responsibilities of state health agencies. As health departments became more involved in issues of environmental protection and regulation of the delivery of medical care, governors and state legislatures concluded that health directors should have more political and administrative skills. As a result, legislatures either combined the health department with other agencies, under a politically appointed secretary or executive, or changed the qualifications for the health director, to allow nonphysicians to serve in this capacity.

As salaries for government service lagged behind the earnings of physicians in other specialties, the pool of public health-trained physicians, particularly those with education or interest in administration, also declined. Today, even in those states requiring the state health director to have a medical degree, the physicians selected often have not had training or prior experience in public health or administration.

Tenure of State Health Directors

Increased turnover in state health directors and changes in their qualifications have occurred as the positions have become more political. In the first half of this century, many state health officers served from 20 to 35 years. They were respected leaders in health affairs in their communities and also were frequently leaders in state medical societies. For example, the terms of the first two state health officers in Virginia covered a total period of 48 years, from 1908 to 1956.

By contrast, the tenure of state health directors has decreased markedly in the past 20 years. In 1992, according to George Degnon, Executive Director of the Association of State and Territorial Health Officials (ASTHO), three-quarters of health directors had been in office for less than five years, a 21 percent increase over the number who were employed for less than five years in 1987.[16] In 32 months from 1991 to late 1993, 36 of the 50 state health officials changed. In fact, five states changed health directors twice during this period.

Those state health directors who are appointed by boards of health generally have longer tenure in office than those appointed by governors, because governors want to appoint department heads who will carry out their policies and initiatives.

IOM Committee Recommendations

The IOM Committee recommended that the director of each department of health be a cabinet level officer, with doctorate level education as a physician or other health professional, education in public health, and extensive public sector administrative experience.[1] Provisions for tenure in office, such as specific terms of appointment, should be enacted, the committee said, to promote needed continuity of professional leadership. In recent years, only four states have had specific terms of appointment for their state health directors, according to George Degnon of ASTHO.

INTERNAL ORGANIZATIONAL STRUCTURE

There is an old expression that form should follow function. One would thus expect state health departments to be organized around the functions they perform. Because many functions are the same in each state, similar organizational structures might be assumed. That assumption is only partially true. Each state health department's internal organizational arrangement has developed over time and represents unique attributes of that state's government, processes, and prevailing culture. In states where the health department is responsible for local services, the structure is more complicated because there are both centralized and decentralized components.

Two Examples: Tennessee and Washington State

Organizational charts for two state health departments are presented in Figures 6.2 and 6.3. The Tennessee Department of Health and Environment, outlined in Figure 6.2, includes both Medicaid and environmental protection functions, has a public health

council rather than a board, and is directed by a commissioner who reports to the governor. The Washington State Department of Health, shown in Figure 6.3, was separated from a merged health and welfare agency in the late 1980s. It includes fewer environmental services, no Medicaid functions, and a board of health. The director is called a secretary and reports to the governor.

In both departments there is also a unit that supports or provides liaison to local health departments. If a state health department is responsible for providing local health services, local or regional offices will appear as an additional major component of the organization.

The Need for Flexibility

As little as possible of the organization's structure should be codified in statutes so that the department may respond to new needs, such as HIV control or injury prevention. Ideally, the state health director can restructure the organization and adjust resources to address emerging problems.

STAFFING

The Public Health Foundation periodically reviews staffing levels in state health departments. In 1990, the 55 state and territorial health departments included approximately 130,000 full-time equivalent positions.[17]

Staff-Population Ratios

Because the ratio of health department staff to population served varies depending on the functions assigned to each state health department, the Foundation groups states by the number of additional programs they provide that are not provided by all states. Ten states provide direct primary care services; 10 provide local public health services to at least 50 percent of the population; 12 administer part of the alcohol, drug abuse, and mental health federal grant; 10 serve as lead environmental agency; and 12 operate institutions, such as hospitals or nursing homes. Of the 48 reporting state health agencies, 37 had one or more of these additional responsibilities, whereas 11 served none of these functions.[17]

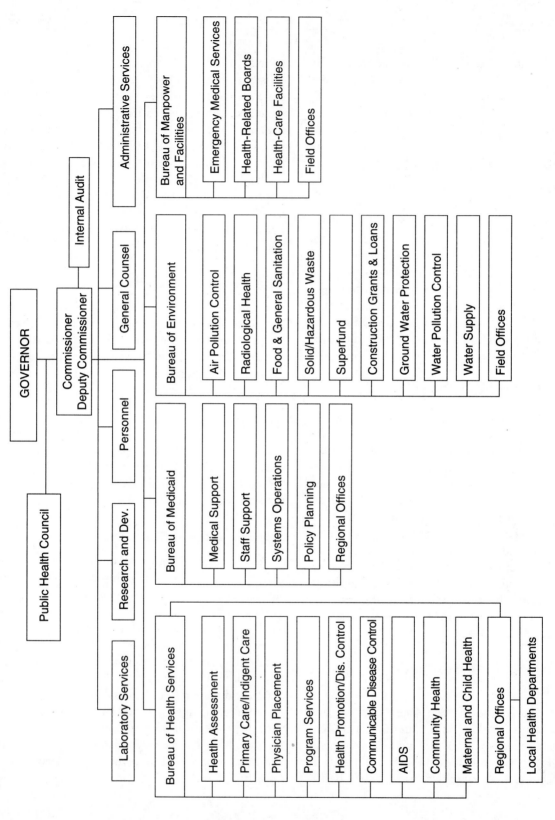

FIGURE 6.2 Tennessee Department of Health and Environment, 1990. Source: Centers for Disease Control and Prevention, Public Health Practice Program Office, Division of Public Health Systems. *Profile of State and Territorial Public Health Systems: United States, 1990.* Atlanta, GA: Centers for Disease Control; 1991.

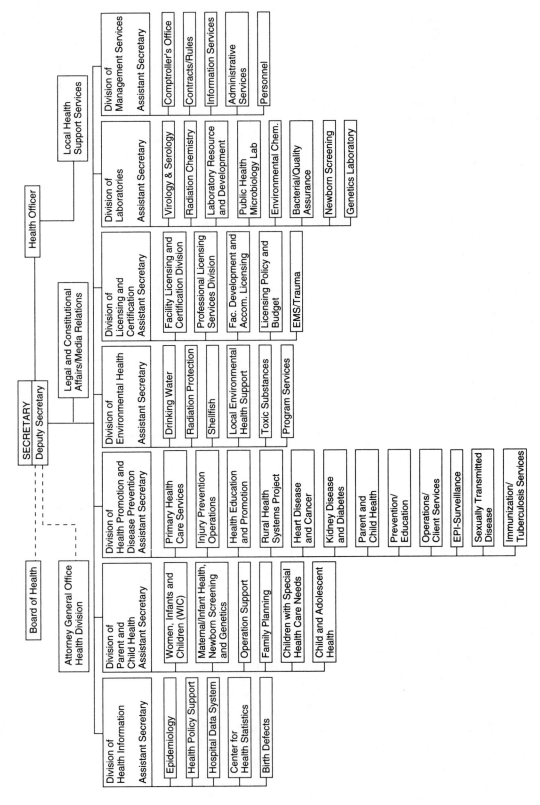

FIGURE 6.3 Washington State Department of Health, 1990. Source: Centers for Disease Control and Prevention, Public Health Practice Program Office, Division of Public Health Systems. *Profile of State and Territorial Public Health Systems: United States, 1990.* Atlanta, GA: Centers for Disease Control; 1991.

Influence of Additional Functions

The median number of staff per population increased with each additional responsibility, from 1.8 to 26.4 employees per 10,000 population. The provision of primary care services and the operation of health care institutions are most strongly related to increased staff size. In general, the lowest ratios of staff to population are in the Great Lakes and Pacific Coast states, and the highest ratios are in the Southeast, where state health departments are more likely to operate institutions and provide local health services.

Problems in Setting Ideal Ratios

Because of the differences in responsibilities assigned to state health departments, it is difficult to determine an ideal ratio of staff to population. In addition, the numbers and kinds of staff needed at the state level will depend on such variables as distances between population centers; types of medical care facilities to be regulated; density and economic status of populations; degree of responsibility for direct delivery of services; and the number, size, autonomy, and sophistication of local health departments. Because most public health agencies are now focusing on how to achieve the National Health Objectives for the Year 2000,[18] models for relating staff to particular activities and outcomes need to be developed. State legislatures are more likely to appropriate additional funds to reach these objectives if staffing models delineate, for example, the ratio of staff needed to provide directly observed therapy to patients with tuberculosis or to immunize all children by age two.

Occupational Groups

Two-thirds of state health agency staff are in the professional, technical, and administrative areas; the remaining one-third are in clerical and other support areas.[17] Registered nurses are the largest single professional group, accounting for 22 percent of the professional, technical, and administrative staff. Environmental and occupational health and safety personnel are the second largest category.

Changes in Numbers of Staff by Occupation

Trends in state health department staffing for the period 1979 to 1989 show a 32 percent decrease in staff devoted to operating institutions and a 23 percent increase in noninstitutional staff. The number of state health agencies operating institutions decreased from 22 to 16 in the same period, due to the closure of many tuberculosis sanatoria and state mental hospitals.[17] The increases in noninstitutional staff reflect the expanded role of state health agencies in chronic disease prevention and control, new activities required by the appearance of the HIV/AIDS epidemic, increases in numbers of pregnant women and children receiving services from the WIC program, a shift from federal to state operation of health programs, and increased involvement with the certification of long-term care facilities.

Changes in Types of Occupations

There have also been changes in specific occupational categories. The number of dentists in state health agencies decreased by 40 percent over the same 10 years, for example, while nutritionists and dieticians almost doubled in number. The decline in dentists reflects a shift in priorities and a reduction in financial support for dental health programs in state health departments. Expansion of the WIC program and increased emphasis on lifestyle changes, particularly those related to diet, have increased the need for nutrition staff.

FUNDING

As with staffing patterns, the expenditures of state health departments are difficult to compare across states because the responsibilities of these departments vary so widely. According to the Public Health Foundation, excluding Medicaid expenditures, in 1991 (the last year for which data are available) state health departments spent $11.2 billion on public health programs. Three-quarters of these expenditures were for personal health services, including $1.5 billion for the operation of institutions. Most of these personal health funds are used at the local level, either through local health departments, subunits of the state health department, or contracts with other service providers.

Sources of Funds

According to the Public Health Foundation, state health agencies receive 50 percent of their funding from state legislatures, 37 percent from federal grants and contracts, 7 percent from fees and third-party reimbursements (excluding Medicaid), 3 percent from local sources, and 3 percent from other sources, such as grants from private foundations. The single largest source of federal funds is the United States Department of Agriculture, which oversees the Supplemental Food Program for Women, Infants, and Children (WIC program). This program accounts for 20 percent of all funds spent by state health departments. The Centers for Disease Control and Prevention (CDC) and the Health Resources and Services Administration (HRSA) are the other major sources of federal funds used by state health departments.

Categorical and Block Grants

Federal funds come to states both as categorical grants, which focus on a particular health problem or population group, and as block grants, which have a broader public health focus. In general, categorical grant programs are controlled by extensive federal regulations and lengthy reporting requirements. They may lack flexibility to meet differing state needs.

New Block Grants

Block grants were created in the early 1980s "to achieve greater flexibility in the use of funds, meaning more efficient use of tax dollars and more cost-effective service to recipients."[19] Of nine new block grants created by the federal government in 1981, four were in the health field in the areas of primary care; prevention; maternal and child health services (MCH); and alcohol, drug abuse, and mental health. Twenty-one previously separate programs were consolidated into these four blocks. Left as categorical programs were childhood immunization, tuberculosis control, family planning, migrant health centers, and venereal disease (now called sexually transmitted disease) control. The MCH and prevention block grants are major sources of financial support for all state health departments. The primary care and alcohol, substance abuse, and mental health block grants are used by other state agencies.

Block Grants in Practice

Initially, the block grants specified no priorities, objectives, or required outcomes. Decisions on how to use the funds were left entirely to state legislatures and governors, who frequently used the grants to fund programs the state was unwilling or unable to support with state revenues.

States favored block grants because they provided more opportunities to meet state priorities or fill gaps in state funding. However, the funds allocated to block grants the year they were created, fiscal year 1981-82, represented a 20 percent reduction in the amounts available for the same programs in the previous year.[20] Thus, states gained authority but lost dollars.

Expenditures

Total state health agency spending is presented, by type of program, in Figure 6.4.

Maternal and Child Health Expenditures

Maternal and child health services are the single largest category of program expenses in state health departments (excluding Medicaid expenditures), accounting for 63 percent of all funds spent for noninstitutional personal health services.[21] Over half (56 percent) of these expenditures are in the WIC program, which provides food vouchers for pregnant women and children. States are dependent on the MCH block grant to cover about one-fourth of the remaining (non-WIC) expenditures for programs to improve the health of mothers and children, including the care of children with disabling conditions. Beginning in the late 1980s, the expansion of Medicaid to cover more pregnant women and children provided an additional source of funding for services to these population groups.

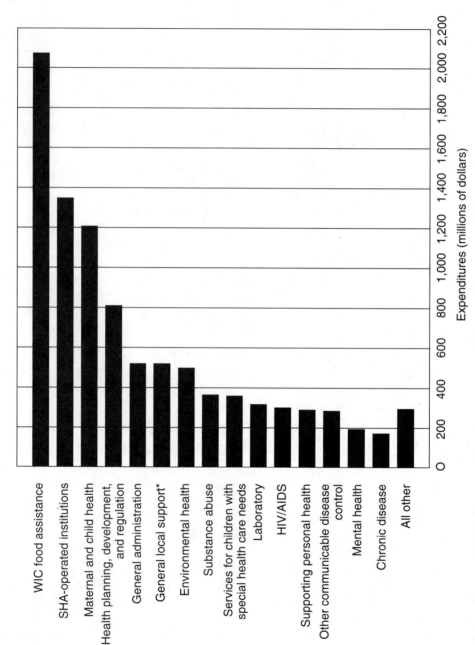

Expenditures (millions of dollars)

* State health agencies provided $1.8 billion to local health departments
in FY 1989. $1.2 billion of which was allocated to the other types of programs displayed here.

FIGURE 6.4 State Health Agency Spending, by Type of Program, Fiscal Year 1989. Source: Public Health Foundation. *1991 Public Health Chartbook.* Washington DC: Public Health Foundation; 1991.

Disease and Disability Prevention Expenditures

The prevention block grant is used by state health departments to support chronic disease prevention, health education and risk reduction, emergency medical services, laboratory testing for communicable diseases and environmental programs, rodent control, dental health, and a variety of other services. Since its inception, this grant has provided the most flexibility of all funding sources used by state health departments. However, the multiplicity of uses of these grant dollars state by state made it hard for Congress to identify exactly which services were being funded with the prevention block, and it failed to increase funding for it at the same rate it did for categorical grants. As a result, the prevention block grant accounts for only one percent of all funds spent by state health agencies.[21]

Recently Congress modified the prevention grant, linking it to the National Health Objectives for the Year 2000. Beginning in 1993, all expenditures from the grant had to be directed toward specific national objectives, as selected by each state. A state level advisory group was required to hold public hearings on proposed uses of the grant.[22] In turn, the federal government required more accountability from states in the use of the funds and removed the decisions from the legislative process.

The preceding chapter describes the changing climate in the federal government regarding block grants. It is likely that there will be substantial efforts to decrease federal funds, put them in block grants, and hold states accountable for how the funds are spent. The pendulum is clearly swinging toward decreased categorical spending, more block grants (though with lower funding), and greater accountability.

State and federal funding for communicable disease control programs increased markedly during the 1980s and 1990s, primarily to prevent and treat HIV/AIDS. Expenditures also increased for the control of tuberculosis, sexually transmitted diseases, and vaccine-preventable diseases. During this period, expenditures on chronic disease programs remained stable. This disparity reflects the willingness of appropriating bodies to allocate money to prevent diseases that spread person-to-person but their relative lack of interest in reducing diseases influenced by lifestyle and behavior, even though the latter are responsible for more morbidity and mortality in the population.

STATE-LOCAL RELATIONSHIPS

A former state health officer once said, "The federal government has most of the money, the state government has most of the legal authority, and the local government has most of the responsibility for protecting the health of the people."[23] To protect the health of citizens, state health departments must have a mechanism for delivering services to people where they live and work. The relationship between state and local health departments reflects the geography, politics, and funding patterns of each state.[24]

Organizational Relationships

One type of state-local organizational relationship is centralized, with either no local health departments or local agencies that are operated by the state health department.[5,25] Eleven states have this type of centralized control, a decrease from eighteen states with such an arrangement in 1974.[24] Of the eleven centralized state health systems, six are in the Southeast and four are in very small states (Delaware, Hawaii, Rhode Island, and Vermont). In another seven states, all in the eastern half of the country, organizational control over local health departments is shared between state and local governments.

Sixteen states have a decentralized organization, in which local government (city, township, county, or some combination) directly operates health departments. This decentralized pattern is more common in the West, where distances between towns are great and local control is popular. An additional sixteen states have some mix of centralized and decentralized control, with local health services provided by the state health department in some jurisdictions, usually rural areas, and by local governments in other jurisdictions, primarily cities and counties with large populations.

Where organizational control is centralized, the state government supplies most of the funds for local health work, so state priorities determine which services are provided at the local level.[5,25] In decentralized situations, local health departments derive a greater percentage of their budgets from local government and tend to be more responsive to local needs.

State Responsibilities for Local Services

Whatever the state-local organizational relationship, state health departments are responsible for establishing standards for local public health functions and holding local agencies accountable to those standards.[1] States may develop requirements for specific services to be offered locally, data to be collected and reported, and minimum staffing requirements to be met. Services inappropriate for smaller units, such as the provision of reference laboratories, or for which there must be statewide consistency, such as the inspection of health care facilities, are usually organized at the state level. The state health department has the additional responsibility of representing the needs of local health units with other state agencies, within both executive and legislative branches of government.

State Funding of Local Health Services

Historically, the state health department has been the recipient of federal public health funds, which it has distributed and monitored at the local level. Beginning in the 1950s, state health departments were bypassed with increasing frequency as the federal government gave grants for local health activities directly to local health departments or to community agencies, particularly in large cities.[3] This new approach was justified by the rationale that state health departments did not have the technical expertise or managerial efficiency to monitor the funds or that state legislatures were dominated by rural interests that had no interest in the new programs.

Whereas the federal government uses block grants to provide flexibility in funding to states, the money distributed by state health departments to local units is usually confined to strict categories, with detailed requirements for data collection and reporting. Claiming

that federal regulations require separate records on all expenditures of federal funds, some states have not attempted to use the block grant concept at the local level. Work is progressing nationally on the development of a uniform data set so that all local and state health departments can provide data in a similar format for national, state, and local decision making. State health departments could monitor funds with such a data set while still providing flexibility in how localities use funds.

CONCLUSION

Although state health departments retain ultimate responsibility for protecting the health of their citizens, their roles, significance, and visibility have frequently been overlooked. More attention is focused on national and local health agencies. The federal government supplies the majority of government funds for health services through the Medicaid and Medicare programs and through categorical and block grants. Local health departments are where citizens actually seek public health services. The state health department is viewed as just a pass-through agency, passing funds and regulations from the federal and state to the local level, but not contributing significantly to the planning, development, and implementation of health services.

To obtain the legal authority and fiscal resources necessary to carry out its mission, a state health department must work with the governor and the state legislature. As noted earlier, the nature of this relationship will depend on where health functions are located in the executive branch and how accessible policy makers are to the state health director. The IOM Committee found that many state health departments did not have the influence necessary to acquire needed resources.[1] Without strong state boards of health or other public health advocacy groups, such as state public health associations, state health departments frequently have been left powerless and impoverished in the competition over state assets.

In the early years of this century, the medical profession was strongly supportive of the creation of state health departments, and members of the medical community often sat on boards of health and served as state health officers. As state health departments have become increasingly involved in the direct delivery of care to persons who cannot afford care in the private sector, however, the relationship between the state health department and the state medical society has frequently deteriorated. Whereas earlier physician health officers were invited to participate in medical society meetings, today's nonphysician health officers are viewed with suspicion by the medical community, and they often do not have the same access to medical colleagues that their predecessors did. Nonphysician administrators are also frequently criticized for not seeking medical advice or not informing the medical society of their plans.[1]

State health departments need the support of the medical profession to help pass key legislation through state legislatures and to provide medical expertise on many public health issues. Strengthening their relationship with state medical organizations is therefore an important challenge for today's state health departments.

The roles and functions of state health departments will continue to evolve as they have in the past. The public increasingly needs protection from new causes of morbidity and mortality, such as violence, drugs, and toxic substances in the environment, while old challenges, including excess infant mortality, remain. The public also expects more regulation of facilities and services that may cause harm. State health departments of tomorrow will be required to meet these expectations with new approaches and new policies.

REFERENCES

1. Institute of Medicine, Committee for the Study of the Future of Public Health. *The Future of Public Health*. Washington, DC: National Academy Press; 1988.

2. McGinnis JM. Setting nationwide objectives in disease prevention and health promotion: the United States experience. In: Holland WH, Detels R, Knox G, eds. *Oxford Textbook of Public Health*. New York, NY: Oxford University Press; 1985.

3. Williams SJ, Torrens PR. *Introduction to Health Services*. 2nd ed. New York, NY: John Wiley & Sons Inc; 1984.

4. Lewis-Idema D, Falik M. Health departments and Medicaid agencies: is the cold war really over? In: *Collaborative Strategies to Improve State and Local Public Health Systems or Is the Cold War Really Over?* Portland, Me: National Academy of State Health Policy; 1990.

5. *Profile of State and Territorial Public Health Systems: United States, 1990*. Atlanta, Ga: Public Health Practice Program Office, Division of Public Health Systems, Centers for Disease Control; 1991.

6. *Responses to the IOM Report: The Future of Public Health*. Washington, DC: Association of State and Territorial Health Officials; 1990.

7. *Services, Expenditures, and Programs of State and Territorial Health Agencies, FY 1978*. Silver Spring, Md: National Public Health Reporting System of the Association of State and Territorial Health Officials; 1980.

8. *Public Health Agencies 1991: An Inventory of Programs and Block Grant Expenditures*. Washington, DC: Public Health Foundation; 1991.

9. Association of State and Territorial Health Officials. By-laws. Washington, DC.

10. *Public Health Agencies 1980. A Report on Their Expenditures and Activities*. Washington DC: Public Health Foundation; 1981.

11. Gossert DJ, Miller CA. State boards of health, their members and commitments. *Am J Public Health*. 1973;63(6): 486–493.

12. *1991 Directory, State Public Health Agencies*. Washington DC: Association of State and Territorial Health Officials; 1991.

13. Gilbert B M MK, Miller CA. State level decision making for public health: the status of boards of health. *J Public Health Policy*. 1982;3(1):51–61.

14. *National Survey of State Boards of Health*. Des Moines, Ia: Iowa Department of Public Health and Health Policy Corporation of Iowa; 1988.

15. Terris M. Letter to all state health officials on results of questionnaire on training and experience. New York Medical College; December 2, 1977.

16. Degnon GK, Morelli V. *1992 Salary Survey*. Washington DC: Association of State and Territorial Health Officials; 1992.

17. *State Health Agency Staffs, 1989*. Washington DC: Public Health Foundation; 1992.

18. *Healthy People 2000. National Health Promotion and Disease Prevention Objectives*. Washington, DC: US Dept of Health

and Human Services; 1990. DHHS Publication No. (PHS) 91–50212.

19. *Health and Human Services Department Block Grants.* Washington, DC: US Dept of Health and Human Services; 1981. HHS Fact Sheet.

20. Dandoy S. Health. In: *Impact of New Federalism on Arizona.* Phoenix, Az: Arizona Academy; 1982.

21. *1991 Public Health Chartbook.* Washington, DC: Public Health Foundation; 1991.

22. Public Law 102–531; 1992.

23. Nitzkin J. Quoted by: Cundiff D. The future of state-local relationships in public health. *Bull Am Assoc Public Health Phys.* 1993;39(2):1–2.

24. Mullan F, Smith J. *Characteristics of State and Local Health Agencies.* Baltimore, Md: The Johns Hopkins University School of Hygiene and Public Health, Health Program Alliance; 1988.

25. DeFriese GH, Hetherington JS, Brooks EF, et al. The program implications of administrative relationships between local health departments and state and local government. *Am J Public Health.* 1981;71(10):1109–1115.

CHAPTER
7

The Local Health Department

Nancy Rawding, M.P.H.
Martin Wasserman, M.D., J.D.

Local health departments have been in operation since the first health departments were formed in Boston, Baltimore, New York City, and Philadelphia during the early 1800s. Today, local health departments carry out public health functions and provide personal health services at the local level, with the goals of safeguarding the public's health and improving community health status.

MISSION OF LOCAL HEALTH DEPARTMENTS

Specifically, the mission of local health departments is to protect, promote, and maintain the health of the entire population of their jurisdiction. They fulfill several functions in pursuit of that mission, including assuring the implementation of statutes and regulations enacted and developed by federal, state, and local governments to protect the public's health. Traditionally, this has involved collecting and analyzing vital statistics, controlling communicable diseases, diminishing environmental risks to health, and providing maternal and child health services, adult personal health services, health education, and other services required by their particular community.

Importance of Local Health Departments

The importance of local health departments is reflected by this recent statement of the National Association of County Health Officials: "Just as all politics is local, all health is local."[1] A 1988 Institute of Medicine report also stresses the importance of local public health services when it states:

> . . . no citizen from any community, no matter how small or remote, should be without identifiable and realistic access to the benefits of public health protection, which is possible only through a local component of the public health delivery system[2]

Current Status of Local Health Departments

Today, in the midnineties, there are 2,888 local health departments nationwide, with almost every area of the country served. Every state either has local health departments, which are entities of city, county, town, and/or district government, or it has divisions of the state health department that operate at the local level. Local health departments employ approximately 192,000 people, of whom about 145,000 are full-time employees,[3] providing direct personal health services to 40 million people annually and carrying out core public health functions in their jurisdictions. The total cost of these activities nationwide is about $8 billion annually.

The midnineties is also a unique time to examine the roles and characteristics of public health service delivery and local health departments because profound changes are occurring in the delivery of both illness care services and public health services. For example, public health departments are affected by the national shift to managed care, the possible development of new block grants, and generally reduced funding from the federal government. As a result, it is widely expected that the role of local health departments will change significantly as the country enters the twenty-first century.

In order to anticipate the changes—and to appreciate their impact on the whole health care system and the nation's health status—it is important to examine the history of local health departments as well as their current roles and capacities. This chapter provides a historical overview and a current survey of local health departments. It then discusses ways in which changes might occur and the potential impact of those changes.

HISTORICAL PERSPECTIVE

The necessity for a governmental agency at the local level to protect, promote, and maintain a community's health has not only been reiterated over the past decade, but it has been confirmed time and again over the past century. For example, a major recommendation of President Hoover's 1931 White House Conference on Child Health and Protection was that:

To make everywhere available these minimum protections of the health and welfare of children, there should be a dis-

trict, county or community organization for health, education and welfare, with full-time officials, coordinating with a statewide program which will be responsive to a nationwide service of general information, statistics and scientific research. This should include: (a) Trained, full-time public health officials, with public health nurses, sanitary inspection, and laboratory workers . . .[4]

Then, in 1945, Haven Emerson, M.D., described the six basic functions of a local health department as follows:[5]

1. vital statistics, or the recording, tabulation, interpretation, and publication of the essential facts of births, deaths, and reportable diseases
2. control of communicable diseases, including tuberculosis, venereal diseases, malaria, and hookworm disease
3. environmental sanitation, including supervision of milk and milk products, food processing, and public eating places, and maintenance of sanitary conditions of employment
4. public health laboratory services
5. hygiene of maternity, infancy, and childhood, including supervision of the health of the school child
6. health education of the general public so far as this is not covered by the functions of departments of education

The primary responsibilities of early health departments were communicable disease control and sanitation. They developed and expanded their scope of service over time in response to the particular needs and characteristics of the community in which they were established. Most of the services developed were of a primary or secondary prevention nature, but many departments also moved to fill gaps left by providers of clinical services. Consequently, there is now a core of programs and services that are common to most local health departments, but there is also wide variation in the type and extent of additional activities that local health departments carry out.

Specifically, the widely disparate needs of urban and rural settings and significant differences in the structure of state and local government services has resulted in wide variation in type and number of services, organizational structure, per capita expenditures, and staffing patterns of local health departments.

CURRENT VIEWS

Today's changing environment of health services has stimulated substantial discussion and redefinition of the roles and responsibilities of local health departments. Nonetheless, committees and work groups of the Institute of Medicine, the Centers for Disease Control and Prevention, the Office of Disease Prevention and Health Promotion, and several national health associations have reaffirmed the importance to community health of the basic mission and services provided by local health departments.

As an example, the National Association of County and City Health Officials has affirmed that local health departments should either provide the following services or assure that they are provided, with high quality, by others in the community:[1]

- conduct community diagnoses
- prevent and control epidemics
- provide a safe and healthy environment
- measure performance, effectiveness, and outcomes of health services
- promote healthy lifestyles and provide health education
- assure access to laboratory testing
- provide targeted outreach and form partnerships
- provide personal health care services
- undertake research and innovation
- mobilize the community for action

The services in this list are very similar to those articulated by Dr. Emerson, providing further evidence that the basic mission and functions of local health departments have remained constant over time.

CHARACTERISTICS OF LOCAL HEALTH DEPARTMENTS

Local health departments vary widely with regard to several important characteristics. These include organizational issues such as jurisdictional type, their size and staffing patterns, the services they provide, and the functions they fulfill.

Organizational Issues

Organizational issues of local health departments refer to jurisdictional type, authority to operate, relationship to the state health department, and governance structure. There are significant variations among departments in all of these factors.

Jurisdictional Type

Local health departments are governmental entities of towns, cities, counties, and/or districts (see Figure 7.1). A sizeable number, 11 percent, are agencies of a town or township jurisdiction. Only 7 percent are single city health departments. Most, 80 percent, of local health departments serve a county or county-related jurisdiction. Over half, 56 percent, are run by a single

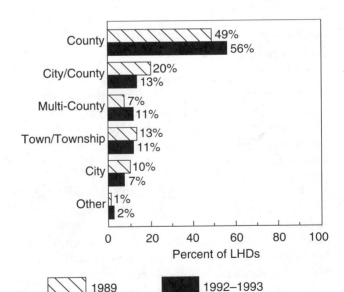

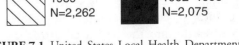

FIGURE 7.1 United States Local Health Departments by Type of Jurisdiction, 1989 vs 1992–1993. SOURCE: *National Association of County and City Health Officials,* 1995.

county government, and another 13 percent are city-county entities,[3] in which case, the local health department may report either to a joint council or commission made up of county and city elected officials or to both county and city boards of health.

Eleven percent of local health departments serve districts, which are jurisdictions made up of several independent counties that have joined together.[3] In Idaho, for example, 44 counties were organized into seven district health departments, each comprised of 4 to 8 counties. This created a larger population and tax base for the new health departments, which allowed them to expand staff numbers and skills and provide a broader and more consistent range of services throughout the state (C. Juntunen, personal correspondence, 1994).

A disadvantage of districts is their longer and more complex system for planning and obtaining approval for program and policy proposals. This is necessary because more governments must be involved in the decision making.

Authority to Operate and State-Local Relationships

Typically, local health departments derive their authority from their state health department and from the county or city government of which they are part. Organizational relationships between local health departments and their state health department vary widely from state to state.

Independent Departments. In California, Michigan, and New York, for example, local health departments operate very independently from the state health department. In these states, the local government develops and/or approves the budget, sets priorities, and hires or appoints the health officer.

An important advantage of this system is that the priorities of local government and the community can be integrated easily into the health department's services. Disadvantages can include a lack of communication among departments, noninvolvement of local health departments in state planning and decision making, and uneven service delivery across the state.

Interdependent Departments. In other states, local health departments are entities of the state, or else they work in a very interdependent fashion with their state health department. In Florida, for example, local health departments are entities of state government and also have a direct reporting relationship to county government. The state health department approves the county health department budget, sets priorities, and determines the programmatic emphasis. The county contributes tax dollars to the state health department budget and, after developing the county budget, contracts with the state for service. The county makes only limited policy and programmatic decisions. The selection of a county health official is begun by the state health department, with review and appointment made by the county board of commissioners. County health department staff are also state employees.

Advantages of this system are that services can be provided uniformly within the state, and priorities can be addressed statewide. Disadvantages include the need for county health departments to "serve two masters" and the limited ability of a county health department to focus on locally determined priorities, programs, and policies.

Importance of Communication. Regardless of the administrative relationship between state and local health departments, efforts must be made by both parties to assure open channels of communication and maximum effectiveness of the system. Problems in these areas are reported by both parties, and a number of efforts have begun in the past five years in some states to further the collaboration between them.

The Washington State Public Health Improvement Committee[6] and the Illinois "I Plan" Project[7] are two examples of concerted effort on the part of state and local health officials to review their mutual goals and systems. In Maryland, an executive advisory committee of local health officials is now being developed to advise the state health official on policy and programmatic issues. All these efforts are being undertaken to improve the level of communication, decision making concerning resource allocation and policies, and the provision of technical assistance from state to local health departments.

The Special Case of City Health Departments. The responsibilities of city health departments operating in charter cities differ somewhat from the authorities and responsibilities of other local health departments because cities generally have broader discretionary powers than other entities of local government. A city charter " . . . empowers them to do almost anything the state does not prohibit them from doing, whereas counties generally can only do the things for which they are specifically empowered."[8]

City health departments differ from county health departments in other ways as well. Many county functions are required by the state, and counties must act as agents of the state in carrying them out. By contrast, cities can choose whether to even have a health department, and theoretically at least, can more readily modify their health department services. For revenue, cities can rely on more types of taxes, including property, sales, and in some cases, income taxes, whereas counties can generally rely only on property taxes. Cities usually act through legislators; counties often function as delegates and subdivisions of the state. As described in the next section, the source of these differences may lie with how and when city and county health departments were formed.

Governance Structures: Local Boards of Health

Boards of health are policy-making or advisory bodies. They were first established in the eighteenth century, when local citizens were appointed by city governments to deal with important diseases and conditions of the time. Today, boards of health govern three out of four health departments in the country.[3] In some states, such as Florida and California, a government council fulfills the functions of a board of health. The composition of boards of health varies according to state law. They usually consist of three to fifteen members. Some states mandate that the members be health professionals.

Roles of Boards of Health. Key roles of boards of health include providing a link between local public health agencies and the community as a whole. In this capacity, the board of health represents the community's interest in developing local health department services and communicates with the community about the activities and goals of the health department. Boards of health can have a great impact on the services and funding of the health department. Members of local boards of health can also serve as a link between the state legislature and the health department. Board members may be able to lobby legislators in a more direct fashion than may be possible for local health officials.[9]

Statutory Authority. As shown in Figure 7.2, almost all boards of health, 88 percent nationwide, have statutory authority to establish local health policies, fees, ordinances, and regulations. About 60 to 65 percent also approve the budget and/or hire the agency head, and 60 to 65 percent establish community health priorities.[3]

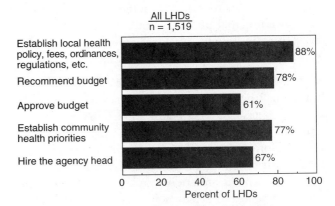

	0 to 24,999 n=650	25,000 to 49,999 n=360	50,000 to 99,999 n=263	100,000 to 499,999 n=203	500,000 + n=43
Establish local health policy, fees, ordinances, regulations, etc.	89%	90%	89%	77%	74%
Recommend budget	82%	82%	75%	69%	58%
Approve budget	63%	66%	64%	48%	35%
Establish community health priorities	77%	79%	81%	72%	58%
Hire the agency head	63%	74%	73%	66%	56%

FIGURE 7.2 Statutory Authority of United States Boards of Health in Jurisdictions with a Board of Health, 1992–1993. SOURCE: *National Association of County and City Health Officials,* 1995.

The Role of Jurisdiction Size. Nationwide, boards of health in smaller jurisdictions (those with populations of fewer than 100,000) tend to have greater statutory authority than those in jurisdictions with larger populations. The size of the population served may also be correlated with the presence or absence of a board of health. Of health departments serving the smallest population, 76 percent are governed by boards of health. Of those serving populations between 25,000 and 50,000, 80 percent are governed by boards of health. Of health departments serving populations over 500,000, only 59 percent are governed by them.[3]

The reason for the higher prevalence and greater role of boards of health in smaller jurisdictions may be historical. In the early twentieth century, few areas of the country with small populations had local health departments, which had developed primarily in the cities. As state health departments developed, legislation often followed to assure that all areas of the state were covered by a governmental public health presence at the local level. In many low-population areas, boards of health were created and given that responsibility.

Future Prospects. In the future, the roles of boards of health may broaden to include enhanced assessment and assurance activities. There is likely to be a change in the number of boards of health as well. Some states, such as Florida, are considering whether a system of local or district boards of health should be created. In other states, plans are under way to consolidate some smaller local health departments, which would lead to a reduction in the number of local boards of health.

Sources of Funding

Health departments may receive funding from several sources: local tax levies; state grants; federal grants, either directly or through the state; reimbursement for personal health care; and fees for licensures, inspections, and certifications. As Figure 7.3 shows, the largest source of funding is from state budgets, including federal pass-through dollars (40 percent of local health department budgets nationwide), followed by local funding (34 percent nationwide). Together, Medicaid and Medicare reimbursement make up 10 percent of funds. Direct federal funding and fees generally contribute a smaller percentage to health department budgets (6 percent and 7 percent, respectively).[3]

The Medicaid Question. Most local health departments (76 percent) bill Medicaid for reimbursement of personal health services delivered to Medicaid clients.[10] An important question is the degree to which local health department service delivery systems should be built around Medicaid's low reimbursement rate. To address this, a very few local health departments have applied to become Federally Qualified Health Centers (FQHC) in order to receive the higher cost-based reimbursement rate available to those entities.

This strategy is a difficult one for many local health departments because FQHC's must provide 24-hour coverage, have a consumer board, and provide comprehensive primary care services. Furthermore, this strategy has proven to be problematic in states that have sought and received section 1115 waivers under the Medicaid program. Among other changes, the waivers relieve the states of the obligation to reimburse FQHC providers on a cost basis.

Some local health officials have questioned the likelihood that the Medicaid program will be viable in local health departments over time, and they have avoided building up the Medicaid system or becoming dependent on it for this reason. The past few years have witnessed a great increase in the number of private Medicaid managed-care providers, and many believe that the provision of primary care services will move out of the public sector as managed-care penetration of the market expands.

Fees. Another important source of revenue, particularly for environmental health programs, is the collection of fees for licenses, certifications, and inspections. Although in many communities it is not acceptable to charge fees for personal health services (because many of the patients are low income), it is usually considered acceptable to charge for environmental services. Fees are charged for the licensing of such facilities as restaurants, barber shops, health-related facilities, recreational facilities, sewage treatment operations, and tanning salons, among others.

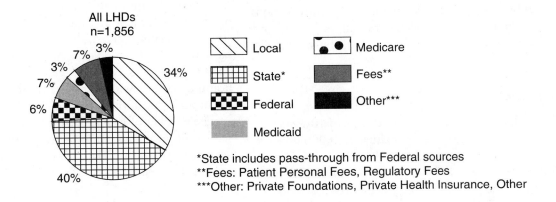

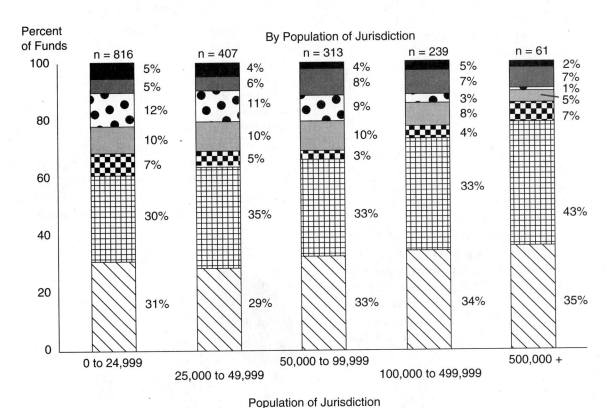

FIGURE 7.3 United States Local Health Department Funds by Source, 1992–1993. SOURCE: *National Association of County and City Health Officials,* 1995.

Size of Local Health Departments

The size of local health departments can be characterized by the size of the population of the jurisdiction served, the size of the department's staff, or its total annual expenditures. Variation in each of these factors is considered next.

Population of Jurisdiction Served

Populations served by local health departments can range from very large—approximately 9,000,000 for Los Angeles County and 8,000,000 for New York City—to very small—just 105 people for the Mount Washington Health Department in Massachusetts in 1989.[10]

Most local health departments serve jurisdictions of relatively small size. For two-thirds (66 percent) of the health departments, the population served is less than 50,000; for 44 percent, less than 25,000.[3] Health departments that serve small populations are likely to have a small tax base, few staff, and a relatively limited configuration of services. For example, for local health departments serving fewer than 25,000 people, the average annual budget is only $295,740, and the average number of staff is just 12. For local health departments that serve populations between 25,000 and 50,000, the average annual budget is $778,688, and the average number of staff is 16.[3]

At the other end of the spectrum, 4 percent of local health departments serve populations of 500,000 or more; 14 percent serve populations between 100,000 and 499,999; and 16 percent serve populations between 50,000 and 99,999. These health departments tend to provide a greater number of services, have an average annual expenditure of $8,338,561, and, on average, employ 152 staff, of whom 117 are full-time and 35 are part-time.[3]

Staffing Size

Almost half, or 42 percent, of local health departments employ fewer than 10 staff, and 20 percent employ fewer than 5 staff. One-quarter of local health departments employ between 10 and 24 staff, and 24 percent employ 25 to 99 staff. Of all local health departments, only 9 percent have 100 or more staff. The very largest health department employs over 5,000 staff.[3]

Overall, the mean and median of total staff size are 63 and 17, respectively. To illustrate how this varies by size of population served, the mean and median of total staff size for health departments serving fewer than 25,000 people are 12 and 8, respectively, whereas for health departments serving populations over 500,000, the mean is 770 and the median 523.[3]

The number of health departments with very small staffs is of great concern to many health professionals. Staffing size is directly related to a department's ability to provide the essential services listed earlier in this chapter.

Total Annual Expenditures

Total annual expenditures of health departments have increased over the past four years for departments in all size categories.[3,10] Nonetheless, many local health departments still operate on very small budgets. Figure 7.4 shows that in 1992 to 1993, 13 percent of local health departments reported expenditures of under $100,000. This was down from 18 percent in 1989. Half of all health departments spend more than $500,000 annually; 34 percent spend more than $1 million; and 10 percent spend more than $100 million. The largest reported annual expenditure for a single local health department in 1992 to 1993 was $360 mil-

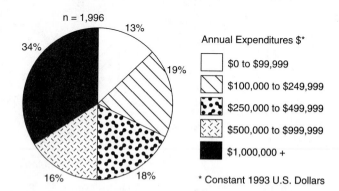

FIGURE 7.4 United States Local Health Departments by Total Annual Expenditures, 1992–1993. SOURCE: *National Association of County and City Health Officials,* 1995.

lion.[3] Detailed information concerning how these funds are spent is not available.

Services and Functions

Local health departments provide a wide range of services that affect nearly all persons in the United States. If public health and prevention services are working well and preventing the occurrence, or reducing the spread, of disease, the public is virtually unaware of their existence. Epidemics are avoided, water quality remains safe, healthy behaviors are adopted, and so on. This relative invisibility of local health departments belies the existence of a wide range of public health activities.

What follows is a broad summary of the major services provided by local health departments. Although data are available on over 50 different services provided by local health departments, descriptions of all of them are not possible here.

Environmental Health

Although in many states the lead responsibility for environmental health lies with an agency other than the health department, 86 percent of local health departments are responsible for environmental health issues.[11]

Traditionally, local health departments have been responsible for assuring the safety of food and milk prod-

ucts. They may conduct restaurant inspections (80 percent of local health departments), provide food and milk control services (56 percent), and offer courses in food handling.[3] Other traditional environmental health services include assurance of the safety of public and private water supplies, solid waste management, management of sewage disposal systems, and vector and animal control.

In response to growing awareness of environmental contamination and the links between human health and the environment, local health departments have taken a leading role in the assurance of indoor air quality, tobacco and second-hand smoke regulation, pollution prevention, emergency response, and management of hazardous materials. Local health departments are increasingly becoming the source of information for the community about environmental risks, and many are initiating programs in occupational health and safety.

Table 7.1 shows the percent of local health departments that provide selected environmental services, by size of the population served. As the size of population increases, more environmental services tend to be provided.

Primary Care and Personal Health Care Services

Local health departments are significant providers of personal health care services. Each year, 40 million

TABLE 7.1   United States Local Health Departments: Selected Environmental Services Provided* by Size of Population Served, 1992–1993

Service	All LHDs	Population of Jurisdiction				
		0 to 24,999	25,000 to 49,999	50,000 to 99,999	100,000 to 499,999	500,000+
Environmental Emergency Response	57%	48%	56%	65%	71%	79%
Groundwater Pollution Control	58%	51%	59%	62%	69%	73%
Hazardous Waste Management	42%	39%	40%	41%	51%	68%
Indoor Air Quality	37%	29%	37%	41%	50%	66%
Private Water Supply Safety	74%	69%	74%	80%	81%	78%
Public Water Supply Safety	52%	47%	48%	55%	61%	70%
Solid Waste Management	46%	41%	50%	46%	55%	60%

*Provided either directly or by contract
SOURCE: *National Association of County and City Health Officials*, 1995

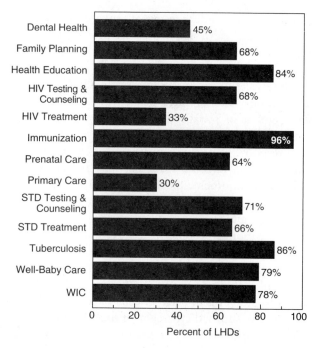

FIGURE 7.5 Percent of United States Local Health Departments Reporting Activity in Selected Service Areas, 1992–1993. SOURCE: *National Association of County and City Health Officials,* 1995.

people receive some type of personal health care from local health departments, including immunizations, well-baby visits, prenatal care, tuberculosis treatment, the treatment of sexually transmitted diseases, as well as many more-discrete services aimed at restoring and maintaining health and preventing transmission of disease. Figure 7.5 shows the percent of local health departments that provide these and other services.

In 47 states, state or local governments are required to provide at least some health care services to the indigent and to others who have no other means of accessing care.[12] Many counties throughout the nation are designated as providers of last resort, often providing more services than they are legally obligated to provide.

Personal Health Care Services. In general, the level of personal health care services provided by local health departments is directly related to their size. About one-quarter of all local health departments provide primary care, which is defined as comprehensive care available 24 hours per day.[3,10,13]

The role of local health departments in the delivery of personal health care services is currently a topic of serious discussion. The cost of these services, their availability elsewhere in the community, and the concern that such services might overshadow a health department's core functions are questions that must be considered and resolved in each community.

In communities where local health departments do not provide primary care services, the health departments still have the responsibility of assuring that needed personal health care services are available and accessible to everyone in the jurisdiction. Indeed, 76 percent of local health departments report that they assess the extent to which clinical preventive services, such as screening, immunization, and counseling services, are provided in the community by others.[3] Local health departments may collect information on a wide variety of indicators of availability of services, including the number of practicing physicians, the existence of ambulatory care centers, the types of community agencies, the number of providers that accept Medicaid reimbursement or have translation services, and others.[3]

In many jurisdictions, local health officials have worked closely with other providers to try to assure that adequate services are accessible to vulnerable populations. Examples of partnerships and linkages that have been developed include subcontracting with hospitals for obstetric services, assisting in the application for federal grants, and working with private providers to accept patients unable to pay for health care services. These are just a few examples of the approaches used by local health officials to try to assure that the people they serve actually get the care they need.

Community Assessment and Involvement

Another very important function of local health departments is to assess their community's health status and to establish priorities for community action. Through a combination of data review (including review of vital records, hospital discharge information, and special epidemiologic studies, among other data sources) and determination of the community's self-perception of its problems and needs, health officials develop plans that address the most pressing needs with their community.

Improvements in health status depend increasingly upon community understanding of, and participation in, community assessment and program development. This awareness is reflected in the models that have been developed to assist health officials in conducting a community health assessment. These include APEX (Assessment Protocol for Excellence in Public Health[14]), PATCH (Planned Approach to Community Health[15]), the Healthy Cities Project,[16] and Healthy Communities 2000: Model Standards.[17]

Staffing Patterns

As previously stated, local health departments currently employ a total of about 192,000 people. These

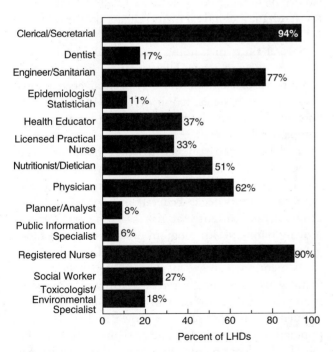

FIGURE 7.6 Percent of United States Local Health Departments that Reported Selected Full- and/or Part-Time Staff, 1989. SOURCE: *National Association of County and City Health Officials,* 1995.

include over 30 distinct professional types. However, according to a study done in 1989, there is no single profession that is represented in every local health department. Clerical/secretarial positions are found in 94 percent of local health departments and registered nurses in 90 percent. Engineers/sanitarians are employed by 77 percent and physicians by 62 percent.[9] Figure 7.6 shows the professions most commonly employed in local health departments nationwide.

As the population of the jurisdiction increases in size, there tends to be more variety in staff composition. As is the case in state health departments, the number of staff in local health departments varies considerably, depending on the scope of services provided and the level of funding in each department.

PROFILE OF AGENCY TOP EXECUTIVES

The characteristics, qualifications, and tenure of agency top executives show considerable variation.

Characteristics of Agency Top Executive

The chief executive officer (CEO) of the local health department usually is also the health official, but in some departments these responsibilities reside in two different individuals. CEOs bear responsibility for administrative issues and management of their agencies, and if they lack public health or medical training, they may have to rely on appropriately trained and licensed health officials or medical advisors in order to make health or medical decisions.

Most health departments (79 percent) are served by a full-time agency executive. Not surprisingly, as the population of the jurisdiction served increases, the likelihood that the job of agency executive will be a full-time position also increases, from 69 percent in the smallest agencies to 96 percent in the largest.[3]

The majority, or 60 percent, of local health directors are male, and over 96% of local health directors are Euro-American. Only 2 percent are African American, but the majority of these serve the largest jurisdictions. The 2 percent identifying themselves as Hispanic are from the largest health departments, with the result that almost one out of every nine health directors serving the largest jurisdictions is Hispanic.[3]

Qualifications of Agency Top Executives

In 1992 to 93, approximately 37 percent of agency top executives held some type of medical doctoral degree (e.g., M.D., D.V.M., D.O.). Of these, 77 percent required the medical degree for the job. Agency top executives in jurisdictions serving populations over 500,000 are much more likely to hold a medical degree than their counterparts in all other jurisdictions—63 percent in the largest areas, as compared with 29 to 40 percent in the smaller jurisdictions. Seventeen percent of all agency heads have graduate public health degrees. In some jurisdictions, there are statutory requirements that the chief health official must have both medical and public health degrees.[3]

It appears that the number of agency top executives with medical degrees is declining somewhat, a change that had been reported anecdotally for several years. It may be due to a move towards professional managers as agency heads.

Tenure of Local Health Directors

The tenure of local health directors has changed little during the years that have elapsed since the first NACCHO survey of local health departments.[3,9] Only 16 percent have been in their positions for fewer than two years, 27 percent for two to five years, 25 percent for five to nine years, 25 percent for ten to nineteen years, and 7 percent for twenty years or more. The majority of the agency top executives (57 percent) have been in their positions for more than five years.[3]

It is interesting to note that the tenure of health directors serving jurisdictions with large populations is shorter than that of health directors serving smaller populations. In jurisdictions of over 500,000 people, 55 percent of the health directors have held their positions for less than five years, and only 17 percent have held their positions for more than ten years. By contrast, in jurisdictions of under 50,000 people, 43 percent have been in their positions for less than four years,

and 29 percent have been in their positions for more than ten years.[3]

The tenure of local health agency heads has remained virtually unchanged for at least the past five years, and it contrasts sharply with the shorter tenure of state health officials. In 1992, for example, 75 percent of state health officials had been in office for less than five years while only 43 percent of local health officials had been in their positions for less than five years. Many attribute the difference in tenure to a lesser degree of politicization of health officer positions at the local level.

THE FUTURE

Local health departments are facing a period of substantial transition in their personal health services especially but also in the environmental services they deliver. Shifts in funding mechanisms, the current national interest in government downsizing, and the possibility of moving more decision-making authority to the states may all have a major impact on the roles and functions of local health departments.

Several shifts in funding are now taking place and more are likely to occur. These include the growing list of approvals of Medicaid section 1115 waivers requested by a number of states, requiring that Medicaid recipients receive medical services through managed-care companies. In those states where such waivers have been granted, health departments must decide whether to become managed-care providers, or to give up Medicaid reimbursement income and shift remaining resources to other community needs. Federal funds for public health programs are currently at risk as Congress discusses moving public health program dollars into large block grant programs with overall reductions in funding.

As mentioned above, local health departments tend to fill gaps in medical services by providing personal health care services to the poor and to other vulnerable populations. If other providers now care for vulnerable populations, such as Medicaid patients, it follows that local health departments can decrease their provision of personal health care services. This will greatly change the staffing, budgets, and service mix of local health departments.

Some health officials are uncertain about how their departments will manage the transition from provision of clinical services by health departments to provision of those services by the private sector. Others welcome the change because it could mean more funds for core public health functions that were described in the beginning of this chapter. Unfortunately, at this time, no dedicated source of funding exists for the provision of these core public health functions, and the lack of such funding lessens the ability of local health departments to provide them.

Some states have begun to plan for a transition from clinical provider to public health core functions provider. The state of Washington, for example, began a statewide effort several years ago to identify funding, staffing, budgets, and other needs for local health departments to provide an adequate level of service for the core public health functions.[6] Legislation was developed and passed to assure the capacity of the state's local public health departments to provide core public health functions. A statewide committee continues to plan public health activities.

The national move to privatize services and functions has also extended to traditional public health services in both personal health care and environmental health. As one example, the entire state of Oklahoma is currently studying how privatization of various core public health services might apply within that state.[18]

The privatization of environmental health services or their transfer to other governmental agencies could result in loss of necessary revenues to local health departments. These revenues help support other important, but uncapitalized, programs. The impact of privatization and/or program transfer to other agencies on the totality of a community's environmental protection efforts must be considered carefully before significant program changes are made. For both environmental and personal health services, careful thought is required to define the role of the health department in monitoring or assuring that services delivered by the private sector are performed well and accountably.

Some have stated that public health is a perspective or an approach and not a set of specific tasks and programs. This suggests that there is no need to continue to assure the existence of local health departments. Clearly, public health services are provided to some degree by institutions and agencies other than local health departments. Managed-care organizations, hospitals, and integrated service networks are beginning, in some cases, to provide public health services. Unfortunately, the services provided tend to be only those for which some form of reimbursement is available.

CONCLUSION

Both NACCHO and many leading health professionals agree that only some of the responsibilities of local health departments can be delegated to others. The NACCHO *Blueprint For A Healthy Community* maintains that, regardless of other responsibilities, local health departments must continue to assure that the essential elements needed to maintain a healthy community are well provided.[1] Local government must retain responsibility for the interpretation of data and the assessment of community health status, the development of public health policy, and the assurance that services needed by the community are available to all its members.

REFERENCES

1. *Blueprint for a Healthy Community: A Guide for Local Health Departments.* Washington, DC: National Association of County Health Officials; 1994:6.

2. Institute of Medicine, Committee for the Study of the Future of Public Health. *The Future of Public Health.* Washington, DC: National Academy Press; 1988.

3. *1992–1993 National Profile of Local Health Departments.* Washington, DC: National Association of County and City Health Officials; 1995.

4. The Children's Charter, President Hoover's White House Conference on Child Health and Protection Recognizing the Rights of the Child as the First Rights of Citizenship Pledges Itself to these Aims for the Children of America; 1931.

5. Emerson H. *Local Health Units for the Nation: A Report of the Subcommittee on Local Health Units, Committee on Administrative Practice, American Public Health Association.* New York: Commonwealth Fund; 1945.

6. *Public Health Improvement Plan.* Olympia, Washington: Washington State Department of Health; 1994.

7. *Project Health: The Reengineering of Public Health in Illinois.* Springfield, Il: Illinois Department of Public Health; 1949: 9,12.

8. Public Hearing on "County Governments and Health Care Reform" held by the National Association of Counties. Testimony presented by Turnock BJ, MD; October 19, 1992.

9. Internal correspondence: Ned Baker, Executive Director, National Association of Local Boards of Health, Bowling Green, OH; 1995.

10. *National Profile of Local Health Departments.* Washington, DC: National Association of County Health Officials; 1990.

11. *Current Roles, Future Challenges of Local Health Departments in Environmental Health.* Washington, DC: National Association of County Health Officials; 1992.

12. *Too Poor to be Sick: Access to Medical Care for the Uninsured.* Washington, DC: American Public Health Association; 1988:39.

13. *Primary Care Assessment: Local Health Department's Role in Service Delivery.* Washington, DC: National Association of County Health Officials; 1992:9.

14. *Assessment Protocol for Excellence in Public Health (APEX/PH).* Washington, DC: National Association of County Health Officials; 1991.

15. *Planned Approach to Community Health (PATCH).* Atlanta, Ga: Centers for Disease Control and Prevention; 1993.

16. *World Health Organization, Five Year Planning Project.* Fadl, Copenhagen: World Health Organization Healthy Cities Project; 1988. WHO Healthy Cities Paper, No. 2.

17. *Healthy Communities 2000: Model Standards.* Washington, DC: American Public Health Association; 1991.

18. Internal correspondence. Oklahoma City, OK: Sara Reed DePersio, MD, MPH, Deputy Commissioner, Personal Health Services, Oklahoma State Department of Health.

CHAPTER

8

Major National Public Health Professional Associations

C. William Keck, M.D., M.P.H.

F. Douglas Scutchfield, M.D.

Two of the more difficult yet important challenges facing public health professionals are keeping up with developments at the state and national level that are relevant to their work and staying connected to a peer network of colleagues. Membership in professional associations can be very helpful in both these areas. Professional associations can be a mechanism for access to such useful items as relevant publications; technical and legislative updates, alerts, and summaries; issue analyses; trend forecasts; career opportunities; and policy development issues.

This chapter provides a description of some of the major national professional associations typically joined by public health workers. There are many other national organizations not listed here that might be of value to some in public health, and the reader is encouraged to search out and explore any group that might be professionally helpful or personally rewarding.

Public health professionals should also explore state-level professional associations in the state in which they work. Many of these associations provide the same benefits and opportunities at the state level that national associations provide at the national level. Indeed, many state associations are affiliated with national ones. Although there are too many to list here, state associations deserve consideration and support.

AMERICAN PUBLIC HEALTH ASSOCIATION (APHA)

Founded in 1872, the American Public Health Association is the oldest and largest organization of public health professionals in the world. (See Table 8.1 on page 107 for address and telephone numbers of this and other health professional associations.) It has more than 32,000 members plus an additional 18,000 members belonging only to state associations affiliated with APHA. More than 75 public health occupations are represented in the membership.

Members can choose to belong to any of 30 special primary interest groups (SPIGs) and sections, which bring together researchers, practitioners, administrators, teachers, and other health workers in a unique multidisciplinary environment of professional exchange, study, and action. The many SPIGs and sections of the APHA offer members substantial opportunities to enhance their standing in the profession through collegial interaction, leadership opportunities, and committee service.

The object of the APHA is to:

> . . . protect and promote personal and environmental health. It shall exercise leadership with health professionals and the general public in health policy development and action, with particular focus on the interrelationship between health and the quality of life, and on developing a national policy for health care and services and on solving technical problems.

The association sponsors an annual meeting and exhibition in the fall of every year. It is the world's largest gathering of public health professionals. The association also helps to set standards; participates in research and matters concerning the profession of public health; influences public health policy, particularly at the federal level, via committees and coalitions with related groups; and publishes a variety of public health-related books and periodicals.

APHA membership includes subscriptions to the association's monthly scholarly journal, *The American Journal of Public Health*, and to the association's newspaper, *The Nation's Health*, which reports on legislation and policy issues affecting all public health professionals. Categories of membership include *regular, contributing*, and a group of special memberships at half price: *student/trainee* (anyone in a full-time college, university, or formal training program preparing for entry into a health career), *retired, special health worker* (anyone employed in community health whose annual salary is below a set minimum), and *consumer* (anyone without income derived from health-related activities).

ASSOCIATION OF SCHOOLS OF PUBLIC HEALTH (ASPH)

The Association of Schools of Public Health was founded in 1940 to represent accredited graduate schools of public health in the United States and Puerto Rico. The association serves the collective needs of its 27 members as they pursue the education and training of professional public health personnel.

The association's mission is to: " . . . improve the public's health by advancing professional and graduate education, research and service in public health." In its efforts to accomplish this mission, ASPH:

- prepares policy studies and other reports on public health personnel issues
- provides a forum for its members and their colleague organizations to consider trends in public health education and practice
- compiles data profiling applicants, students, graduates, and faculty
- acts as a clearinghouse for available public health education resources
- provides consultation, technical assistance, and training from the schools to federal, state, and local health agencies, private non-profit organizations, and industry
- facilitates the capacity for federal agencies to utilize the capabilities of the schools for health promotion and disease prevention activities
- maintains liaisons with other national and international associations and government agencies
- monitors congressional activities
- represents the concerns of schools of public health to Congress and the executive branch.

Each member school is represented in the association by its dean. Categories of membership include: *active* (schools that are pre-accredited and accredited by the Council on Education for Public Health); *associate* (schools that have actively begun the accreditation process); and *affiliate* (organizations or programs associated with graduate educational institutions, which have specialty interests in common with the purpose of the association). Only active members can vote and serve as officers, but any member can serve on the association's many councils and committees.

ASSOCIATION OF STATE AND TERRITORIAL HEALTH OFFICIALS (ASTHO)

The Association of State and Territorial Health Officials was founded in 1942. Its members consist of the directors of public health in each state, the District of Columbia, and the United States territories and possessions. ASTHO also has 17 affiliated groups that represent directors of divisions within state health departments. These groups function independently of, yet cooperate very closely with, ASTHO to develop and promote sound public health policy.

The purpose of the association is to:

> . . . formulate and influence, through collective action, the establishment of sound national public health policy and to assist and serve state health departments in the development and implementation of state programs and policies for the public's health and prevention of disease.

ASTHO's staff works with its members to formulate and present public health recommendations to the Congress, the administration, and other national organizations. The association conducts numerous projects, some funded by federal agencies, to promote public health program development at the state level. It also sponsors meetings and serves as an informational resource to state agencies on public policy developments through its publications, including the biweekly *Washington Report*, which provides an update of legislative activities and concerns of state health departments, and *Action Alerts*, which seek membership support for ASTHO positions on particular issues before Congress.

ASTHO provides opportunities for its members to serve on its executive committee, task forces, and other committees. In 1981, the association established the

Public Health Foundation, a private, nonprofit organization that monitors developments in public health and facilitates the exchange of information among public and voluntary health agencies, researchers, and educators.

ASSOCIATION OF TEACHERS OF PREVENTIVE MEDICINE (ATPM)

Founded in 1942, membership in the Association of Teachers of Preventive Medicine is open to any professional engaged in or interested in the education of students in the professions of preventive medicine and public health. Its approximately 500 members include teachers, researchers, practitioners, administrators, residents, and students who are affiliated with schools of medicine, schools of public health, other health professional schools, and various health agencies.

The mission of the association is to: " . . . ensure the primacy and excellence of individual and community health promotion and disease prevention in the education of physicians and other health professionals." In pursuit of that mission, the association:

- sponsors meetings, especially *PREVENTION*, the premier annual conference on preventive medicine cosponsored with other groups
- represents the interests of its members to Congress, federal agencies, and related professional organizations
- sends its members the bimonthly scholarly journal, *The American Journal of Preventive Medicine*, published in cooperation with the American College of Preventive Medicine
- provides opportunities for individuals and institutions to obtain financial support for research and curricular projects
- provides opportunities for professional responsibility and recognition through service on committees and councils and in elective office.

ATPM also strives to highlight and foster the role of units in preventive medicine within medical schools and offers institutional membership opportunities to medical school departments and divisions of preventive medicine.

Categories of membership in ATPM include: *regular individual member, sustaining member* (those giving tax-deductible donations to the ATPM Foundation, which awards grants to preventive medicine students and faculty), *associate member* (full-time health professions students, residents, and fellows), *retired member* (members who have reached full retirement and age 62), *emeritus member* (selected members who have been given dues-free status by the board), and *institutional member* (academic institutions, health agencies, and other organizational entities that are engaged in teaching preventive medicine, disease prevention and health promotion, and public health).

AMERICAN COLLEGE OF PREVENTIVE MEDICINE (ACPM)

The American College of Preventive Medicine, founded in 1956, is the professional organization of 2,000 physician specialists who practice preventive medicine. The mission of ACPM is to: " . . . advance the science and practice of disease prevention and health promotion and provide leadership in research, professional education, development of public policy and enhancement of standards." Members include physicians certified by the American Board of Preventive Medicine or by another American board of medical specialties, under criteria established by ACPM in 1993.

In support of its mission, ACPM develops educational initiatives including:

* cosponsorship of the annual conference on preventive medicine, PREVENTION
* a review course
* the development and publication of materials to support postgraduate training in the specialty, such as a residency program directory and training manual
* the development of competencies.

ACPM also advocates public policies consistent with scientific principles of the discipline, collaborates with United States Public Health Service agencies with similar interests, and works on behalf of the specialty to improve and expand financing for graduate medical education. ACPM communicates through the scholarly journal, *The American Journal of Preventive Medicine,* which is published jointly with the Association of Teachers of Preventive Medicine. It also produces a newsletter and other publications.

Categories of membership in ACPM include *member, fellow* (those who have been members for three years and have demonstrated contribution to the field and/or organization), *associate member, affiliate member, resident,* and *emeritus.*

AMERICAN ASSOCIATION OF PUBLIC HEALTH PHYSICIANS (AAPHP)

The American Association of Public Health Physicians was organized in 1954 as the national organization that represents physicians in all public health fields. The association's 160 members are doctors of medicine or osteopathy who are engaged in activities related to public health. The members elect officers and a board of trustees to manage the association's affairs. There is no central office or paid staff.

The objectives of AAPHP include:

* promoting cohesive leadership in health by public health physicians
* serving as a forum for public health physicians on proposed legislation
* encouraging placement of qualified public health physicians in health department leadership positions
* working with other professional organizations to develop solutions to the nation's community health needs
* stimulating continuing public health and preventive medicine educational programs for its members.

In pursuit of these objectives, AAPHP:

* cosponsors the annual PREVENTION meeting
* holds business meetings twice each year, once at PREVENTION and once at the Annual Meeting of the American Public Health Association
* has direct representation in the House of Delegates and Section of Preventive Medicine of the American Medical Association as well as on the Board of Regents of the American College of Medicine

- publishes its monthly newsletter, the *Bulletin*
- provides a reduced subscription rate to the *American Journal of Preventive Medicine* for its members.

NATIONAL ASSOCIATION OF COUNTY AND CITY HEALTH OFFICIALS (NACCHO)

Founded in 1994 through the combination of the National Association of County Health Officials (NACHO) and the United States Conference of Local Health Officers (USCLHO), the National Association of County and City Health Officials represents all of the nation's approximately 3,000 local health departments and serves as the national voice of local health officials. NACCHO seeks local health departments as sustaining members and has more than 650 on its roster. Service (membership) fees are set on the basis of the size of the population served by the member health department.

NACCHO aims to improve the health of people and communities by:

> . . . assuring an effective local public health system; being the voice of local public health officials at the national level to promote the local perspective on national health program and fiscal policies; developing technical competence, managerial capacity and leadership potential of local public health officials and the local public health workforce; building partnerships and collaborative relationships with state and federal health agencies and other national organizations with an interest in health; and maintaining communications with local health officials to serve as an exchange point for information and ideas.

In pursuing its mission, NACCHO communicates actively with county, city, and district health departments, as well as with numerous federal officials and agencies and with other health professional organizations. The association's bimonthly newsletter, *NACCHO News,* is distributed to these groups. Special reports and periodic *Fact Sheets* are prepared on issues relevant to local health departments.

NACCHO convenes five national meetings of local public health officials each year. Its annual meeting is the country's major gathering of these individuals. Its four other meetings are held in conjunction with the annual meeting of the American Public Health Association, the annual PREVENTION conference (which NACCHO cosponsors), the annual meeting of the National Association of Counties (NACo), and the NACo Legislative Conference.

NACCHO publishes the *National Directory of Local Health Departments* and pursues projects designed to help health departments accomplish their tasks. Projects have included development of the *Assessment Protocol for Excellence in Public Health (APEX/PH),* development of the *National Profile of Local Health Departments,* and the *Blueprint of Healthy Communities: A Guide for Local Health Departments.* The association has also been externally funded to review the public health areas of access to care, environmental health, maternal and child health, primary care, and multicultural health.

Membership in NACCHO provides local health officials with opportunities to participate as board members and officers, serve on a variety of project committees, and interact with colleagues and peers. Each member belongs to one of three *Forums*—the Big City/Metro Forum (serving populations in cities of more than 350,000), the City-Based Forum (serving populations principally located within cities and towns), or the County-Based Forum (serving populations within the jurisdictional boundary of a county or counties).

NATIONAL ENVIRONMENTAL HEALTH ASSOCIATION (NEHA)

Established in 1937, the National Environmental Health Association is comprised of professionals in the field of environmental health and protection from private and public sectors, academia, and the uniformed services. Its approximately 5,600 members represent more than 50 different countries. They participate in NEHA through an array of committees that are organized within nine distinct technical sections. Members can also participate as officers or as members of the association's board of directors.

NEHA is dedicated to: " . . . advancing the environmental health and protection professional for the purpose of providing a healthful environment for all." It works to foster cooperation and understanding among professionals in the environmental health and protection field and to contribute to the resolution of worldwide environmental health issues. In pursuit of these purposes, NEHA:

- sponsors the credentialing of four categories of environmental health professional
- offers a program and registry for continuing education
- develops environmental educational products
- sponsors educational conferences, including a four-day annual educational conference
- sponsors regional workshops and the four-day exam review workshops for the Registered Hazardous Substances Professional and Registered Environmental Health Specialist preparing for the credentialing examination
- publishes the *Journal of Environmental Health* ten times a year
- publishes more than 125 other, regularly updated offerings intended to assist members seeking continuing professional education.

Membership categories in NEHA include: *regular member, sustaining member* (corporations), *institutional member* (academic institutions), and *student member.*

SOCIETY FOR PUBLIC HEALTH EDUCATION, INC. (SOPHE)

Founded in 1950, the Society for Public Health Education is a national organization of educators that is devoted exclusively to the interests of public health education and health promotion. Its members choose among seven special interest group sections that bring colleagues together in specialty education areas including medical care/patient; international health; school health; community health; work site health; university faculty; and health communications/social marketing for networking, study, and action. Eighteen regions have local affiliated chapters.

SOPHE aims to promote the health of all people by:

- stimulating research on the theory and practice of health education
- supporting high-quality performance standards for the practice of health education and health promotion
- advocating policy and legislation affecting health education and health promotion
- developing and promoting standards for professional preparation of health education professionals
- promoting contact among health education professionals.

SOPHE sponsors annual and midyear meetings, certifies continuing education contact hours, and promotes professional preparation and practice standards. Members receive the society's journal, *Health Education Quarterly*; its quarterly newsletter, *News and Views*; and an annual membership directory.

Society governance, advocacy, and educational efforts offer members opportunities to enhance their standing in the profession. Categories of membership include: *active fellow, student member* (those enrolled full-time in a health education training program), and *emeritus* (retired persons).

THE AMERICAN ASSOCIATION OF PUBLIC HEALTH DENTISTRY (AAPHD)

Established in 1937, the American Association of Public Health Dentistry seeks as members all individuals concerned with improving the oral health of the public. Its 850 members worldwide are largely dentists and dental hygienists whose primary commitment is to dental public health.

The purpose of AAPHD is to: " . . . provide leadership for improving the oral health of the public based on the principles of dental public health." In support of that purpose, the association sponsors an annual meeting held just prior to and in conjunction with the annual meeting of the American Dental Association. It also publishes quarterly both *The Journal of Public*

Health Dentistry and a newsletter, the *Communique*. The association also produces an educational fluoridation brochure, curricular guidelines for such subjects as dental sealants, and position papers and resolutions on various issues affecting oral health and dentistry. The American Board of Dental Public Health, which certifies dentists as specialists in dental public health, is sponsored by the association.

Members of AAPHD are encouraged to participate by serving on a wide variety of committees established to address issues of importance to the profession and to community oral health. They are also encouraged to run for election for the association's officer and executive council positions. Categories of membership include: *voting* (those who possess a degree in dentistry or in an allied dental field), *associate* (those without degrees in dentistry or allied dental fields, but who engage in public and preventive oral health programs), and *student* (students enrolled full-time in an accredited school of dentistry, dental hygiene, or public health).

TABLE 8.1   Major National Public Health Professional Associations

American Public Health Association (APHA) 1015 15th Street N.W. Washington, D.C. 20005 TEL: 202-789-5600 FAX: 202-789-5681	*American Association of Public Health Physicians (AAPHP)* *National Association of County and City Health Officials (NACCHO)* 440 First Street, N.W., Suite 500 Washington, D.C. 20001 TEL: 202-783-5550 FAX: 202-783-1583
Association of Schools of Public Health (ASPH) 1660 L Street, N.W. Suite 204 Washington, D.C. 20036-5603 TEL: 202-296-1099 FAX: 202-296-1252	*National Environmental Health Association (NEHA)* 720 South Colorado Boulevard South Tower, 970 Denver, Colorado 80222-1925 TEL: 303-756-9090 FAX: 303-691-9490
Association of State and Territorial Health Officials (ASTHO) 415 Second Street, N.E. Suite 200 Washington, D.C. 20002 TEL: 202-546-5400 FAX: 202-544-9349	*Society for Public Health Education, Inc. (SOPHE)* 2001 Addison Street, Suite 220 Berkeley, California 94704 TEL: 510-644-9242 FAX: 510-845-4113
Association of Teachers of Preventive Medicine (ATPM) 1660 L Street, N.W. Suite 208 Washington, D.C. 20036-5603 TEL: 202-463-0550 FAX: 202-463-0555	*The American Association of Public Health Dentistry (AAPHD)* 10619 Jousting Lane Richmond, Virginia 23235-3838 TEL: 804-272-8344 FAX: 804-272-0802
American College of Preventive Medicine (ACPM) 1660 L Street, N.W., Suite 206 Washington, D.C. 20036-5603 TEL: 202-466-2044 FAX: 202-466-2662	

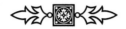

PART THREE

TOOLS FOR PUBLIC HEALTH PRACTICE

CHAPTER

Leadership in Public Health Practice

Dennis D. Pointer, Ph.D.
Julianne P. Sanchez, M.A.

*"Think like a person of action,
Act like a person of thought."*
Aristotle

This chapter is intended to help you gain an understanding of *leadership*, one of the most important organizational and management concepts. The chapter first explores the concept of leadership. Then it summarizes what is known about the factors related to leadership effectiveness and posits an integrative model of leadership that blends together different perspectives on leadership. The chapter ends with suggestions for improving leadership knowledge and skills.

Before reading the chapter, first think about these questions. They will help clarify your thinking about the issue.

- What is leadership? Write a one or two sentence definition that captures the essence of the term.
- Is leadership synonymous with management, or is leading just one of many things a manager does? In what ways are they different, or how are they the same?

- Think of several individuals you feel are really exceptional leaders. What, if anything, do they have in common?
- Think of several individuals who are truly poor leaders. What, if anything, do they have in common?
- How does leadership affect the performance of what's being led (whether it's an individual, a group or an organization)? That is, in what ways can leadership make a difference?
- Have you ever known people who were successful leaders in one situation and failures in others? Why is this the case?

WHAT IS LEADERSHIP?

Leadership is the means by which things get done in organizations—and all organizations exist to get things done. A manager can establish goals, strategize, relate to others, communicate, collect information, make decisions, plan, organize, monitor, and control; but without leadership, nothing happens.

111

Leadership is one of the most highly valued management abilities. Public health agencies and their divisions, departments, units, and programs can thrive under superior leadership. They can face considerable difficulty or even fail when their leadership is poor. Managers who have the ability to lead are therefore in demand.

Defining Leadership

As important as leadership is, however, it is a difficult concept to define. Here's how one major textbook in the field describes the situation:

> It is neither feasible nor desirable at this point in the development of the discipline to resolve the controversy over the appropriate definition of leadership. For the time being, it is better to use the various conceptions of leadership as a source of different perspectives on a complex, multifaceted phenomenon.[1]

Nonetheless, it is important to define leadership in order to study it, learn about it, and improve one's leadership skills. Thus, here is a simple definition of leadership that includes only the essential attributes about which most scholars working in the field would have little disagreement:

> Leadership is the process through which an individual attempts to intentionally influence another individual or group in order to accomplish a goal.

The core concepts embedded in this seemingly simple definition warrant emphasis and elaboration.

- Leadership is a *process*. It is a verb, an action word, not a noun. Leadership manifests itself in doing; it is a performing art.
- Only individuals lead. The *locus* of leadership is in a person. Inanimate objects do not lead, groups do not lead, organizations do not lead, only people do. When looking for and at leadership, our subject is the individual.
- The *focus* of leadership is other individuals and groups. A leader cannot exist without followers. Followers might be individuals, groups, members of an organization, or the population of a nation.
- Leadership entails *influencing* followers—their thoughts (the cognitive target of influence), their feelings (the affective target), and/or their actions (the behavioral target). Influence is leadership's center of gravity and most critical element.
- The objective of leadership is *goal accomplishment*. Leadership is instrumental; it is done for a purpose.
- Leadership is *intentional*, not accidental. All of us *unknowingly* influence others hundreds of times each day, but those are not acts of leadership.

Leadership is exercised in a lot of different places and in a wide variety of situations, not just by managers in the workplace. Persuading a friend to have dinner at one's favorite restaurant, for example, requires leadership. All the key elements are there: a locus of leadership, a follower, and an act of intentional influence undertaken to accomplish a goal.

ORGANIZATIONAL LEADERSHIP

All organizations exist to accomplish tasks that are too large and/or complex to be undertaken by individuals or small groups working alone. Organizations do this by sequentially subdividing work, over and over again. All organizations sequentially subdivide tasks in a similar way until they are small enough and simple enough to be performed by an individual. In the process, the organizations are partitioned into a series of departments, divisions, sections, or programs, all of which must be managed.

Leadership in a Public Health Agency

The provision of public health services in a community is a task that is so large and complex that an organization must undertake it. A public health agency assumes this task and proceeds to subdivide it: a department of environmental health does some parts of it; maternal and child health does other parts; laboratory services does other parts; and so on. The provision of services in environmental health, to cite just one example, in turn, is so large and complex a task that it, too, must be subdivided. It is parceled out among different divisions (for example, water and air).

Figure 9.1 presents a schematic organizational chart of a typical public health agency. The figure focuses

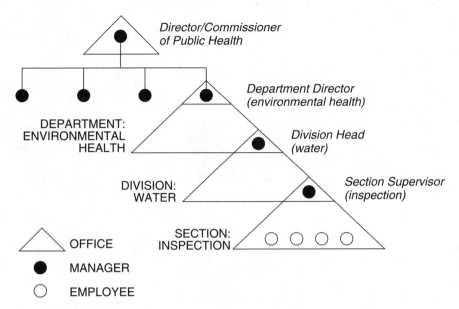

FIGURE 9.1 Public Health Organizations: Components and Managerial Offices

on just one of four segments of a much larger organizational structure. In each component there is a managerial office, associated with which are sets of expectations called **roles**. Roles are constellations of things the manager is expected to do.[2] Roles are attached to the office, not the particular person occupying it. Occupants of the office may come and go, but the roles remain the same.

Leadership Versus Management

There are many different roles for managers, and leadership is only one of them. Leadership and management are not synonyms. A manager is an individual who holds an office to which multiple roles are attached whereas leadership is one of the roles attached to the office of manager. This is a point that causes considerable confusion.

Performance of the leadership role is the way managers get things done; without leadership or with poor leadership, the organization is impaired. Although leadership is not the only role of the manager, it is certainly the central one. All of the other roles of the manager, such as formulating goals, developing strategies, communicating, making decisions, and resolving conflicts are converted into tangible results through leadership.

Leadership Role of the Manager

Put Figure 9.1 under a magnifying glass and you have Figure 9.2. It focuses on one managerial office in the public health agency's chain of command. The manager is a subordinate of the director and a peer of other department directors having the same reporting relationship. Simultaneously, the manager holds a superordinate position within the department of environment health services.

There are several key points that can be illustrated by focusing on the leadership role of the manager in Figure 9.2.

Multidirectionality

Leadership is **multidirectional**. The department director leads subordinates not only in the component of the agency of which he or she is the manager, but also leads peers, superiors, and individuals and groups outside the agency.

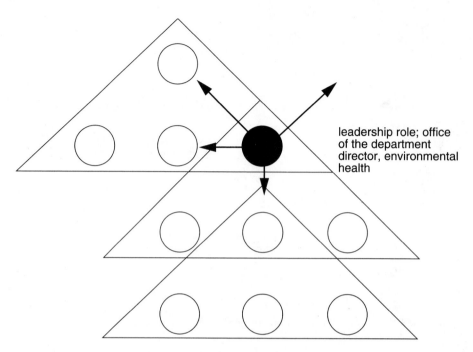

leadership role; office of the department director, environmental health

FIGURE 9.2 Directionality of the Manager's Leadership Role

Only when leadership is conceptualized as intentional influence is the proper distinction between managing and leadership made. The director of the department of environmental health services intentionally influences or leads but does not manage peers, for example, in chairing a committee to implement Assessment Protocol for Excellence in Public Health (APEX) standards. The director also may lead a superior by providing direction prior to an upcoming budget review meeting with the governor, county supervisors, or city council. Additionally, the director might engage in the leadership role when working with other units of government and community organizations. The department director leads in all directions simultaneously. Thus, leadership's arrows of influence point in several directions at once.

The Focus Downward

Although leadership is multidirectional, it is the **downward focus** that has received the greatest amount of attention and study. When thinking of leadership,

the first thing that generally comes to mind is the relationship between managers and their subordinates. The vast majority of leadership research has this focus. Most acts of leadership are pointed downward, primarily towards direct subordinates but secondarily towards subordinates in lower and lower layers of the agency.

Leading Other Managers

When engaging in leadership, irrespective of the direction of influence, the focus is generally other managers. In general, it is only at the level of the section supervisor that nonmanagers are led. For the most part, managers lead other managers.

Power

The extent to which leadership attempts are successful depends on the amount of *power* associated with a particular managerial office and the person holding it. Power can be defined as the potential to influence. The more power managers possess, the greater the potential that they will be able to influence other individuals and groups. The key concept here is potential; one can have power and not use it. Leadership, on the other hand, is the use of power to exert influence.

Power can come from many sources. An important source of power in organizations is the office held. There, power is the result of formal authority. Some other sources of power include:

- information, knowledge, skills, abilities, and experience (expert power)
- connections with other individuals and groups who possess influence (referent power)
- control of incentives (reward/coercive power)
- one's own persona (charismatic power)

LEADERSHIP EFFECTIVENESS

All managers are not equally effective or successful as leaders. It is important to understand why in order to select good leaders and improve leadership skills.

What Influences Leadership Effectiveness?

There has been a raging debate for the last 50 years regarding what makes a successful leader, but there are still three very different points of view. These can be summed up as nature, nurture, and situational factors.

Nature

According to this view, which is illustrated by Figure 9.3, leadership effectiveness is primarily a result of traits and dispositions that individuals are endowed with at birth or develop very early in life. By the time a person assumes a management position, these charac-

teristics are set and nearly impossible to change in any significant way. In short, some people have traits that predispose them to be successful leaders, whereas others do not.

Nurture

According to this view, shown in Figure 9.4, leadership effectiveness is primarily due to abilities and behaviors that can be learned. Personal traits and dispositions provide the foundation upon which abilities are acquired and behaviors are developed, but they are only the foundation. Individuals who are exceptional leaders make themselves, they are not born that way.

Situational Factor

Figure 9.5 illustrates the argument that leadership effectiveness is primarily due to the characteristics of the situation in which managers find themselves. Inborn traits, abilities, and behaviors are important, but they are very situation specific. In one situation, certain traits, abilities, and behaviors may predispose a manager to be an effective leader; in a different situation, the result could be ineffectiveness and failure instead.

Discussion

To underscore the practical importance of these different perspectives, consider the following questions:

- If you agree with the nature argument, which personal traits and dispositions do you think are most associated with leadership effectiveness and success?
- If you agree with the nurture argument, which abilities and behaviors do you think are most associated with leadership effectiveness and success? What do you think are the best ways to acquire these abilities and develop these behaviors?
- If you agree with the situational argument, which factors do you think are most important for leadership effectiveness and success?
- Do you think that nature, nurture, and/or situational factors work together to influence leadership effectiveness? If so, why?

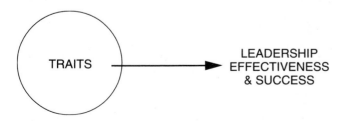

FIGURE 9.3 The Nature Argument

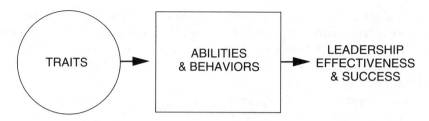

FIGURE 9.4 The Nurture Argument

The importance of this issue is further underscored by these two questions that scholars have been trying to help practicing managers answer for almost half a century:

- If you wanted to select an effective and potentially successful leader, what traits, abilities, and behaviors would you look for?
- If you wanted to improve your own leadership effectiveness, what traits, abilities, and behaviors would you focus on developing or improving?

Review of the Research

What follows is not a thorough review of the literature because the objective is to provide an introduction only. To explore the area further, consult the key references that have been provided. It is interesting to note that none of the basic work in this area has been conducted in public health organizations.

The vast majority of theorizing and research on leadership effectiveness can be classified into three different perspectives: **trait, behavioral,** and **contingency.**[3] In the next sections, these perspectives are described, some of their major studies reviewed, and key findings highlighted. Additionally, several emerging leadership theories and concepts are introduced.

The Trait Perspective

Because it is individuals who lead, it is natural and reasonable to look for those characteristics of individuals that might separate effective leaders from ineffective ones. Indeed, this is where early research began. It focused almost exclusively on military commanders and those holding political office.

In the late 1930s, psychologists became interested in leadership and began investigating relationships between individual characteristics and leadership effectiveness in organizations. Even though as early as the 1940s it was suggested that these relationships were weak and not generalizable across different situations,[4] the research continued. Just about every attribute imaginable has been studied in this regard.[5]

The most comprehensive review of this literature was conducted by Roger Stodgill in his classic work *Handbook of Leadership.*[6] Stodgill examined 287 studies undertaken from 1904 through 1970. Stodgill's review, and the earlier review of Sartle[7] identified a small number of traits that seemed to be present in leaders (as compared to followers) and in good leaders (as compared to poor ones). These included intelligence, dominance, self-confidence, high energy level, and task-

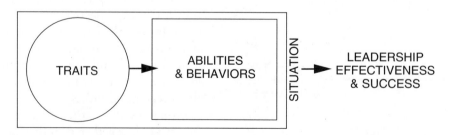

FIGURE 9.5 The Situational Argument

relevant knowledge. However, the findings were inconsistent and the relationships were very weak, suggesting that there are no individual traits that consistently predict leadership effectiveness or that always differentiate those who lead from those who follow.[8]

It is difficult to argue that individual traits have no effect whatsoever on leadership effectiveness. Such a conclusion runs counter to experience, logic, and common sense. Researchers began to appreciate that traits had an impact, but not in the way originally imagined. Instead, researchers concluded that

- Traits are best thought of as predispositions. A particular trait or set of traits tends to predispose (though not cause) an individual to engage in certain behaviors that may or may not result in leadership effectiveness.
- Multiple traits can be associated with a given behavior, and more than one behavior can be linked to an individual trait.
- It is behavior and not traits per se that is most closely related to leadership effectiveness.

These three observations help explain why a set of universal leadership traits has yet to be discovered. Nonetheless, research in this area continues.[9]

The Behavioral Perspective

Interest in leadership behaviors emerged as it became apparent that individual traits were inadequate to explain variations in leadership effectiveness. Researchers reasoned that if variation in individual traits could not explain such differences, perhaps the behaviors that flowed from them could. Most of this research has focused on:

- identifying dimensions that can be used to describe and categorize different leadership behaviors
- developing models of leadership style, where a style is defined by a combination of behaviors
- examining how specific leadership styles are related to effectiveness
- developing more rigorous ways to conceptualize and measure leadership effectiveness

Early Work. The first study employing a behavioral perspective was conducted by Kurt Lewin and his associates at the University of Iowa in the 1930s.[10] These researchers compared three styles of leadership—autocratic, democratic, and laissez-faire—in groups of preteen boys. Leaders of the groups were confederates of the researchers and were instructed on how to perform in the various styles.

Democratic leaders coordinated activities of the group and facilitated majority rule and decision making on important matters. Autocratic leaders directed the activities of the group and made important decisions without input from members. Laissez-faire leaders, who accidentally emerged during the course of the study, provided neither facilitation nor direction. This work was significant because it focused on behavior rather than traits, identified and described different leadership styles, and found that variations in style had an impact on followers.

Ohio Studies. Several major studies of leadership were undertaken immediately after World War II. One of the most widely cited was conducted by a group of investigators at Ohio State University.[11] These researchers addressed the question of how behavior of a leader impacts upon work, group performance, and satisfaction. Instruments were designed to measure leadership behavior as perceived by managers themselves, as well as by their peers, superiors, and subordinates.

Two dimensions of leadership behavior were identified: *initiating structure,* or the degree to which a manager defined and organized the work that was to be done and the extent to which attention was focused on accomplishing objectives established by the manager; and *consideration,* or the extent to which the manager exhibited concern for the welfare of the group and its members, stressed the importance of job satisfaction, expressed appreciation, and sought input from subordinates on major decisions.

Initiating structure and consideration were not conceptualized as opposite ends of the same continuum but rather as separate and independent dimensions. A manager's behavior could range from high to low on both dimensions. As depicted in Figure 9.6, the two dimensions combine to form four distinct leadership styles.

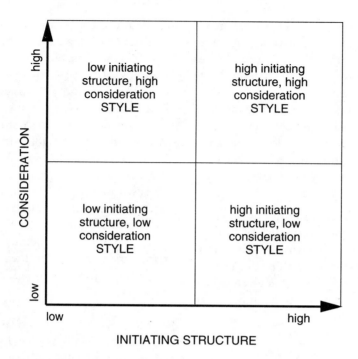

FIGURE 9.6 Ohio Leadership Study: Behaviors and Styles

Researchers hypothesized that group performance would be maximized when a manager had a leadership style that was high in both consideration and initiating structure. However, numerous follow-up studies have found little consistency between these leadership styles and group satisfaction or performance.[12,13] As with the trait research, it appeared that other factors were confounding results.

Michigan Studies. In related work, Rensis Likert and his colleagues at the University of Michigan specified two leadership behaviors: job centered and employee centered.[14] They were defined similarly to consideration and initiating structure in the Ohio studies. Investigations conducted in a wide variety of industries found that effective supervisors were employee centered. They focused on needs of the group and also established high performance goals that were determined jointly with their followers.[15,16]

The Managerial Grid. While the Ohio and Michigan studies provided the theoretical underpinnings for

the behavioral perspective, several other works are frequently referred to in most reviews of this literature. Blake and Mouton, for example, formulated the managerial grid, which they popularized in their book of the same name.[17] Their model, originally developed as a consulting tool, was extensively employed in leadership development programs during the 1960s and 1970s. The grid has two dimensions: *production orientation* and *people orientation*.

In production orientation, leadership behaviors are directive and focused on accomplishing assigned objectives or tasks. In a people orientation, by contrast, leadership behaviors are focused on enhancing the quality of manager-follower and follower-follower interactions. A manager's behavior can range from low to high in both dimensions, resulting in five different leadership styles:

1. *high production and low people orientation,* in which leadership behavior focuses exclusively on goal/task accomplishment and maximizing productivity through explicit direction and tight control

2. *high production and high people orientation*, in which leadership behavior is goal/task centered but seeks a high degree of subordinate involvement
3. *low production and high people orientation*, in which leadership behavior focuses on creating fulfilling relationships even if goal/task accomplishment and productivity suffer
4. *low production and low people orientation*, in which leadership behavior is focused on neither goal/task accomplishment nor fulfilling the needs of subordinates, and minimal energy is expended on execution of the leadership role
5. *moderate production and moderate people orientation*, in which leadership behavior focuses on balancing goal/task accomplishment with subordinate need fulfillment

Blake and Mouton contended that the high production- and high people-oriented style was most effective and resulted in the best outcomes in terms of group productivity and satisfaction, irrespective of the situation faced. Little research supports their assertion, but there is some evidence that this style is preferred by managers and perceived by them to be most effective.[18]

Bipolar Model. Robert Tannebaum and Warren Schmidt portrayed leadership behavior as a continuum that ranged from manager centered to follower centered.[19] In the manager-centered style, considerable authority is exercised and followers have little opportunity to participate in making decisions that affect them. Leadership behavior is autocratic and directive. In the follower-centered style, by contrast, the manager exercises a minimum of authority, and followers have considerable freedom to set their own goals and determine how tasks should be executed. Leadership behavior is democratic and participatory.

Contrary to previous models, Tannebaum and Schmidt, conceptualized leadership behavior as bipolar. One was either manager centered, follower centered, or somewhere in between. The authors explicitly stated that there was no one style that would be equally effective in all situations. Additionally, they noted that the effectiveness of a particular style depended upon three factors: characteristics of the manager (such as their traits/dispositions, skills, and values); characteristics of followers (such as their skills/knowledge/experience, readiness to assume responsibility, understanding of goals and tasks); and characteristics of the situation (such as time availability, nature of the problem). This model underscored the point that leadership effectiveness depended on contingencies, and they suggested some important ones. However, the model did not specifically indicate how a manager should select the most effective style in specific circumstances.

The Contingency Perspective

Beginning in the early 1960s, it became increasingly apparent that variations in leadership effectiveness and success could not be adequately explained by either traits or behaviors. Attention turned to incorporating situational characteristics, or contingencies, into leadership models. Recall that this notion was first introduced in the 1940s. A number of leadership contingency models have been developed, but only three are discussed here: leadership match, path-goal, and leadership effectiveness and adaptability (LEAD). The first two models have been the subject of considerable empirical research, and the last has been extensively employed as a teaching and leadership development tool. The section concludes with a discussion of attribution theory, which deals with the manager as a contingency.

Leadership Match Model. The first comprehensive contingency model of leadership was developed by Fred Fiedler.[20–22] His model is complex, and only a highly simplified description of it is provided here. The underlying notion is that managers are unable to alter their style to any appreciable degree. Leadership effectiveness thus depends not on fitting one's style to the situation but rather on selecting a situation that is conducive to one's style.[23]

Based on previous behavioral studies, two leadership styles were specified: task oriented and employee oriented. Fiedler developed a unique and controversial way to measure them. After completing a 20-item questionnaire, subjects were assigned a least-preferred coworker (LPC) score. The LPC score reflected the degree of regard a respondent held for the coworker whom she preferred least. Managers with low LPC scores (disregard for the least-preferred worker) were classified as having a task-oriented leadership style. Managers with a high LPC score (favorable evaluations of the coworker who was least preferred) were classified as possessing an employee-oriented style.

Fiedler also identified three situational factors: manager-follower relationship, which could be good or poor; task structure, which could be either high or low; and manager position power, which could range from strong to weak. The combined effect of these three factors is to produce situations that are favorable, moderately favorable, or unfavorable to the manager.

Based upon studies conducted with hundreds of groups in a variety of organizations, it was determined that managers with a task-oriented leadership style were most effective in situations that were either favorable or unfavorable. Managers with an employee-oriented leadership style, on the other hand, did better in situations that were moderately favorable. It is important to note that there have been several criticisms of this work, including questions regarding the validity of the LPC questionnaire and concerns that situational factors and leadership style may not be independent of one another.[24,25]

Path-Goal Model. The path-goal leadership model is based on the expectancy theory of motivation,[26,27] which addresses why someone is motivated to do one thing rather than another. Expectancy theory focuses on effort, performance, rewards, and the relationships between them, which are referred to as expectancies, instrumentalities, and valences.

An **expectancy** is the relationship between effort and performance. Sometimes a given amount of effort results in a high level of performance, at other times it does not. **Instrumentality** is the degree to which a person perceives that performance will lead to rewards. Finally, a **valence** is the strength of a person's preference for different types of rewards. According to expectancy theory, a person will be highly motivated when effort results in performance (high expectancy) and when performance leads to rewards (high instrumentality) that are valued (high valence).

Whereas expectancy theory describes these relationships, the path-goal model of leadership is interested in the factors that affect them. This model was formulated initially by Martin Evans[28,29] in the early 1970s and then refined by Robert House and Terrance Mitchell.[30,31] It has undergone constant revision over the years.

According to the path-goal model, the manager exercises influence to increase the motivation of a follower attempting to accomplish a specific goal, in a particular context, during a finite period of time. As depicted in Figure 9.7, a follower's level of motivation is a result of her perceptions of expectancies, instrumentalities, and valences. Such perceptions are affected by three sets of contingencies: leadership behavior/style, features of the work environment, and characteristics of the follower.

In most leadership situations, follower characteristics and features of the work environment are not under the direct control of the manager; in the short run they are fixed. Follower characteristics include such things as:

- needs and motives (for example, the degree to which they value achievement, power, and affiliation)
- ability to perform the task (their knowledge, skills, and experience)
- the extent to which they feel they have control over critical contingencies that affect their performance in a given situation

Features of the work environment include, among others, the extent to which the task is structured or unstructured, the amount of time available to complete the task, the nature and degree of interdependence among work group members, and a host of organizational characteristics.

The contingency most under a manager's control is his own leadership style. The dimensions that define leadership style are presently conceptualized as instrumental behavior (defining objectives and specifying the task to be performed), participatory behavior (seeking follower input on decisions that affect them), and achievement-oriented behavior (establishing goals and setting expectations that challenge followers).

Some of the implications of the path-goal theory of leadership include the following:[32]

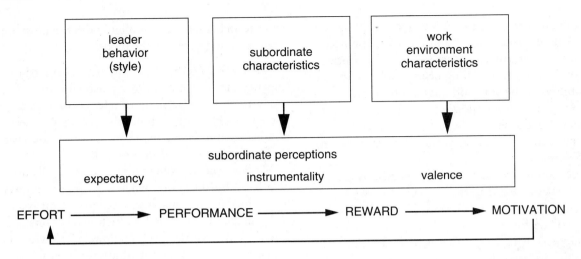

FIGURE 9.7 The Path-Goal Model

- One of the most important aspects of leadership behavior is stimulating the release of, and focusing on, follower effort and motivation.
- Often the path between effort, performance, and rewards is difficult. The manager must do everything possible to turn what is often a cow path into a well-designed, high-speed freeway.
- In leading, the manager should appreciate that individuals' valences are heterogenous, that is, people value various rewards differently. The manager should understand what a follower values and construct rewards accordingly.
- Leadership behavior should help followers define expectancies. Questions that need to be addressed include how a follower directs her effort so that it results in adequate, if not exemplary, performance and what additional knowledge, skills, and experiences a follower needs to perform assigned tasks.
- Leadership behavior should focus on clarifying instrumentalities. It is important that followers understand the specific type and amount of reward that will flow from a given level of performance.
- The manager should be mindful of how work environment characteristics affect follower expectancies, instrumentalities, and valences and the implications of these effects for the selection of a leadership style. For example, when a task is very unstructured, a fol-

lower may not know how to perform the job successfully (instrumentality is low). In such instances, a higher level of instrumental leadership behavior may be required.

The LEAD Model. The leadership effectiveness and adaptability (LEAD) model was developed by Paul Hershey and Kenneth Blanchard while they were affiliated with the Center for Leadership Studies at Ohio University.[33] According to this model, differing degrees of task- and relationship-oriented behavior (defined in a way similar to the Ohio and Michigan studies) produce four different leadership styles:

1. *high task, low relationship*
2. *high task, high relationship*
3. *low task, high relationship*
4. *low task, low relationship*

Hershey and Blanchard argued that the single most important contingency in selecting an effective leadership style is the follower's task-relevant maturity. Maturity, in turn, is a function of three traits: motivation, or energy and the will to expend it, to accomplish the assigned task; responsibility, or the willingness and ability to plan, organize, and complete the task; and competence, or the necessary knowledge, skills, and/or experience, to perform the task proficiently.

A mature follower is highly motivated, is willing and able to assume responsibility, and possesses the necessary competencies. An immature follower, by contrast, lacks motivation, is not willing or is unable to assume responsibility for the task, and does not have the necessary competencies. It is important to note that maturity is situational and task specific; a follower may be very mature performing one task yet quite immature performing another.

Hershey and Blanchard provide suggestions regarding which styles are most effective with followers having varying degrees of task-relevant maturity. If the maturity of the follower is very low, for example, the model suggests using a style that is high task- and low relationship-oriented. In this case, the follower is unmotivated, is not willing or able to assume responsibility, and does not possess the competencies necessary to perform the task. Therefore, to get the task done, leadership must be very directive. A low degree of relationship-oriented behavior is recommended so as not to reinforce the follower's state of immaturity.

If the maturity of the follower is exceedingly high, on the other hand, the model suggests using a low task- and relationship-oriented leadership style. Here the follower is extremely motivated, is very responsible, and possesses all the competencies necessary to perform the task. The follower does not need (and, in fact, would likely not appreciate) task directiveness; he or she knows what to do and how to do it. High relationship-oriented behavior is not needed because the follower gets reinforcement from other followers and from performance of the task itself. In this case, task and relationship responsibilities are totally delegated to the follower.

This is a highly abbreviated and simplified description of a model that has many more features than can be discussed here. For example, the authors provide a dynamic interpretation that focuses on sequences of leadership behaviors to enhance follower maturity. They have designed a package of questionnaires that provide feedback regarding the extent to which leaders perceive themselves employing the four different leadership styles; how others (subordinates, peers, superiors) perceive their leadership styles; and how selection of different leadership behaviors aligns with the most appropriate style suggested by the model.

Attribution Theory. One important leadership contingency factor is a manager's personal frame of reference. Attribution (sometimes referred to as perceptual or cognitive) theory[34,35] holds that a manager's selection of a leadership style depends on the way follower behavior is perceived and interpreted.

Managers notice some things and are totally unaware of others. Furthermore, what is noticed is always filtered through the manager's unique cognitive frame and reshaped by it. Based on such perceptions, a manager attributes causes to the follower's behavior. There are two general types of attributions: internal (such as lack of follower effort and/or ability) and external (such as bad luck, inadequate task design by others, and poor supervision).

According to attribution theory, a manager's choice of leadership behavior is significantly influenced by such attributions. For example, a manager might employ one leadership style if a follower's poor performance is attributed to task overload but a different one if the cause is laziness.

Attribution theorists argue that in many cases, a manager's choice of leadership style may be due more to the perceptual and cognitive frame than the "reality" of the situation itself. Indeed, reality is only what one perceives it to be. To reiterate, the basic notion of attribution theory is a simple one: an important determinant of leadership style is the manager's perceptions and attributions.[36] The resulting admonition is important: managers need to be aware of these inherent biases and develop ways to minimize them.[37]

Implications of the Contingency Perspective. There are several implications that transcend the specific models of leadership described in this section but arise from a general contingency perspective. First, the contingency perspective underscores the fact that leadership effectiveness is situational. Leadership behaviors and styles focus on influencing specific followers (whether individuals or groups), in a specific context, performing a specific task in order to accomplish a specific objective at a particular point in time. All of these contingencies vary from one situation to another. Thus, the most effective leadership style in one situation is unlikely to be the most effective in another. Three sets of contingencies seem to be most closely related to leadership effectiveness: (1) characteristics of the manager; (2) characteristics of the followers; and (3) characteristics of the immediate context in which the manager and followers interact.

Much of leadership behavior has to do with stimulating and then focusing follower motivation. Leadership effectiveness, in turn, depends more than anything else on a manager having a full and diverse repertoire of styles and being able to move flexibly among them. A manager must also possess the ability to diagnose the most critical contingencies of a given situation and select an effective leadership style for that situation based on the diagnosis. The way a specific leadership situation is diagnosed depends in no small measure on the manager's perceptions and attribution of causes to follower behavior. Finally, to be an effective leader, a manager must have ability to execute the chosen style well.

Taken to the extreme, contingency-driven leadership may appear erratic and arbitrary because the leader behaves differently toward the same followers in different situations or differently toward different followers in the same situation. This can be confusing and frustrating for followers unless the manager is very explicit about the reasons for behaving in a particular way.

A final implication from the contingency perspective relates to the theory itself. Given the large number of contingency factors and the complex ways in which they are interrelated, it is highly unlikely that a general theory of leadership effectiveness will be formulated anytime soon.

Emerging Theories and Concepts

The trait, behavioral, and contingency perspectives form the basis for most leadership theory, research, and practice. However, in the past decade, some new perspectives have been developed. In this section the transactional/transformational and charismatic theories of leadership are described. A collection of concepts that broaden the thinking regarding leadership effectiveness are also introduced.

Transactional and Transformational Leadership

James McGregor Burns, in his classic work *Leadership*, identified two types of politicians—*transactional* and *transformational*.[38] There is a growing body of literature that draws a distinction between these two leadership orientations in organizations.[39] Whereas transactional leadership attempts to preserve and work within the constraints of the status quo, transformational leadership seeks to upset and replace it.

For the most part, models of leader behavior examined up to this point view managers as involved in exchange relationships with followers. The defining characteristic of these relationships is transactional: "I'll provide what you want if you'll give me what I want." Transactional leadership entails recognizing what followers want and giving it to them if their performance warrants it. As Kuhnert and Lewis note, "In these exchanges transactional leaders clarify the roles followers must play and the tasks they must complete in order to reach their personal goals while fulfilling the mission of the organization."[40]

This sounds very much like the path-goal model of leadership, in which the manager attempts to influence follower expectancies, instrumentalities, and valences. The objective of leadership is to get followers to comply with the rules of the game as it is currently being played. The result of such transactions, proponents of the theory contend, is ordinary levels of performance.[41] Performance improvements, if they occur at all, are marginal and achieved incrementally over a long period of time.

Transformational leaders, on the other hand, are more concerned with changes than exchanges. Seeking to alter both the objective and the nature of manager-follower interactions, they motivate followers to take on difficult goals they normally would not pursue and to adopt the value that work is far more than the performance of specific duties for specific rewards. The relationship between transformational managers and their

TABLE 9.1   Transactional and Transformational Leadership

Dimension	Transactional	Transformational
Goal	maintain status quo	upset status quo
Activity	play within the rules	change the rules
Locus of reward	self (maximize personal benefits)	system (optimize systemic benefits)
Nature of incentives	tit for tat	the greater good
Manager-follower interaction	mutual dependence	interdependence
Needs fulfilled	lower level (physical, economic, and safety)	higher level (social- and self-actualization)
Performance	ordinary	extraordinary

followers is not contractual but empowering. Advocates of the transformational orientation suggest that it produces extraordinary levels of performance that flow from enrollment in a cause rather than compliance with a set of rules.[42]

Transactional and transformational modes of leadership are differentiated by the type of goals pursued, the nature of manager-follower relations, and the values to which managers and followers adhere. Table 9.1 compares the two modes of leadership with regard to these and other characteristics.

Charismatic Leadership

Charisma is derived from a Greek word meaning *divinely inspired gift* or *state of grace*. It is a characteristic that has been attributed for centuries to those with truly exceptional leadership abilities. The concept was first introduced into the organizational literature by Max Weber who defined charismatic authority as being based on " . . . devotion to the specific and exceptional sanctity, heroism, or exemplary character of an individual person . . . "[43] The concept has received renewed interest by leadership scholars who have focused on a small subset of individuals able to exercise extraordinary levels of influence.[42,44] Charismatic leadership is

> . . . a distinct social relationship between the leader and follower, in which the leader presents a revolutionary idea, a transcendent image . . . the follower accepts this course of action not because of its rational likelihood of success, but because of an effective belief in the extraordinary qualities of the leader.[45(p315)]

It has been increasingly recognized that charisma is not a characteristic of the manager per se, but rather a result of the interaction of many factors: manager and follower traits; manager and follower behaviors; the relationship between the manager and followers; situational dynamics; and the nature of the goal being sought. Table 9.2 shows a list of characteristics that have been identified in the literature.

It is clear that the present notion of charisma weaves together concepts from the trait, behavioral and situational perspectives. Because charisma is, by definition, rare as well as dynamically complex, it is exceedingly difficult to study. As a result there has been little empirical research in this area.[46]

Toward a Broader Conceptualization of Leadership Effectiveness

There has been a trend over the last decade to reconceptualize what constitutes leadership effectiveness and the factors that account for it.[47] The contention, although not always explicitly stated, is that past theorizing and research, in its quest for methodological rigor and empirically testable relationships, has been far too narrow. Writers such as Warren Bennis,[48] James Kouzes and Barry Posner,[49] Gareth Morgan,[50] Tom Peters,[51] Peter Senge,[52] and Peter Vail[53] suggest that high performance leadership depends on such things as systems thinking, visioning, facilitation of learning, and follower empowerment.

Systems Thinking. Managers lead in systems, and all systems have a number of attributes in common, even though their surface features may vary. Effective leaders possess a highly refined understanding of systems—their form, operating dynamics, and the way they achieve stability and undergo change.

TABLE 9.2 Characteristics of a Manager

Nature of the goal manager traits	• revolutionary/transformational • self-confidence • dominance • need for influence/power • strong conviction in beliefs • creativity • high energy level • enthusiasm
Leadership behaviors	• ability to conceptualize and convey transcendent vision/ideology • ability to inspire and build confidence • use of unconventional means • rhetorical fluency
Follower traits	• dependence • need to transcend self and situation
Follower behaviors	• dedication • commitment
Manager-follower interaction	• projection of idealized traits/behaviors on the leader by followers • identification (psychological fusion) of followers with leader • empowerment of followers by leader
Nature of the context	• crisis • uncertainty • transformation • deprivation

SOURCES: Dow TE. The Theory of Charisma. *Sociol Q.* 1969;10: 306–318.
Shils EA. Charisma, order and status. *Am Sociol Rev.* 1965; 30:199–213.
Wilner AR. *The Spellbinders: Charismatic and Political Leadership.* New Haven, Ct: Yale University Press, 1984.

It is difficult to think systemically. As Peter Senge notes, ". . . since we are part of the lacework ourselves, it's doubly hard to see the whole pattern . . . Instead we tend to focus on snapshots of isolated parts of the system and wonder why our deepest problems never get solved."[52(p7)] Systems thinking requires mastering a conceptual framework and associated set of analytical tools and techniques that enhance understanding of system patterns and how they can be changed.

Visioning. In order to lead, one must be going somewhere and accomplishing something that is worthy of a follower's effort. A vision is the target that beckons so that the most effective manager can lead by pulling, not pushing. Effective managers have the ability to formulate rich images of future states that are both possible to achieve and highly desirable. Ideas for the images, ranging from general dreams to specific goals, may be the product of the manager, the followers, or both.

When communicated powerfully (often through symbols and metaphors) and shared by all members of a system, a vision releases and focuses huge amounts of energy. It fosters genuine commitment and enrollment and not simply compliance.

Facilitating Learning. Organizations and the environments in which they operate are not static but constantly undergo change. Increasingly such change is revolutionary rather than evolutionary. Change of the revolutionary variety has been characteristic of health services, both public and private, during the last decade.

In periods of revolutionary change, ways of thinking and doing that have been very successful in the past rapidly lose much of their value. In such instances, organizations face two supreme challenges if they are to thrive. First, they must unlearn what is no longer relevant. Second, they must develop new mental maps, acquire new knowledge, and develop new sets of skills. Effective leaders facilitate this follower unlearning and relearning.

Empowering Followers. Rosabeth Kanter observes that, "Powerlessness corrupts. Absolute powerlessness corrupts absolutely."[54(p285)] The essence of leadership is getting things done, yet there is pitifully little that managers can do by themselves.

Followership is the reciprocal of leadership. Effective and successful leadership is dependent upon effective, successful, and empowered followers. For example, team-oriented approaches to continuously improve quality, such as total quality management (TQM) and continuous quality improvement (CQI), have attracted increasing attention; both require high levels of follower empowerment to be successful.

The effective leader views followers as the primary source of organizational creativity, energy, and value added. The effective leader creates a climate that empowers followers, so they are willing and able to make their maximum potential contribution.

An Integrative Framework

Over half a century of research has identified a number of factors that seem to be related to leadership effectiveness. Figure 9.8 shows an integrative framework that summarizes and interprets these findings. Given the concepts that have been covered in previous sections of this chapter, the model should be relatively self-explanatory. Accordingly, only selected aspects of it are highlighted here.

Leadership Style

A manager's leadership style is the pattern of behavior in which he or she engages to intentionally influence followers to accomplish a specific goal in a particular situation. Leadership style can be specified by three sets of behavioral dimensions: focus, objective, and approach.

Focus. Focus is the direction of a manager's influence. External leadership is directed outward, outside the boundary of the organizational component for which the manager is responsible (that is, toward superiors, peers, and/or individuals and groups outside the organization). Internal leadership is directed downward, toward subordinates within the manager's organizational component.

Objective. Objective is what a manager hopes to accomplish in exercising influence. A transformational leader seeks to alter the nature of both the goals sought and manager-follower interactions; the objective is to change the status quo. A transactional leader, by contrast, attempts to optimize the outcome of manager-follower exchange relationships by achieving stated goals in the most efficient manner within the "rules" as presently defined.

Approach. Approach is the way in which a manager influences followers. In exercising *directive* leadership, a manager defines the task and specifies how it is to be performed. The focus is on goal accomplishment, and little attention is paid to manager-follower or follower-follower relationships. In exercising *facilitative* leadership, a manager involves followers in making decisions that affect them, and considerable attention is paid to fulfilling their needs.

Determining Style. A manager's behavior can vary between high and low on each of these three sets of dimensions, the specific combination of which defines one's leadership style in a given situation. This is influenced by two sets of factors: the manager's traits and dispositions, knowledge and skills; and the characteristics of the followers and the situation, which are filtered through the manager's distinctive cognitive frame.

The manager's leadership style, in turn, affects the motivational dynamics (expectations, instrumentalities, and valences) of followers, who are mediated by their own cognitive frame. Leadership style affects follower efficiency, effectiveness, creativity, satisfaction, turnover, and absenteeism. The feedback loops depicted in Figure 9.8 can be either positive (reinforcing a given characteristic) or negative (dampening or extinguishing it).

All models leave out more than they include, in addition to overly simplifying complex relationships and dynamics. This one is no exception. The model is admittedly crude and incomplete. Its purpose is to stimulate thinking about how pieces of the leadership jigsaw puzzle fit together.

DEVELOPING LEADERSHIP SKILLS

There are several ways to develop leadership skills: mentoring, reflection, understanding self and followers, and continued learning.

Mentoring

Identify and work with a mentor. Leadership is a performing art; becoming proficient at it requires continual and intensive coaching from an experienced practitioner who is invested in the student's development. There is a growing body of evidence to suggest that establishing an effective mentoring relationship is one of the most important factors separating successful from unsuccessful leaders.[55] To learn more about how to work with a mentor, read *Mentoring at Work: Developmental Relationships in Organizational Life.*[56]

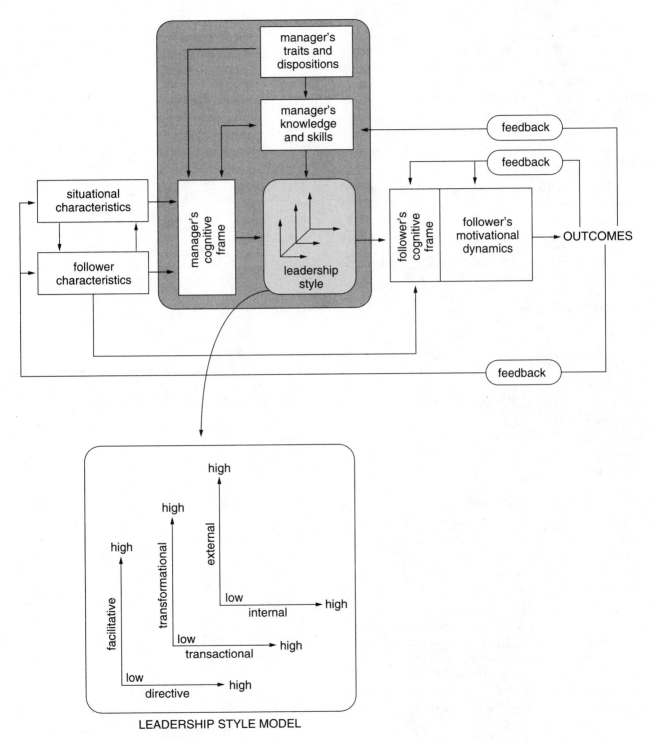

FIGURE 9.8 Leadership: An Integrative Framework

Reflecting

Become a reflective leadership practitioner. Reflection is the key to really learning from experience. Just as a winning sports team reviews its game films, so should the manager get in the habit of replaying and analyzing the leadership situations in which he or she has been involved. Schedule some time for reflection before each day ends. Reflect on both your successes and your failures. Ask yourself questions such as:

• Did you get the result anticipated? If so, why? If no, why not?
• What could or should you have done differently?
• What lesson have you learned from this experience?

Such reflection requires considerable discipline, but the effort pays off in more effective leadership.

Understanding Self

Continually seek to understand yourself better. All accomplished artists have an intimate knowledge of their tools. The primary tool of the leader is himself or herself. One particularly efficient way to gain enhanced self-understanding is through the feedback provided by self-administered leadership questionnaires, instruments, and inventories. Many are available, and much can be gained by getting feedback on leadership behaviors and style.

Understanding Followers

It is virtually impossible to lead if you don't have an in-depth understanding of your followers. Which of my actions create road blocks and sap your energy or enthusiasm? Invest the time and energy in getting to know each follower upon whom your effectiveness and success depends. Find out their aspirations, their wants and needs. Ask what they view as their most important competencies (that is, knowledge, skills, and experiences) and how the organization could make better use of them. Find out what motivates them most.

Constantly seek feedback from followers. Our perceptions of ourselves are always somewhat at odds with how others perceive us. To be an effective and successful leader you must understand the impact you are having on others. The best way to gain such understanding is to ask questions. How am I coming across? What am I doing that helps you to be as effective, creative, or satisfied as you can be?

Continued Learning

Keep reading and studying. Experience is the single best teacher of leadership, but there are not enough hours in the day to acquire all the needed experience. Some has to be gained vicariously through reading.

Reading provides the essential models, concepts, and ideas that promote much more effective and efficient learning. There are thousands of books on leadership, and hundreds of new ones are published every year. Each puts forth its own recipe for success. No one has the time, energy, patience, or money to consume even a small proportion of what is being written. The following books are recommended without reservation:

• Bennis W and Nanus B. *Leaders.* New York, NY: Harper and Row; 1985.
• Covey SR. *Principle Centered Leadership.* New York, NY: Simon and Schuster; 1990.
• DePree M. *Leadership Is an Art.* New York, NY: Doubleday; 1989.
• Gardner J. *On Leadership.* New York, NY: The Free Press; 1990.
• Kelley R. *The Power of Followership: How to Create Leaders People Want to Follow, and Followers Who Lead Themselves.* New York, NY: Doubleday/Currency; 1991.
• Kouzes JM and Posner BZ. *The Leadership Challenge: How to Get Extraordinary Things Done in Organizations.* San Francisco, Ca: Jossey-Bass; 1990.
• Senge P. *The Fifth Discipline: The Art and Practice of the Learning Organization.* New York, NY: Doubleday/Currency; 1990.
• Vail PB. *Managing as a Performing Art: New Ideas for a World of Chaotic Change.* San Francisco, Ca: Jossey-Bass; 1989.

CONCLUSION

A vital tool for the success of a public health agency is leadership. Without leadership the agency will not accomplish its mission or achieve its potential. This review illustrates some features of leadership and provides some suggestions for improving the leadership (or followership) you will provide. The key to success continues to be your commitment to being the best possible leader you can.

REFERENCES

1. Yuki GA. *Leadership in Organizations.* Englewood Cliffs, NJ: Prentice-Hall; 1981:5.

2. Katz D, Kahn RL. The taking of organizational roles. In: *The Social Psychology of Organizations.* New York, NY: John Wiley and Sons; 1966.

3. Jago AG. Leadership: perspectives in theory and research. *Management Science.* 1982;28:315–336.

4. Jennings WO. A review of leadership studies with a particular reference to military problems. *Psychol Bull.* 1947;44:540–579.

5. Stodgill RM. Personal factors associated with leadership: a survey of the literature. *J Appl Psychol.* 1948;32:35–71.

6. Stodgill RM. *Handbook of Leadership.* New York, NY: The Free Press; 1974.

7. Sartle CL. *Executive Performance and Leadership.* Englewood Cliffs, NJ: Prentice-Hall; 1956.

8. Lord AG, et al. A meta analysis of the relation between personality traits and leadership: an application of validity generalization procedures. *J Appl Psychol.* 1986;7:402–410.

9. Coska LS. A relationship between leader intelligence and leader rated effectiveness. *J Appl Psychol.* 1984;14:22–34.

10. Lewin K, et al. Patterns of aggressive behavior in experimentally created social climates. *J Soc Psychol.* 1939;10:271–276.

11. Stodgill R, Coon A, eds. *Leader Behavior: Its Description and Measurement.* Columbus, Oh: Bureau of Business Research, the Ohio State University; 1957.

12. Fleishman EA. Twenty years of consideration and structure. In Fleishman EA, Hunt JG, eds. *Current Developments in the Study of Leadership.* Carbondale, Il: Southern Illinois University; 1973:1–37.

13. Halpin AW. The leadership behavior and combat performance of airplane commanders. *J Abnorm Soc Psychol.* 1954;39:82–84.

14. Likert R. *New Patterns of Management.* New York, NY: McGraw-Hill; 1961.

15. Katz D, et al. *Productivity, Supervision and Morale in an Office Situation.* Ann Arbor, Mi: Institute for Social Research, University of Michigan; 1950.

16. Katz D, et al. *Productivity, Supervision and Morale Among Railroad Workers.* Ann Arbor, Mi: Institute for Social Research, University of Michigan; 1951.

17. Blake J, Mouton R. *The New Managerial Grid.* Houston, Tx: Gulf Publishing; 1978.

18. Blake RR, Mouton JS. Theory and research for developing a science of leadership. *J Appl Behav Sci.* 1982;18:275–291.

19. Tannebaum R, Schmidt W. How to choose a leadership pattern. *Harvard Business Review.* 1973;51(3):162–180.

20. Fiedler FE. *A Theory of Leadership Effectiveness.* New York, NY: McGraw-Hill; 1967.

21. Fiedler FE, Chemers MM. *Leadership and Effective Management.* Glenview, Il: Scott, Foresman; 1974.

22. Fiedler FE, et al. *Improving Leadership Effectiveness.* New York, NY: John Wiley; 1976.

23. Hall DD, Norgaim KE. The leadership match game: matching the man to the situation. *Organizational Dynamics.* 1976;4:6–16.

24. Stinson JE, Tracy L. Some disturbing characteristics of LPC scores. *Personnel Psychology.* 1974;27:477–485.

25. Nebeker DM. Situation favorability and perceived environmental uncertainty: an integrative approach. *Admin Sci Q.* 1975;20:281–294.

26. Vroom VH. *Work and Motivation.* New York, NY: John Wiley; 1964.

27. Porter LW, Lawler EE. *Managerial Attitudes and Performance.* Homewood, Il: Richard D. Irwin; 1968.

28. Evans MG. Leadership and motivation: a core concept. *Acad Manage J.* 1970;13:91–102.

29. Evans MG. The effects of supervisory behavior on the path-goal relationship. *Org Behav in Human Perf.* 1970;5:277–298.

30. House RJ. A path-goal theory of leader effectiveness. *Admin Sci Q.* 1971;16:321–323.

31. House RJ, Mitchell TR. Path-goal theory of leadership. *J Contem Bus.* 1974;3/4:81–98.

32. House RJ, Baetz ML. Leadership: some empirical generalizations and new directions. *Res Org Behav.* 1979;1:385–386.

33. Hershey P, Blanchard KH. *Management of Organizational Behaviors: Utilizing Human Resources.* Englewood Cliffs, NJ: Prentice-Hall; 1977.

34. Shaver KG. *An Introduction to Attribution Processes.* Hillsdale, NY: Eribaum Books; 1983.

35 Mitchell TR, et al. An attributional model of leadership and the poor performing subordinate: development and validation. *Res Org Behav.* 1981;3:197–234.

36. Lord RG, et al. A test of leadership categorization theory: internal structure, information processing and leadership perception. *Org Behav and Human Perf.* 1984;34:343–378.

37. Mitchell TR. Attributions and actions: a note of caution. *J Manage.* 1982;8(1):65–74.

38. Burns JM. *Leadership.* New York, NY: Harper and Row; 1978.

39. Tishy NM, Devanna MA. *The Transformational Leader.* New York, NY: John Wiley; 1986.

40. Kuhnert KW, Lewis P. Transactional and transformational leadership: a constructive/ developmental analysis. *Acad Manage Rev.* October 1987;12:649.

41. Liden RC, Dienesch RM. Leader-member exchange model of leadership: a critique and further development. *Acad Manage Rev.* 1986;11:618–634.

42. Bass BM. *Leadership Beyond Expectations.* New York, NY: The Free Press; 1985.

43. Eisenstadt SN. *Max Weber: On Charisma and Institution Building.* Chicago, Il: University of Chicago Press; 1968:46.

44. House RJ. A 1976 Theory of Charismatic Leadership. In: Hunt JG, Larson LL, eds. *Leadership: The Cutting Edge.* Carbondale, Il: Southern Illinois University Press; 1977: 189–207.

45. Dow TE. The theory of charisma. *Sociol Q.* 1969;10:315.

46. Conger JA, Kanungo RN. Toward a behavior theory of charismatic leadership in organizational settings. *Acad Manage Rev.* 1987;12:637–647.

47. Management's new gurus. *Business Week.* August 31, 1992: 44–52.

48. Bennis WG, Nanus BI. *Leaders.* New York, NY: Harper and Row; 1985.

49. Kouzes JM, Posner BZ. *The Leadership Challenge: How to Get Extraordinary Things Done in Organizations.* San Francisco, Ca: Jossey-Bass; 1988.

50. Morgan G. *Riding the Waves of Change: Developing Managerial Competencies for a Turbulent World.* San Francisco, Ca: Jossey-Bass; 1988.

51. Peters T. *Thriving on Chaos: Handbook for a Management Revolution.* New York, NY: Alfred A. Knopf; 1987.

52. Senge PM. *The Fifth Discipline.* New York, NY: Doubleday/ Currency; 1991.

53. Vail PB. *Managing as a Performing Art: New Ideas for a World of Chaotic Change.* San Francisco, Ca: Jossey-Bass; 1989.

54. Kelley RE. *The Power of Followership: How to Create Leaders People Want to Follow and Followers Who Lead Themselves.* New York, NY: Doubleday/Currency; 1991.

55. Dreher GF, Ash RA. A comparative study of mentoring among men and women in managerial professional and technical positions. *J Appl Psychol.* 1990;75:539–546.

56. Kram KE. *Mentoring to Work: Developmental Relationships on Organizational Life.* Glenview, Il: Scott, Foresman; 1985.

CHAPTER

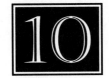

Defining Mission, Goals, and Objectives

J. Michael McGinnis, M.D.
Deborah R. Maiese, M.P.A.

The 1980s could be described as a decade-long experiment in using a form of management by objectives to foster improvements in public health. Monitoring, tracking, and publicly reporting on the first set of national health objectives[1] laid the foundation to continue the process through the 1990s with year 2000 targets.[2] By measuring health status and health outcomes over the past 15 years, the public health community, in collaboration with the private and voluntary sectors, has established a framework for action based on realistic opportunities to improve the health of the American people.

Seeking long-term improvement through the assessment of current activities and outcomes and designing actions to enhance performance are integral components of management practices traditionally used in the private sector. With the development of national health objectives, parallel processes have been put in place for monitoring and reporting on morbidity and mortality in the public sector. This chapter discusses the influence of such private sector management techniques on the nation's public health agenda. It describes efforts since 1979 by the United States Public Health Service (PHS) to develop, monitor, and track goals and objectives to improve the health of all Americans.

INTRODUCTION

The nation's health promotion and disease prevention agenda lays out a long-term plan of what can be achieved. It charts a course with enough breadth but sufficient specificity that groups throughout the country have joined in an unprecedented collective effort. Constituencies not often traditionally involved in health were engaged in setting the goals and objectives and now work on their attainment. Consider the following examples:

- Transportation departments, highway safety groups, and advocates of safe and drug-free driving have joined forces with state and local health departments to achieve tremendous success in reducing fatal motor vehicle crashes, particularly those involving alcohol.
- In schools and on college campuses across the country, students are being educated about risky behaviors that lead to both current and future morbidity in an effort to prevent disease, disability, and premature death.
- In work sites, employers are instituting policies for smoke-free workplaces and offering blood pressure and cholesterol screenings.
- National organizations of health professionals, agencies that focus on specific diseases, and organizations that represent specific population groups are using the nation's health objectives to frame program activities, conferences, publications, and strategic plans.

In short, the goals and objectives included in *Healthy People 2000* provide a sense of what can be accomplished collectively if Americans apply themselves to health promotion and disease prevention.

GUIDING MANAGEMENT THEORY

Since the 1950s, **management by objectives (MBO)** techniques have been applied and pursued by the private sector. During the 1980s, governments at all levels—federal, state, and local—began using MBO techniques to guide their activities and measure their performance. At the same time, **total quality management (TQM)** techniques began to emerge from the private sector, influencing public sector management systems. The release of the *National Performance Review Report* in 1993 introduced a new lexicon of management principles for reinventing government.[3]

Management by Objectives

The phrase *management by objectives* was first introduced by Peter Drucker in 1954 in his book *The Practice of Management*.[4] As a consultant to General Motors

and in his lectures at New York University and before management groups, Drucker, a political scientist, refined the concept of management by objectives. As corporate organizations grew in size, he reasoned, the need for decentralizing work occurred. In fact, as George Odiorne later observed, "MBO [is] a natural product of decentralization."[5]

The widespread use of the MBO concept ensued among large firms throughout the United States in the 1960s and 1970s. With the increasing size and complexity of government, MBO was introduced in the public sector in the 1970s and 1980s to improve efficiency in operations.

According to Odiorne, MBO is

. . . a process whereby the superior and subordinate managers of an organization jointly identify its common goals, define each individual's major areas of responsibility in terms of results expected, and use these measures as guides for operating the unit and assessing the contribution of each of its members.[5]

As a framework, MBO lays out the steps necessary to achieve a desired outcome. Even the objective-setting process, in and of itself, has merit. Creating the objective through the involvement of senior management can establish acceptance. In turn, assignments, strategies, program activities, and tasks undertaken to accomplish the objective can be more efficiently organized and performed with greater focus through the application of MBO. Odiorne also stated that "objectives start at the top of the organization and that people understand what is expected of them, where their help and resources will come from, how much freedom they have, and what reporting relationships are necessary."[5] He went on to emphasize that MBO "enhances the possibility of obtaining coordinated effort and teamwork."[5]

In addition to "stating what is expected for everyone involved, MBO measures what is actually achieved."[5] Defining the outcome, beyond the expenditure of resources to achieve it, makes for meaningful program reviews. "Three forms of review are important in MBO—the periodic audit, the continuing review, and the annual review."[5]

Financial accounting and program operations audits comprise one component of review. Continuing reviews are done on a frequent basis (for example, daily, weekly, monthly, or quarterly) and involve an examination of results with the objectives. Annual reviews encompass all objectives. Taking stock of whether objectives were met or fell short of the target helps in setting objectives for the next year.

The Influence of Engineering Quality Control

In 1950, in post-World War II Japan, Dr. W. Edwards Deming, a statistician, lectured on statistical quality control to the Union of Japanese Scientists and Engineers. His ideas on quality found widespread acceptance in Japan. Now, in the United States, Deming's theories are being practiced in both public and private sectors.

Dr. Deming identified 14 obligations of top management, one of which was that goals and objectives "create a constancy of improvement."[6] They provide a new philosophy for leadership by helping to "break down barriers between staff areas" and "put everybody . . . to work to accomplish the transformation."[6] His management approach combines planning, scientific study, and measurement with the human side of leadership—respect, empowerment, and involvement of the workforce.

Total Quality Management

Another American, Joseph M. Juran, also took the engineering concept of statistical quality control and transformed it into what has come to be called total quality management. Together the teachings of Deming and Juran have spurred quality circles and quality improvement activities throughout private industry and government.

For example, in 1987 Congress created the Malcolm Baldrige National Quality Award to stimulate American businesses to strive for quality performance. As another example, in 1988 the Federal Quality Institute began awarding the Presidential Quality Award for quality performance in the federal government. The criteria for these awards are leadership, information and analysis, strategic quality planning, human resource development and management, management of process quality, quality and operational results, and customer focus and

satisfaction. The current literature is also full of references to quality improvement and quality management.

Total Quality Management In Health

In 1987, a quality improvement project with a specific health focus was begun, called the National Demonstration Project (NDP) on Quality Improvement in Health Care. Teams from 21 health care organizations paired with 21 experts in quality management for a yearlong effort at answering the question, "Can the principles and techniques of industrial quality control be applied successfully to health care?"[7]

In the initial two-day meeting in Boston, the "arranged marriages"[7] between health care and quality management began with the health care participants sharing a problem in their organization, one they thought could be addressed through quality management techniques. Over an eight-month period, the NDP teams designed 21 projects and organized staffs, of from two to twenty people to address the problem and monitor and report on their performance.

Of the 21 projects, 15 were successful. A common element of successful projects was that top managers were engaged in the quality improvement effort. Such high-level participation was a stronger predictor of success than the size or structure of teams, such as steering committees and working groups. NDP tackled "nonclinical processes, such as business systems, information systems, registration and access systems, and systems for deploying staff"[7]—systems for which TQM had already been tried. At the end of the initiative, 11 of the projects had made "some form of institutional commitment to continuing quality improvement as an operating strategy."[7]

Based on his experience with NDP, Dr. Donald Berwick called on leaders in health—providers, health care institutions, and purchasers—"to establish and hold on to a shared vision of a health care system undergoing continuous quality improvement."[8] In a 1989 article, Dr. Berwick pointed out that:

> . . . developing sound measurement tools that represent common values . . . aggregating data centrally to help caregivers learn from each other . . . and continuously

reviewed statements of how one intends to behave are essential to quality improvement.[8]

In 1992, Drs. Kaluzny, McLaughlin, and Simpson from the University of North Carolina observed that "TQM applications in the public sector and particularly in public health agencies have been limited."[9] They note exceptions, however: the Model Standards Program, the Assessment Protocol for Excellence in Public Health, and the national health objectives are all tools for public health agencies "to assess their potentials and goals for health outcomes."[9]

Clinical Practice Guidelines. Another tool for health providers and managers to use in rendering high quality care is clinical practice guidelines. Jencks and Wilensky noted that "the federal government and professional groups have started an expanding process of developing and publishing practice guidelines, which provide a potential focus for quality improvement efforts."[10]

In this same article, Jencks and Wilensky observe that "modern quality management methods are statistically oriented and data intensive . . ."[10] The *Guide to Clinical Preventive Services,*[11] published in 1989 by the United States Preventive Services Task Force, continues to provide guidance for clinicians in determining the medical effectiveness and appropriateness of interventions. Recently published guidelines by the Agency for Health Care Policy and Research on benign prostate hyperplasia[12] and the management of cancer pain[13] have consumer versions and quick reference guides for clinicians that accompany the complete practice guideline.

In releasing the 1994 Joint Commission on Accreditation of Health Care Organizations (JCAHCO) Accreditation Manual for Hospitals, Dr. Dennis S. O'Leary said, "this represents the initial and long-awaited transition of Joint Commission standards from those that focus on capability to those that focus on actual performance."[14] He called this a "radical change in the framing of standards based expectations."[14] The title of the education program of JCAHCO is Continuous Quality Improvement Tools and Techniques for Patient Care and Process Improvement and the manual is called *Using Quality Improvement Tools in a Health Care Setting.* With the introduction of continuous quality improvement by the largest accrediting organization, widespread use of TQM in the private health care sector is likely.

Conclusions

Two conclusions emerge from this discussion of management theory and practice. First, setting goals and measurable objectives is essential for guiding an organization. The agenda-setting function is critical to providing vision and ongoing direction. To be successful, the mission statement should be set through a participatory process with high-level management providing leadership but with all affected parties engaged in the process. Second, the goals must be measurable, broadly understood, and communicated to the participants involved. Continuous feedback vis-à-vis the targets serves to motivate the participants toward achieving the agreed-upon goals.

APPLYING MANAGEMENT THEORY TO HEALTH

Setting the framework is the first obligation of management. Thus, the process of establishing goals and objectives is the starting point of this section.

Setting Specific Goals and Objectives

The 1990s health objectives set forth general prerequisites that pertain to the successful application of the process of setting objectives.[15] The prerequisites include the ability to define a problem clearly, the existence of a discrete constituency, the availability of an effective intervention methodology, the social acceptability of that methodology, and a means to track progress.[12]

Five types of objectives are used in business—**outcome, strategy, productivity, marketing,** and **innovation.** These business objectives are applied to health in Table 10.1 and elaborated on in the following sections.

Outcome Objectives

For business, the outcome, or bottom line, is measured in profits. For the health care sector, it is mea-

TABLE 10.1 Comparison of Management Objectives in Business and Health Sectors

Objective Classes	Business Applications	Health Applications
Outcome	Profits	Morbidity and mortality reduction
Strategy	Product type and mix	Risk factors
Productivity	Labor/capital mix	Scope of services
Marketing	Client attitudes and awareness	Public/professional attitudes and awareness
Innovation	Product improvement	Surveillance, evaluation, and research

SOURCE: McGinnis JM. Setting nationwide objectives in disease prevention and health promotion: The United States experience. In: Holland WW, Detels R, Knox G, eds. *Oxford Textbook of Public Health.* Vol. 3. New York, NY: Oxford University Press; 1985.

sured in reduced morbidity and mortality. In order to attain these goals, programs must be designed to take the organization step-by-step towards them.

Strategy Objectives

This, in turn, requires that strategies be constantly reviewed and modified. For a car manufacturer to increase profits, for example, the types of automobiles produced may need to be revised to meet the demographics and demands of consumers. A production strategy that results in more vans and fewer station wagons, or more sports cars and fewer sedans, may help to increase profits.

In health, the strategies pursued to reduce premature death, disease, and disability depend on the identification of risk factors. The research literature has established, for example, that smoking, fatty diets, and exposure to environmental hazards are risk factors for cancer. Therefore, to minimize the risk of developing cancer, strategies might involve messages to teens not to start smoking and cessation programs for people who have already taken up smoking; promoting dietary changes, such as reducing calories from fat and increasing intake of fruits and vegetables; and educating the public on measures to protect themselves from potentially hazardous materials, such as asbestos.

Productivity Objectives

Productivity objectives in business address the mix of labor and materials used in the production of goods and services. The unit cost of a particular product

must be kept at a particular level in order to sell at a competitive market price that still provides the company with coverage of their costs and a margin of return on investment.

In health, productivity addresses the scope of the interventions and services that are offered, the extent to which they reach the targeted audience, and the appropriateness and the acceptability of the services to the clients. These health objectives encompass both services offered on a one-to-one basis and population-based services.

Marketing Objectives

Marketing objectives have been widely used by business to create demand for products. The power of advertising has steered consumer taste and product purchases for years. With the advent of public service announcements, the public health community started conveying messages to impact on risky behaviors, such as not driving drunk and not using illegal drugs. Similarly, in the personal care delivery arena, the advertising of health plans and the services of individual hospitals and practitioners has become commonplace in the 1990s.

Innovation Objectives

Innovation objectives for business involve investments in research and development. Examples include the automation of product assembly, the use of computer-controlled manufacturing systems, and the adoption of information technologies that link work sites and speed the transfer of information among them. Investment in technology enhances the efficiency of process and reduces the unit costs of products. Such is also the case in the health sector, where health services research, biomedical research, and prevention research are expanding the science and knowledge base for clinicians, scientists, and public health practitioners.

Agreeing on Important Issues

Applying these objective-setting principles to public health began at the federal level in 1979, when the first national health goals were set. With the publication of *Healthy People: The Surgeon General's Report on Health Promotion and Disease Prevention,*[1] national goals for mortality reductions by 1990 were established for four age groups:

1. a 35 percent reduction in infant mortality (under the age of one year);
2. a 20 percent reduction in childhood deaths for children ages 1 through 14
3. a 20 percent death rate reduction for ages 15 through 24 years
4. a 25 percent death rate reduction for ages 25 through 64 years

For those over age 65, the goal was a reduction of the number of disability days and improvements in the quality of life.

Moving beyond mortality reductions, the Public Health Service began examining factors that determine health status. Biological, behavioral, environmental, and social risk factors were identified, along with interventions and services that had been shown scientifically to be effective in reducing morbidity and mortality. This analysis was performed by a government planning group charged with developing background papers on 15 disease prevention/health promotion areas.

The papers were reviewed by 167 experts from outside the government, including health care providers, academics, state and local health officials, and staff members of voluntary health associations. These experts and PHS officials were also invited to participate in a 1979 conference in which the first draft of objectives for the 15 priority areas were developed. The pa-

pers and draft objectives were published in the *Federal Register* and circulated to more than 2,000 groups and individuals for review and comments.

The result of this collaboration was *Promoting Health/Preventing Disease: Objectives for the Nation.*[16] This 1980 publication set 226 objectives with targets for achievement by 1990. The objectives addressed:

- improvement in health status
- reduction of risks to health
- increases in public and professional awareness
- improvement and expansion of health services and protective measures
- enhancement of surveillance measures and research efforts.

Consensus had been reached on what could be achieved through health promotion and disease prevention interventions.

Broadening Ownership

The 1990 objectives laid the foundation for a similar agenda for the year 2000. Over a three-year period beginning in 1987, the year 2000 objectives were developed. The Institute of Medicine of the National Academy of Sciences, under a cooperative agreement with PHS, established the Healthy People 2000 Consortium. National membership organizations from across the country were invited to join in the development of the nation's prevention agenda. Initially, the Healthy People 2000 Consortium consisted of 157 organizations and all state and territorial health departments.

These groups were invited to present testimony at seven regional hearings held in Los Angeles, Birmingham, Houston, Seattle, Denver, Detroit, and New York City. A panel consisting of PHS regional health administrators, other PHS officials, and members of the Association of State and Territorial Health Officials heard both the invited testimony and testimony from the public. Another 18 minihearings were held in conjunction with annual meetings of national health organizations. Through these hearings, a total of some 800 pieces of written and oral testimony were collected.

The testimony was used by PHS lead agencies to draft prevention objectives for the year 2000. The objectives were developed in accordance with the following principles:

- They had to be credible, reflecting available scientific evidence.
- They had to continue to track the 1990 objectives.
- They had to be compatible with goals already adopted by federal agencies and health organizations.
- They had to be relevant and understandable to a broad audience.
- They had to be measurable.

A draft of the objectives, entitled *Promoting Health/ Preventing Disease: Year 2000 Objectives for the Nation,* was released in September 1989. The cover letter to this working document noted that "more than 7,000 people have contributed to the process of developing the year 2000 objectives."[17] Public comment continued to flow into PHS on this draft and was used by the lead agencies to create a consensus document that has come to be known as the nation's prevention agenda.

Healthy People 2000

This unprecedented collaboration of states, academics, private and voluntary organizations, and interested members of the public built *Healthy People 2000: The National Health Promotion and Disease Prevention Objectives.*[2] Released on September 6, 1990, *Healthy People 2000* launched a ten-year national initiative to improve the health of Americans. Clearly, the goals and objectives in *Healthy People 2000* are not simply those of the federal government. They are national in scope and will require the combined efforts of the public and private sectors if they are to be achieved.

Goals

The three goals of *Healthy People 2000*[2] are to:

1. increase the span of healthy life
2. reduce health disparities among Americans
3. achieve access to preventive services for all Americans

Objectives

The 300 objectives of *Healthy People 2000* are organized into 22 priority areas. They address health promotion, health protection, and preventive services. Health promotion relates to individual lifestyle choices, such as exercise, diet, and other behaviors. Health protection refers to environmental and regulatory measures, such as occupational safety and food and drug safety. Preventive services include counseling, screening, and other interventions in a clinical setting. Surveillance and data systems, in which ongoing efforts to achieve the objectives are tracked, provide the foundation for all of the priority areas and thus become priority area number 22, as shown in Table 10.2.

The order of the 22 priority areas shown in the table does not reflect difference in their importance.

There are also four age-related mortality objectives, for infants, children, adolescents and young adults, and adults, which continue to track the objectives for these age groups that were set in 1979. For older adults, a new measure called *years of healthy life* has been developed. This measure incorporates self-reported assessments of disabilities and injuries and concentrates on extending that portion of life that is free of impairments.

The *Healthy People 2000* objectives are of three types:

1. **health status**—objectives to reduce death, disease, and disability
2. **risk reduction**—objectives to reduce the prevalence of risks to health or to increase behaviors known to reduce such risks
3. **services and protection**—objectives to increase comprehensiveness, accessibility, and/or quality of preventive services and preventive interventions

In *Healthy People 2000,* there is explicit recognition that "progress toward a healthier America will depend substantially on improvements for certain populations that are at especially high risk."[2] High risk was defined in terms of worse rates or a differing trend in rates than for the overall population. To this end, *Healthy People 2000* sets specific targets to narrow the gap between the overall population and those population subgroups

TABLE 10.2 *Healthy People 2000* Priority Areas

Health Promotion

1. Physical Activity and Fitness
2. Nutrition
3. Tobacco
4. Alcohol and Other Drugs
5. Family Planning
6. Mental Health and Mental Disorders
7. Violent and Abusive Behavior
8. Education and Community-Based Programs

Health Protection

9. Unintentional Injuries
10. Occupational Safety and Health
11. Environmental Health
12. Food and Drug Safety
13. Oral Health

Preventive Services

14. Maternal and Infant Health
15. Heart Disease and Stroke
16. Cancer
17. Diabetes and Chronic Disabling Conditions
18. HIV Infection
19. Sexually Transmitted Diseases
20. Immunization and Infectious Diseases
21. Clinical Preventive Services

Surveillance and Data Systems

22. Surveillance and Data Systems

Age-related Objectives

Children
Adolescents and Young Adults
Adults
Older Adults

SOURCE: *Healthy People 2000: National Health Promotion and Disease Prevention Objectives.* Washington, DC: US Dept of Health and Human Services; 1990. PHS publication 91-50212.

that now experience above-average incidence of death, disease, and disability.[2]

Race-, ethnic group-, gender-, and age-specific population targets were set in *Healthy People 2000* to focus the attention of the nation on eliminating health disparities among Americans. Targets for people with low incomes and people with disabilities were also established. A total of 223 specific population targets were developed based on national data indicating that

a particular population group was at greater risk than the overall population.

An example of a special population target can be found in the maternal and infant health priority area addressing prenatal care. As shown in Table 10.3, this is a service and protection objective. The 1987 baseline showed that, overall, 76 percent of pregnant women were receiving first trimester care. However, African-American, Native American, Alaskan Native, and Hispanic women all had lower rates of prenatal care. The year 2000 target is to increase prenatal care in the first trimester of pregnancy to 90 percent for *all* women.

Keeping Leadership Active

Leadership goes beyond setting and implementing goals. Leaders must also assure that progress towards achieving goals is monitored. This is the only route to success in health as it is in business.

Beginning with the 1990 health objectives for the nation, an agency of the Public Health Service was assigned by the assistant secretary for health with lead responsibility for each of the 15 priority areas. Lead agencies regularly reported to the assistant secretary on their efforts to achieve the 1990 targets.

TABLE 10.3 Prenatal Care Targets

Services and Protection Objective

14.11 Increase to at least 90 percent the proportion of all pregnant women who receive prenatal care in the first trimester of pregnancy. (Baseline: 76 percent of live births in 1987)

Special Population Targets

Proportion of Pregnant Women Receiving Early Prenatal Care

		Percent of Live Births	
		1987 Baseline	2000 Target
14.11a	Black women	61	90
14.11b	American Indian/ Alaska Native women	60	90
14.11c	Hispanic women	61	90

SOURCE: *Healthy People 2000: National Health Promotion and Disease Prevention Objectives.* Washington, DC: US Dept of Health and Human Services: 1990. PHS publication 91-50212.

Lead agencies in the PHS continue to coordinate each *Healthy People 2000* priority area. Each lead agency forms a work group with representatives from federal and state governments as well as private and voluntary agencies. In collaboration with the National Center for Health Statistics at the CDC, each work group explores data sources, assuring that surveillance systems are in place to track the objectives. Approximately every two years, the lead agency presents a progress review to the assistant secretary for health.

Reviewing Progress Towards Healthy People 2000 *Objectives*

At the annual progress review, every objective is reviewed. Baseline data are presented and compared with the most current statistics available to show whether progress is being made or whether the nation is losing ground. Such data are indispensable for tracking the objectives. Following each progress review, a report summarizing the meeting with the assistant secretary for health is prepared and widely distributed. This report gives the current data on the objectives as well as the strategies that PHS will pursue to overcome barriers and make progress on reaching the objectives.

To complement priority area progress reviews, the assistant secretary began in 1992 cross-cutting progress reviews on special populations. In these reviews, the focus has been on narrowing health status disparities among population groups. The first was on Native Americans and Alaska Natives. This was followed by reviews on women, Hispanics, and adolescents and young adults.

Other Leadership Activities

PHS agency heads have been asked by the assistant secretary for health to support the national objectives in all appropriate grant announcements. To this end, PHS grant announcements describe the PHS commitment to achieve the objectives and reference the specific priority areas supported by the grant.

Healthy People 2000 is a promissory note to the nation from the PHS, with states and other levels of government and the private sector to provide needed services and resources. The national health objectives

process is a nonpartisan effort guided by five assistant secretaries for health. As the coordinator of *Healthy People 2000*, the PHS has the obligation of developing and implementing strategies to achieve the objectives and of identifying barriers to success. Part of the PHS role is to monitor, track, and report, on a periodic basis, the results of these collaborative efforts, informing the nation of the health status of the American people.

Building in Accountability

An important component of any management-by-objectives approach is regular monitoring and reporting. PHS began its public reporting with *The 1990 Health Objectives for the Nation: A Midcourse Review,* which was published in November 1986. The preface to this review states that "having passed the midpoint of the decade, we are in a position to take our bearings, to assess our progress to date, and to consider necessary midcourse corrections."[18] The publication provided a report card on each of the 226 objectives, showing both the good news—where improvements in health were being made—and the bad news—where increasing incidence of disease required redoubled efforts to reach the targets. Indeed, the introduction to the report suggested that the review serve as the "raw material for agenda-setting for the next five years."[18] Thus, the report not only celebrated successes, but it also called attention to preventable conditions that could be reduced, if not eliminated, by further action.

Specific Results of the 1990 Objectives

The results of the 1990 objectives were released in an article[19] in the *Journal of the American Medical Association,* which was co-authored by the five assistant secretaries for health involved in the national health objectives process. The results are noteworthy in that the nation met or exceeded three out of the four mortality goals for 1990.

For infant mortality, the 1990 rate (based on provisional data) was 9.1 per 1,000 live births, which is very close to the target of 9.0. This is an impressive 34 percent decline over the decade of the 1980s.

For children ages 1 through 14, the goal was exceeded—30.1 deaths per 100,000 population as compared to a target of 34.0 per 100,000. This achievement is partly due to reduced motor vehicle crash deaths, in turn the result of increased use of seat belts and child safety seats.

For adolescent and young adults ages 15 through 24 years, the nation fell short of the 20 percent mortality target, in part because of unintentional injuries, particularly fatal motor vehicle crashes, and, in part, because of increases in intentional injuries, particularly violent ones. Homicides and suicides did not decline as much as had been projected. The decade ended with a reduction in mortality of 11 percent for adolescents and young adults.

For adults ages 25 through 64 years, the 1990 data showed the death rate to be reduced to 400.4 per 100,000 population, which essentially achieves the target of 400. Behavioral changes that reduced cigarette smoking, high blood cholesterol, and high blood pressure contributed to the declines in heart disease and stroke.

The goal of reducing the days of disability for persons over 65 years of age was not met. Restricted activity days totaled on average 31.4 days in 1990, compared with the goal of 30 days.

In June 1992, *Health, United States, 1991, and Prevention Profile*[20] provided an overall summary of the results of the 1990 objectives:

- Thirty-two percent of the 1990 targets were attained.
- Progress was made on another 30 percent of targets.
- Fifteen percent declined or showed no progress.
- The remaining 23 percent could not be evaluated because of insufficient data.

Thus, the decade ended with successes but with some important challenges for the 1990s as well.

Specific Results of the Year 2000 Objectives

Health, United States, 1992, and Healthy People 2000 Review[21] provided the first of what will be a decade-long series of annual profiles on the nation's year 2000 health objectives. A section for each priority area presents the baseline data, target figures, and the most current data available for each objective. Data issues are also discussed. The first year report indicates that of the 332 objectives, the nation:

- met 4 percent of the targets
- made progress on another 28 percent
- lost ground on 15 percent
- had mixed results on 4 percent
- had data for baselines for 4 percent
- had no new data within which to evaluate progress on 28 percent
- had no data for the baseline on 10 percent

Another publication that helps describe national progress is *Prevention '91/'92*,[22] a series of biennial reports of the Department of Health and Human Services on prevention-related activities of the federal government. The series provides comprehensive listings of the prevention programs of the Department of Health and Human Services—the Administration on Aging, the Administration for Children and Families, the Health Care Financing Administration, and the nine agencies of the Public Health Service.

Beginning with the 1991/1992 edition, *Prevention* used the national health promotion and disease prevention objectives from *Healthy People 2000* as the framework for presenting federal prevention efforts. The resources spent on prevention by the Department of Health and Human Services are organized by *Healthy People 2000* priority areas. This inventory shows fiscal years 1989 and 1990 actual spending and fiscal year 1991 estimated spending for prevention to be nearly $15 billion.[22]

In addition, other agencies of the federal government report on their own prevention programs. Prevention activities are broadly defined. They include, for example, environmental programs of the Environmental Protection Agency; the Women, Infants and Children (WIC) program of the Department of Agriculture; and the Occupational Safety and Health Program of the Department of Labor.

Lessons from Objective Setting

Many valuable lessons have been learned from the process of setting objectives. The year 2000 objectives, for example, have given the nation a realistic sense of what can and ought to be achieved in health. The objectives have provided a vehicle for reporting current status, trends, and ultimately whether success or failure results. Public accountability is probably the most noteworthy feature of the management-by-objectives approach.

The objectives have helped to unify the public health community and have served as a stimulus for long-range planning at the federal, state, and local government levels, as well as in the private and voluntary sectors. The objectives-setting process has also helped decision makers identify priorities in the management of scarce resources.

Continuous quality improvement in health has proven to be useful and a worthwhile part of the national agenda. Individuals are taking personal responsibility for their behaviors—including wearing seat belts, practicing safer sex, and not drinking and driving. Health providers are increasingly aware of the importance of providing counseling, screening, testing, and appropriate referrals for clinical preventive services. Health care institutions, public health agencies, and community health agencies are adopting their own objectives to guide their actions and unify their purposes.

In addition, national objectives help promote interactions with new constituencies. For example, the public health community has made great progress with the transportation sector in reducing fatal traffic accidents through the use of child safety seats and seat belts. As another example, nutrition objectives have created new partners in the food processing industry, leading to food-labeling reform. New linkages are also being made in school health, and, of course, work site health promotion continues to strengthen the link between health and business.

State Actions

Objective setting and monitoring have been ongoing in state health departments for the past 15 years. A 1985 survey by the George Washington University Intergovernmental Health Policy Project found that 18 states had developed their own objectives for 1990.[23] By the end of the 1980s, nearly all of the states had adopted health objectives. As of July 1994, 37 states and the District of Columbia had completed their own disease prevention and health promotion objectives for the year 2000. Another 15 states and Puerto Rico continue to pursue the development of year 2000 objectives.

Each state has developed its own plan with its own emphasis. Rhode Island and Illinois, for example, have undertaken extensive baseline assessment to document the current health status of residents and circulated these assessments for public review and comment. New Jersey conducted a telephone survey to ascertain directly from residents their own health status and health priorities for the state, leading to development of *Healthy New Jersey 2000.*[24]

Some states have drafted documents that parallel the 22 priority areas. *Healthy Arkansans 2000,*[25] for example, includes all 22 of the national priority areas. Other states have adopted only selected priority areas and objectives. In some instances, the states share the same year 2000 targets as the nation; in others, they have set their own targets, sometimes seeking a greater amount of change, at other times a slightly less ambitious target, than the *Healthy People 2000* objectives. The various uses of the objectives and the multitude of approaches that the states have pursued are indicative of the flexibility and versatility of the national prevention agenda.

State Action Contacts

A network of healthy people 2000 state action contacts was established to serve as liaisons between the Public Health Service and the states, in order to foster communication among states and to serve as the central point of contact for residents on year 2000 activities. In some states, the state health official serves as the contact point; in others, this responsibility is held by staff in the health statistics or planning branch.

Healthy People 2000 State Action,[26] a PHS publication, highlights the scope of activities in the states relating to the year 2000 objectives and lists all the action contacts. Making the objective setting and monitoring processes accessible to the public helps to increase citizen participation.

Grants to States

To enhance state capacity to assess progress toward *Healthy People 2000* objectives, in 1992 the CDC's

National Center for Health Statistics (NCHS) awarded five-year grants to Maine, Oregon, Texas, Ohio, Iowa, North Carolina, and Utah. Through funding of the Kansas Health Foundation, Kansas is also participating in this state assessment initiative. Grant programs are based on the recognition that data for policy development and program management is a critical component of any objectives process.

Community Actions

Healthy People 2000 has also provided a framework for communities to undertake their own health status measurements and establish year 2000 objectives. Local objective setting is taking place throughout the country in cities big and small. In California, for example, Los Angeles, San Francisco, Pasadena, Chico, and Escondido are participating in *Healthy Cities 2000* initiatives. Through the framework of their community-planning efforts, health needs of the community's people are identified, and interventions that are acceptable to the community are publicized. *Healthy People 2000* offers a blueprint for communities to effectively bring together their resources to make a difference in health.

Healthy Communities 2000

To assist communities in planning and implementing prevention agendas, the American Public Health Association and CDC jointly developed *Healthy Communities 2000: Model Standards, Guidelines for Community Attainment of Year 2000 National Health Objectives*[27] and a *Guide to Implementing Model Standards.*[28] Linked to *Healthy People 2000* objectives, the model standards provide public health agencies with a tool for determining a community's priority health issues. In its preface, *Model Standards* calls for public health to be accountable for its shortfalls as well as its successes.[28] The Institute of Medicine, in its 1988 publication, *The Future of Public Health,* also called on state public health agencies to establish statewide health objectives, appropriately delegate power to localities, and hold the localities accountable.

APEX/PH

The Assessment Protocol for Excellence in Public Health (APEX/PH)[29] was developed by the National Association of County Health Officials in collaboration with the American Public Health Association, the Association of Schools of Public Health, the Association of State and Territorial Health Officials, and the United States Conference of Local Health Officers, with support from CDC. APEX/PH provides public health agencies with a tool for assessing their organizational capacity to meet community needs, assessing community health status, setting priorities for action, and monitoring progress toward achieving established objectives.

Healthy Community Program

The National Civic League offers a Healthy Community Program, which includes workshops and printed materials, such as a *Healthy Communities Directory, Healthy Communities Handbook,* and *Radon Action Handbook.*

Summary and Examples

All of these tools were designed to help public health leaders work with citizens to develop and implement their own community health objectives. These activities are under way on a statewide basis in Indiana, Colorado, California, North Carolina, and South Carolina. For example, the Colorado Trust awarded $4.5 million to 13 cities in that state to undertake a healthy communities effort. In California, there are 10 charter healthy cities participating in the California Healthy Cities Project. Both North Carolina and South Carolina have county coalitions coordinating health promotion and disease prevention efforts throughout their states.

Healthy People 2000 Consortium Actions

All 50 states and more than 300 national organizations in the Healthy People 2000 Consortium are working with their local chapters and members to reduce preventable death and disability, enhance the quality life years of the American population, and greatly reduce health disparities. Organizations such as the National Medical Association, the American Indian Health Care Association, and the National Coalition of Hispanic Health and Human Services Organizations (COSSMHO) are examples of consortium members who are using their expertise, contacts, and resources to contribute to national efforts to improve the health of all Americans.

Will the federal government meet the year 2000 objectives? Certainly not on its own. The resources of government are insufficient to set in motion the changes that need to take place in America's homes, classrooms, clinics, and work sites if the objectives are to be achieved. The Healthy People 2000 Consortium, membership organizations, and the health departments of all 50 states and U.S. territories are needed to achieve the nation's prevention agenda.

In 1992, the Healthy People 2000 Consortium Action report showed the diverse mix of activities being sponsored by some 140 organizations, almost half of them private and voluntary sector members, in their efforts to achieve the year 2000 objectives.[30] The theme of the 1993 meeting of the Healthy People 2000 Consortium and a PHS publication, *Turning Commitment into Action,* attempts to communicate ideas on how consortium members are using the national health objectives to stimulate their members.[31]

The National Association of Children's Hospitals and Related Institutions (NACRI), for example, had as its 1992 theme *Give It a Shot,* a year-long effort to increase the number of immunized children. In 1991, NACRI's work centered on a campaign to reduce unintentional injuries. September was bicycle safety month, for example, with safety tips for children riding their bicycles to school. The colder months had a theme of fire safety.

As another example, the American Indian Health Care Association has transformed *Healthy People 2000* into a user-friendly handbook entitled *Promoting Healthy Traditions.*[32] Using Indian artwork, quotations, and references to tribal healing traditions, the book raises such questions as: Who are the healers in your community? How would you describe the concept of wellness? What are the healthy traditions of your community? The handbook is a very positive example of a communication tool that has been adapted to reach Native Americans, emphasize the importance of health, and help them develop their own health objectives.

Congressional Actions

Congress has enacted three laws that incorporate *Healthy People 2000* objectives:

1. the Maternal and Child Health Block Grant that required reporting of the amount of money spent for each of the national objectives for maternal and infant health
2. the Indian Health Care Improvement Act (Public Law 94-437), which directs the Indian Health Service to annually report the allocation of resources to the 61 year 2000 objectives on the health status of Native Americans
3. the 1993 authorization of the Preventive Health and Health Services Block Grant, in which Congress linked activities undertaken by the states with these grants to year 2000 health objectives.

The last law requires each state to have a plan that specifies the populations to be served by its activities and programs and estimates the number of personnel and resources that will be used. States must also agree to measure the extent of progress being made toward improving the health status of the population. In consultation with the states, DHHS is developing sets of data for uniformly defining health status for purposes of the year 2000 health objectives.

The Minority Health Improvement Act

Although not specifically tied to *Healthy People 2000,* the Minority Health Improvement Act of 1990 (Public Law 101-527) has provisions for improving the level of racial and ethnic health data obtained through national surveys conducted by NCHS. The act also requires states to increase the amount of information obtained from vital records and to establish grant programs to improve minority statistics.

Seven cooperative agreement grants were awarded under this section of the act on September 30, 1992.

These include such projects as one to improve the collection of health data for northwest Native Americans, another to establish an oral health database in South Texas, and a third to examine whether national health data systems accurately portray the health status of Asian-Americans.

Next Steps

As the midpoint of the decade approaches, the PHS has begun a review of the nation's disease prevention and health promotion objectives. The review consists of target revisions based on selected baseline revisions, new special population subobjectives, language modifications in existing objectives, and new objectives. Incorporating new science, new information, and new data will help to strengthen the nation's prevention agenda by making it more relevant to today's health issues. Announced at an October 1993 Healthy People 2000 Consortium meeting, the midcourse review provides consortium members with an opportunity to continue to work together to make the necessary midcourse revisions that will enhance the nation's prevention agenda.

Reinventing Government

The emphasis for government in the 1990s is customer satisfaction—identifying the customers the government is serving and determining whether the customers' needs are in fact being met. This focus on the customer is found in Deming's 14 management principles discussed earlier. An executive order from President Clinton directs agencies of the federal government to conduct customer surveys to identify, from the perspective of the recipient, both strengths and weaknesses in products or services.

National Performance Review

The September 1993 release of The National Performance Review report, *Creating a Government that Works Better & Costs Less,*[3] was the culmination of a government-wide effort at "creat[ing] a culture of public entrepreneurship."[3] With more than 1,000 recommendations, this report, produced largely through the input

of government employees, charts a course for the federal government based on TQM principles:

> First, we will require that all federal agencies put customers first by regularly asking them how they view government, what problems they encounter and how they would like services improved. We will ensure that all customers have a voice and that every voice is heard.[3]

In addition, the National Performance Review recommends that government processes be examined and evaluated. To this end, the Department of Health and Human Services established a Continuous Improvement Steering Committee chaired by a deputy secretary. The committee identified its work as strategic planning, human resources management, and customer services integration. It has surveyed employees for their suggestions and created a database assuring the confidentiality of employees' suggestions for improvements. It has also published a newsletter to keep its constituents, the employees of DHHS, informed.

A State-Level Example

The Alaska Native Medical Center of the Indian Health Service is working to deliver medical services more efficiently and in ways that better serve and satisfy their customers, using a National Performance Review rationale: "Without a performance target, managers manage blindly, employees have no guidance, policymakers don't know what's working, and customers have no idea where they may be served best."[3]

A Final Example

The Government Performance and Results Act of 1993 required that ten federal agencies begin in 1994 a three-year strategic planning pilot. At the end of this demonstration period, all federal agencies were required to develop strategic plans.

CONCLUSION

As the National Performance Review report stated, "governance means setting priorities, then using the immense power of the federal government to steer what happens in the private sector."[3] Improving the health of Americans is an enormous challenge requiring renewed and ongoing effort. Every state and organization needs to continue to be a partner with the United States Public Health Service to attain the *Healthy People 2000* goals.

Through a consensus development process, the nation has a disease prevention and health promotion agenda for the year 2000. *Healthy People 2000* has charted a course for improved health for all Americans. It provides individuals, public health workers, health care providers, schools, and employers with the opportunity to develop local objectives intended to change behaviors, cultures, and environment. Through the Healthy People 2000 Consortium there is the potential for reaching millions of Americans with effective disease prevention and health promotion messages and activities, and thereby making a profound impact on the health of the American people.

REFERENCES

1. *Healthy People: Surgeon General's Report on Health Promotion and Disease Prevention.* Washington, DC: US Dept of Health, Education and Welfare; 1979. PHS publication 79-55071.

2. *Healthy People 2000: National Health Promotion and Disease Prevention Objectives.* Washington, DC: US Dept of Health and Human Services; 1990. PHS publication 91-50212.

3. *Creating a Government that Works Better and Costs Less.* Washington, DC: National Performance Review; September 1993.

4. Drucker, P. *The Practice of Management.* New York, NY: Harper & Row; 1954.

5. Odiorne GS. *MBO II. A System of Managerial Leadership for the 80s.* Belmont, Ca: Fearon Pitman Publishers, Inc.; 1979.

6. Deming E. *Out of Crisis.* Cambridge, Massachusetts. Massachusetts Institute of Technology Center for Advanced Engineering Study; 1982.

7. Berwick D, Godfrey A, Roessner J. *Curing Healthcare.* San Francisco, Ca: The Jossey-Bass Publishers Health Series; 1991.

8. Berwick D. Continuous improvement as an ideal in healthcare. *N Engl J Med.* January 5, 1989;320:53–56.

9. Kaluzny A, McLaughlin C, Simpson K. Applying total quality management concepts to public health organizations. *Public Health Rep.* May-June 1992;107:257–264.

10. Jencks S, Wilensky G. The health care quality improvement initiatives, a new approach to quality assurance in Medicare. *JAMA.* August, 1992;268:900–903.

11. US Preventive Services Task Force. *Guide to Clinical Preventive Services.* Baltimore, Md: Williams & Wilkins; 1989.

12. *Prostate Hyperplasa: Diagnoses and Treatment.* Rockville, Md: Agency for Health Care Policy and Research; February 1994. Publication No. 94-0582.

13. *Management of Cancer Pain.* Rockville, Md: Agency for Health Care Policy and Research; March 1994. Publication No. 94-0592.

14. Press Release of the Joint Commission on Accreditation of Healthcare Organizations: Accreditation Manual for Hospitals. Oakbrook Terrace, Illinois; 1992.

15. Holland WW, Detels R, Knox G, eds. *Oxford Textbook of Public Health.* Second edition. Volume 3. New York, NY: Oxford University Press; 1985.

16. *Promoting Health/Preventing Disease: Objectives for the Nation.* Washington, DC: US Dept of Health and Human Services; 1980.

17. *Promoting Health/Preventing Disease: Year 2000 Objectives for the Nation.* Washington, DC: US Dept of Health and Human Services; September 1989.

18. *The 1990 Health Objectives for the Nation: A Midcourse Review.* Washington, DC: US Dept of Health and Human Services; 1986.

19. McGinnis JM, Richmond J, Brandt E, Windom R, Mason J. Health progress in the United States. Results of the 1990 Objectives for the Nation. *JAMA.* November 1992;268:2545–2552.

20. *Health, United States, 1991 and Prevention Profile.* Hyattsville, Md: National Center for Health Statistics, US Dept of Health and Human Services; 1992. PHS publication 92-1232.

21. *Health, United States, 1992 and Healthy People 2000 Review.* Hyattsville, Md: National Center for Health Statistics, US Dept of Health and Human Services; 1993. PHS publication 93-1232.

22. *Prevention '91/'92.* Washington, DC: US Dept of Health and Human Services; 1992.

23. *Status Report: State Progress on 1990 Health Objectives for the Nation.* Washington, DC: Public Health Foundation; 1988.

24. *Healthy New Jersey 2000.* Trenton, New Jersey: New Jersey Department of Health; 1993.

25. *Healthy Arkansas 2000.* Little Rock, Arkansas: Arkansas Department of Health; 1991.

26. *Healthy People 2000 State Action.* Washington, DC: US Dept of Health and Human Services; 1992.

27. *Healthy Communities 2000: Model Standards, Guidelines for Community Attainment of Year 2000 National Health Objectives.* Washington, DC: American Public Health Association; 1991.

28. *Guide to Implementing Model Standards.* Washington, DC: American Public Health Association; 1991.

29. *APEX/PH, Assessment Protocol for Excellence in Public Health.* Washington, DC: National Association of County Health Officials; 1990.

30. *Healthy People 2000 Consortium Action.* Washington, DC: US Dept of Health and Human Services; 1992.

31. *Turning Commitment into Action.* Washington, DC: US Dept of Health and Human Services; 1993.

32. *Promoting Healthy Traditions Workbook: A Guide to the Healthy People 2000 Campaign.* St. Paul, Minnesota: American Indian Health Care Association; 1990.

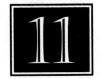

CHAPTER

11

Community Assessment and Empowerment

Martha F. Katz, M.P.A.
Marshall W. Kreuter, Ph.D.

In 1923, C.E.A. Winslow offered this remarkably comprehensive and visionary definition of public health (emphasis added by authors of the present chapter):

> Public health is the science and the art of preventing disease, prolonging life, and promoting physical health and efficiency through organized community efforts for the sanitation of *the environment,* the control of *community infection,* the education of the individual in the principles of personal hygiene, *the organization of medical and nursing services* for the early diagnosis and preventive treatment of disease *and the development of the social machinery* which will ensure to *every individual in the community* a standard of living adequate for the maintenance of health.[1]

The phrases have been put in italics to accentuate Winslow's obvious understanding of public health's interdependence with the community institutions and community members it is obliged to serve.

This chapter addresses the role of the community in public health by:

- examining the rationale for greater attention to community participation in public health practice,
- providing an overview of four well-documented public health approaches, each of which is designed to strengthen a particular aspect of community-based strategies to promote health and prevent disease
- recommending specific actions that can be taken at the national, state, and community levels to enhance community participation in the planning and implementation of public health programs

WHY TAKE A COMMUNITY PARTICIPATION APPROACH?

Consider the events that ultimately give rise to the development of public health intervention programs.

For example, an outbreak or unexpected increase in the incidence of a health problem is detected, the problem is studied, and special efforts are made to identify the **causal chain** of factors associated with the problem. Then efforts are made to determine what links in that chain, if modified, will prevent, control, or end the problem.

Epidemiologic studies of heart disease, cancer, injuries, suicide, homicide, alcohol and drug abuse, teen pregnancy, preventable problems associated with aging, and AIDS do reveal causal chains, but they are very complex chains. The precursors of health problems such as these are characterized by a convoluted combination of biological, behavioral, environmental, political, and economic factors. Although policy and program planners may propose scientifically sound solutions, they are unlikely to become reality if they do not take into account the role that values, beliefs, and similar intangible factors play in the development and resolution of public health problems in individuals and communities.

Conceptualizing the Community

For some, the word **community** conjures up images of formal political structures governing an area with geographic boundaries—a village, town, or city. This geopolitical view is appropriate when the primary concern is to delimit areas of service coverage or to establish the parameters for an epidemiologic study. However, in the context of public health practice, community is a much more complex concept. It also must take into account the people who live within those boundaries and their many attributes—their formal and informal social networks and support systems, the norms and cultural nuances that define their uniqueness, their institutions, their politics, their belief systems.

The Role of Intangible Factors in Health

In our approach to preventive or curative health planning, we must take into account the character of the community. We must be cognizant of the intangible factors which bind communities together or that separate one community from another. The knowledge of these

intangibles is critical to successful community empowerment. They profoundly influence health status, risk factors, health behavior and community characteristics.

What we know, what we think, what we feel, what we believe, whom we believe in, whom we trust, our personal capacities, our role models, our resources and means, our environment and conditions of living—all of these factors influence our health status. Furthermore, few if any of these factors are constant. Not only do they vary over time, but they also vary from country to country, state to state, community to community, neighborhood to neighborhood, and person to person.

The Significance of Community Participation

Modern philosophers and ethicists have argued that solutions to the complex problems of the 1990s and the twenty-first century demand a shift in perspective from individual rights to community responsibilities.[2,3] The commitment to shared values and common goals empowers a group to tackle complex issues that seem insurmountable when faced by individuals. This is why the community, or more specifically, the dynamic interplay required to generate a legitimate community approach, must play a central role in the way we approach planning, for either preventive or curative health services.

The justification for making community participation an essential ingredient for effective public health practice can be summed up as follows:

- Nonmedical factors, including volitional behaviors, social conditions, and community values, have a major influence on health status.
- Because improvements in health status are not likely to yield to medical interventions alone, planners and policy makers must actively engage the public in the development of solutions to health problems.
- Policy development, one of the three core functions of public health,[4] requires active involvement of the people who are affected by public health programs and policies.

STANDARDIZED APPROACHES FOR COMMUNITY-ORIENTED PUBLIC HEALTH PROGRAMS

The scientific literature is rich with studies in community-based chronic disease prevention and control.[5–10] Some of these studies have documented measurable reductions in morbidity and mortality;[5,7,11,12] others have documented desired decreases in specific health risks.[13,14] The health benefits of community-based approaches are by no means limited to populations with means; positive outcomes have been detected from community interventions targeting a variety of ethnic and socioeconomic population groups.[15–17]

As the encouraging results from these demonstration studies surfaced at international, national, state and provincial, and local professional meetings, public health workers wanted to know more in order to integrate the strategies into their own local practices. Several organized efforts were made to create standardized approaches to meet the practical needs of those responsible for community health.

In this section, four such standardized approaches are reviewed. Each of the four addresses an important but complementary element of community-based public health approaches:

1. *Healthy Communities 2000: Model Standards:* develops consensus on measurable outcome and process objectives for public health programs.
2. *APEX/PH:* organizes a collaborative health infrastructure.
3. *PATCH:* expands community participation in setting health priorities and the design and implementation of outcome-oriented intervention programs.
4. *Healthy Cities:* activates political and organizational institutions for public health promotion.

Healthy Communities 2000: Model Standards

Shared values and goals are a valuable magnet for drawing together diverse community groups that have different missions and obligations. By working together to set health targets for the whole community, leaders from different community organizations can find common ground that enhances their ability, individually and collectively, to improve the health of their communities. *Healthy Communities 2000: Model Standards*[18] was developed to provide an understandable set of health status and process objectives that a group of local health leaders could easily adapt to the needs of their community.

Published in 1991, *Healthy Communities 2000* is the product of a collaborative effort by the American Public Health Association, the Association of State and Territorial Health Officials, the National Association of County Health Officials, the United States Conference of Local Health Officers, the Association of Schools of Public Health, and the Centers for Disease Control and Prevention. The current (3rd) edition is designed to be a community guidebook for achieving the national health objectives for the year 2000. It is a tool that can be used by local leaders to engage a whole host of players in setting achievable health priorities.

Some of the key features of *Healthy Communities 2000* include:

- fill-in-the-blank format that allows community leaders to use local data to set local targets
- topics and chapters that match the priority areas and age groups used in *Healthy People 2000*
- a summary of 11 practical steps for using the model standards (See Figure 11.1)
- a set of objectives for community implementation, using the framework recommended in the 1988 Institute of Medicine report, on *The Future of Public Health*[4]
- sample indicators for measuring achievement of the objectives, using data sources likely to be available at the local level

Healthy Communities 2000 is unique because it provides practical tools for applying the national health objectives to local needs and priorities. The report strongly encourages a consensus process to involve community leaders in developing local goals, outcome and process objectives, and implementation plans to achieve the objectives. Rather than prescribing a unique

11. Monitor and evaluate the effort on a continuing basis

 10. Develop and implement a plan of action

 9. Develop community-wide intervention strategies

 8. Select outcome and process objectives that are compatible with local priorities and Healthy People 2000 objectives

 7. Determine local priorities

 6. Assess health needs and available community resources

 5. Organize the community to build a stronger constituency for public health and establish a partnership for public health

 4. Assess the community's organizational and power structures

 3. Develop an agency plan to build the necessary organizational capacity

 2. Assess the lead health agency's organizational capacity

 1. Assess and determine the role of one's health agency

FIGURE 11.1 The Eleven Steps of Model Standards. SOURCE: *Guide to Implementing Model Standards.* Washington, DC: American Public Health Association; 1993:8–9.

process for establishing these objectives, it recommends that local public health leaders use and adapt as necessary the proven models for building relationships within the community—tools such as APEX/PH, PATCH, and Healthy Cities.

APEX/PH: Assessment Protocol for Excellence in Public Health

The complexity of contemporary health problems makes it virtually impossible for any single health entity to effectively protect and promote the public's health. For this reason, all public sector health agencies need to join forces with other private and voluntary health organizations to achieve the common goal of improved public health. APEX/PH was designed to facilitate that process.[19]

APEX/PH was developed under the joint leadership of the National Association for County Health Officials and the Centers for Disease Control and Prevention to assist local health departments in assessing their ability

to meet the public health needs of their communities. Its key features include:

- strong leadership by the local health officer to insure successful implementation of the process
- internal evaluation of the organizational capacity of the health department
- involvement of community representatives in identifying their health problems and priorities
- development of a community plan for improving the ability of the health department to meet the community health needs that were identified through the assessment process

Users of APEX/PH are encouraged to undertake a three-part process: (1) organizational capacity assessment, (2) community process, and (3) completing the cycle.

Organizational Capacity Assessment

During this first part of the process, the health department director and an internal self-assessment team study their authority to operate, carry out community assessment and policy development, and manage major administrative areas, such as financial, personnel, and program management. Through this process, the health department creates an organizational action plan, that includes setting priorities for correcting perceived weaknesses.

Community Process

The second part of the APEX/PH process calls for the formation of a community advisory committee to identify priority health problems and set health status goals and objectives. Following collection of community health data, the advisory committee can develop objectives tailored to local needs. This is done by adapting the national health objectives identified in *Healthy People 2000* and the sample community-level objectives in *Healthy Communities 2000: Model Standards.* The product of this community advisory committee is a community health plan that is data-based and represents the concerns of members of the community.

Completing the Cycle

The third part of the APEX/PH process is the implementation of the community health plan by the local health department. To complete the cycle, the local health officer must pull together the results of the organizational action plan and the community health plan to assure that the local health department's capabilities match the needs identified by community leaders. The overall goal is for the health officer to use these two plans to improve the management of the health department and enhance its ability to serve the community.

Overview

APEX/PH provides a practical, step-by-step process for local health departments to assess their capacity to build stronger partnerships with their community. It focuses on administrative capacity, basic organizational structure, and the role of the agency in the community. The health department's involvement with members of the community is institutionalized through the establishment of the community advisory committee and periodic evaluation of the community health plan.

PATCH: Planned Approach to Community Health

In the early 1980s, public health literature reported that community-based prevention programs were effective in the reduction of population risks associated with coronary heart disease.[5,7,16,20,21] Based on these encouraging findings, the Centers for Disease Control and Prevention developed PATCH as a means of translating the methods reported in these studies into a protocol that state and local health agencies could use to plan, deliver, and assess the progress of community-based health promotion programs.[22]

Conceptually, PATCH was influenced by:

1. PRECEDE, the health education planning framework[23]
2. literature on community organization and community development[24-26]
3. guidelines outlined in the second edition of *Model Standards: A Guide for Community Preventive Health Services*[27]
4. CDC's traditional modus operandi of working through state health agencies in the application of health promotion and disease prevention programs

An overriding concept in both the development and continuing evolution of PATCH has been the commitment to make the process practical. It was to address this need for practical, health-promotion field training that shaped the original design of PATCH as a skills-based training program. The goal was for health education leaders in state health agencies to work in concert with their local level counterparts to establish community health education programs.[22] Based on accounts of applications since 1986, the time required from initiation to implementation of specific interventions in a PATCH program is from eight to twelve months.

Before reviewing PATCH further, it is useful to raise a caveat. Breaking a dynamic process into its component parts sometimes helps to understand that process. However, in such a dissection, it is easy to lose sight of the interdependence and synergy that makes the process work. When applying PATCH—or, indeed, any of the four approaches discussed in this section—recall the wisdom of the familiar aphorism, "don't miss the forest for the trees."

Phases of PATCH

There are five general phases in the PATCH process:

1. *mobilizing the community:* establishing a strong core of representative local support and participation in the process
2. *collecting and organizing data:* gathering and analyzing local community opinion and health data for the purpose of identifying health priorities
3. *choosing health priorities:* setting objectives and standards to denote progress and success
4. *interventions:* designing and implementing multiple intervention strategies to meet objectives
5. *evaluation:* continuous monitoring of problems and intervention strategies to evaluate progress and detect need for change

The PATCH System

The PATCH program itself can be seen as a system, as a working partnership among the CDC, the state health agency, and the community.

Role of the CDC. The CDC provides resource materials, training, and technical assistance concerning PATCH to providers of health promotion, such as state health agencies. The CDC also maintains a national network so that information can be readily shared among communities using PATCH.

Role of the State Health Agency. The state health agency provides training and technical assistance to communities that use PATCH. It also provides a PATCH state coordinator who:

1. establishes a team within the state health agency with expertise in chronic disease prevention, health education, epidemiology, statistical analysis, and other areas pertinent to community health
2. identifies actual and in-kind resources for each community

3. assists the community with data issues
4. reports progress to the CDC
5. serves as the state contact for the national PATCH network

Organizational Infrastructure

Within the community, the organizational infrastructure of PATCH consists of three partners: the community group, the steering committee, and the local coordinator.

The Community Group. The community group collects data, selects health priorities and objectives, and helps with program implementation. The ideal group is composed of 20 to 40 members, including private citizens, political office holders, lay leaders, and representatives of service and social organizations, health organizations, private companies, and other community groups.

The Steering Committee. The steering committee is composed of six to twelve members of the community group. It helps the local coordinator guide the PATCH process and identifies resources to support the priorities specified by community members.

The Local Coordinator. The local coordinator is generally a health educator from a local health agency. The coordinator guides PATCH activities for the community, and helps with many tasks, particularly working towards building skills among the community members participating in PATCH and thereby fostering community ownership of the process.

Overview

Although participation in PATCH is voluntary, it has formidable coverage in the United States. Thirty-nine states and territories have received PATCH training, and there are 130 community programs operational (oral communication from Nancy Watkins, National Center for Chronic Disease Prevention and Health Promotion, March 16, 1994). A listing of detailed PATCH program descriptions are available in several published sources.[28]

Healthy Cities

The *healthy cities* concept emerged in the mid-1980s as a demonstration project of the European office of the World Health Organization. Against the backdrop of two important WHO initiatives, the Alma Ata Declaration and the health for all strategy, the original healthy cities project used six cities as sites to test the feasibility of creating public, private, and voluntary partnerships. The goal was to coalesce the collective energies of these intersectoral groups into coordinated, broad-based approaches to the resolution of health-related problems.[29] The intuitive merits of the healthy cities approach created great interest internationally as work of the process was communicated through the normal health communication channels.

Descriptions of the key elements of the healthy cities project, including recommended strategies for implementation, are described in a series of three documents, the *WHO Healthy Cities Papers*.[29] The general goal of healthy cities is to enhance the health of cities, their environments, and their people. The philosophic heart of the process is grounded in two key principles of *Global Strategy of Health for All by the Year 2000*:[30] multisectoral collaboration and public participation.

Participation Criteria

To participate officially in the healthy cities program, applicant cities must gain approval from the appropriate WHO infrastructure according to their general criteria.[31] Specifically, cities must:

- have a specific political commitment at top city level to develop and implement a healthy cities strategy
- be prepared to secure the necessary resources to pursue and implement their healthy cities strategies
- be prepared to participate actively in the exchange of experiences within the European healthy cities network
- be prepared to actively support the development of a national healthy cities network

Healthy City Actions

Each healthy cities project is expected to have a strategy and the capacity to carry out interrelated actions in order to attain four major goals: assure organizational capacity, enhance information, establish initiatives, and create networks.

Assure a Strong Political Managerial Organizational Capacity. The major task here is to recruit and bring together high-level groups of decision makers who represent the main agencies and organizations within the city. This action will enable planners to establish contact with the political power base of the city.

Enhance the Production and Dissemination of Relevant Information. This task is usually manifested by carrying out a community diagnosis with an emphasis on detecting inequalities in health status within the city. The WHO recommends that a variety of local area data be collected, including the public perception of the community's health.

Establish Intersectoral Initiatives. The primary action here is to build sound, working links among local institutions, including all levels of schools, health organizations (public, private, and voluntary), and all organizational entities with a direct or indirect interest in health.

Create Effective Networks and Secure Mutual Aid. The theme of networking is omnipresent in healthy cities. An important premise is that by creating connections between a wide variety of health-related institutions around a common theme of *health for all,* organizational interdependence will be nurtured, and both human and material resources for health that are often underutilized can be enhanced.

Healthy Cities Projects in Action

Although originating in Europe, the healthy cities model has been applied in cities and communities the world over. In a 1992 publication edited by Ashton,[32] accounts of healthy cities case studies are chronicled in Europe, Canada, the United States, Australia, and several South American countries.

In the United States, the project has been implemented in Indiana and California. Healthy Cities Indiana uses both the Canadian and WHO models; the

California Healthy Cities Project is very similar to the original WHO model.

Healthy Cities Indiana. The ultimate goal of Healthy Cities Indiana is to provide data-based information to policy makers and to promote healthy public policies. The project attempts to promote a public-private partnership in public health through a process of community leadership development and social change. Several communities in Indiana participate in the process and have implemented action plans.

The California Healthy Cities Project. The California Healthy Cities Project is a statewide effort to improve the health status of the state's residents through the promotion of a public policy approach to health. The project has been implemented in seven cities. Each city has focused on health priorities and implemented interventions that address these priorities. The next challenge will be to move beyond initial interventions to institutionalizing the healthy cities concept within the cities' continuing practices. It is anticipated that the project will be institutionalized at the statewide level to continue providing services while reaching other cities.

Toronto's Healthy City Project. In Canada, the city of Toronto's Healthy City Project has been under development since the Healthy Toronto 2000 Workshop was held in 1984. In 1986, a strategic planning committee began developing a strategy to make Toronto a healthy city. The overall goals of the Toronto strategy are to:

- reduce inequities in health opportunities
- create physical environments supportive of health
- create social environments supportive of health
- advocate a community-based health services system.

The primary objectives of the Toronto project are communication (to both city government staff and the public), project development, and research and analysis.

Healthy Cities and PATCH: Similarities and Differences

It is useful to compare the healthy cities and PATCH approaches. Even though they appear quite similar, they are based on different underlying assumptions.

Similarities

The processes followed by the healthy cities and PATCH strategies share many common threads. For example, both emphasize the importance of creating a supportive infrastructure. In addition, the role of the Healthy Cities Project office within the WHO regional office in Copenhagen is somewhat analogous to the role played by the Division of Chronic Disease Control and Community Intervention at the Centers for Disease Control and Prevention in Atlanta, Georgia. Both offices:

- have the responsibility for providing program guidelines and support materials
- promote intersectoral collaboration (the strengthening of collaboration among health organizations and agencies horizontally within the community)
- promote active participation among community members
- emphasize the importance of collecting site-specific data, including perceptions of health status among residents of the target population
- provide guidelines and technical support for data collection
- provide opportunities for training
- provide guidelines and support for program evaluation

Differences

The major differences between the two models become clear when the assumptions that underlie each approach are examined.

Healthy Cities Assumptions. Originators of the Healthy Cities Project were influenced by the historical reality that 75 percent of Europeans reside in large cities or towns that collectively bear the largest burden of ill health. It was argued that large cities typically are ineffective and inefficient in responding to health problems because their public sector health organizations are compartmentalized and disjointed. For this reason, the healthy cities approach places a clear, a priori emphasis on two conceptual issues: that inequity is a universal deterrent to health and that changes in both public policy and health policy should be a first priority.

This emphasis is reflected in the healthy cities themes. From 1988 to 1992, the Healthy Cities Project proposed annual themes. The purpose of these themes was to give direction to project cities as they formulated and carried out the activities of their respective programs. The themes were

- inequities in health
- strengthening community action and developing personal skills
- supportive physical and social environments
- reorienting health and environmental services and public health
- healthy policies for healthy cities

PATCH Assumptions. PATCH, on the other hand, has tended to focus on smaller population entities, either small-to-moderate communities or neighborhoods within cities. In some instances, PATCH has been applied in larger populations, but only when there was evidence that sufficient intersectoral collaboration was in place to give the program a chance for success.

PATCH begins by combining the principle of community participation with the diagnostic steps of applied, community-level epidemiology. This approach is understandable given that epidemiology is the science foundation of the Centers for Disease Control and Prevention. The PATCH process may begin at one of two points: (1) when community members analyze health problems within their community and determine which of those problems pose the greatest threat to the health of the community and are amenable to health promotion/disease prevention actions; or (2) when community members are mobilized to address preselected health problems. The issues of inequity and policy formation then surface as the community assesses its problems and determines the root causes.

CONCLUSION: FINDING SYNERGY BY PLAYING TO STRENGTHS

Each of the approaches discussed in this chapter is often associated with a particular aspect of community-based health promotion and disease prevention. For example:

- The healthy communities 2000 approach provides detailed guidance on how to construct practical, clear objectives that address priority public health problems.
- APEX/PH promotes the use of the healthy communities 2000 process and offers a guide for local leadership to assess their resource and regulatory readiness in preparation for delivery of programs and interventions to the community.
- The PATCH program features a theory-based planning road map for practitioners to use in the development of community interventions. The approach acknowledges the importance of community member involvement in the decision-making process.
- Healthy cities provides a clarion call for acknowledging that the root causes of health problems can be found in social conditions and that a political presence and action is, in most cases, an essential ingredient for redressing health problems.

As important as these individual features are, it is paramount that practitioners realize that all four approaches share two common assumptions: (1) that the community is the nexus for effective health promotion and disease prevention; and (2) that direct, unencumbered communication with the public is critical for health promotion success. The word communication is seminal here because it requires engagement, participation, and shared understanding.

Thus, as practitioners review these approaches as well as other effective community-based strategies reported in the literature, the question should not be which approach is the best one. Rather, it should be how can one draw from the collective strengths of all the approaches? The challenge to develop a working knowledge of contemporary community-based strategies and apply creative energy to selecting the approach, or component thereof, that is most appropriate will vary depending on the unique needs and circumstances of the community in question.

ACKNOWLEDGMENT

The authors with to thank Kathy Cahill, Brick Lancaster, and Charles Nelson of the National Centers for Disease Control and Prevention for their thoughtful suggestions and critique of the manuscript. Thanks also to Susan Arduino and Patti Foote for their preparation of the manuscript. Finally, a special thanks to Dexiu Zhang for her very capable research assistance on the PATCH and healthy cities portions of the chapter.

REFERENCES

1. Winslow CEA. *The Evolution and Significance of the Modern Public Health Campaign.* New Haven, CT: Yale University Press; 1923. (Reprinted in: *J Public Health Policy;* 1984)

2. Callahan D. *What Kind of Life: The Limits of Medical Progress.* New York, NY: Simon and Schuster; 1990.

3. Etzioni A. *The Spirit of Community: Rights, Responsibilities, and the Communitarian Agenda.* New York, NY: Crown Publishers Inc; 1993.

4. Institute of Medicine, Committee for the Study of the Future of Public Health. *The Future of Public Health.* Washington, DC: National Academy Press; 1988.

5. Kotchen JM, McKean HE, Jackson-Thayer S, et al. The impact of a high blood pressure control program on hypertension control and CVD mortality. *JAMA.* 1987;257:3382–3386.

6. Centers for Disease Control. Increasing breast cancer screening among the medically underserved, Dade County, Florida. *MMWR.* 1991;40(16):261–263.

7. Puska P, Missinem A, Tuomilento J, et al. The community-based strategy to prevent coronary heart disease: conclusions from the ten years of the North Karelia Project. *Annu Rev Public Health.* 1985;6:147–193.

8. Vartiainen E, Pusko P, Tossavainen K, et al. Prevention of non-communicable diseases: risk factors in youth—the North Karelia Youth Project (1984–1988). *Health Prom.* 1986;1(3); 269–283.

9. Lando HA, Loken B, Howard-Pitney B, Pechacek T. Community impact of a localized smoking cessation contest. *Am J Public Health.* 1990;80:601–603.

10. Pierce JP, Macaskill P, Hill A. Long term effectiveness of mass media led antismoking campaigns in Australia. *Am J Public Health.* 1990;80:565–569.

11. Morisky DE, Levine DL, Green LW, Shapiro S, Russell RP, Smith CR. Five year blood pressure control and mortality following health education for hypertensive patients. *Am J Public Health.* 1983;73:153–162.

12. Heath GW, Leonard BE, Wilson RH, Kendrick JE, Powell KE. Community based exercise intervention: Zuni Diabetes Project. *Diabetes Care.* 1987;10:579–583.

13. Altman DG, Flora JA, Fortmann SP, Farquhar JW. The cost effectiveness of three smoking cessation programs. *Am J Public Health.* 1987;77:1562–1565.

14. Forsyth MC, Fulton DL, Lane DS, Burg MA, Krishna M. Changes in knowledge, attitudes and behavior of women participating in a community outreach education program on breast cancer screening. *Patient Education and Counseling.* 1992; 19(3):241–250.

15. Lacey LP, Phillips CW, Ansell D, Whitman S, Erbie N, Chen E. An urban, community based cancer prevention screen and health education intervention in Chicago. *Public Health Rep.* 1989;104(6):536–541.

16. Fortmann SP, Williams PT, Hulley SB, et al. Does dietary health education reach only the privileged? The Stanford three community study. *Circulation.* 1982;66(1):77–82.

17. Michielutte R, Dignan MB, Wells AB, et al. Development of a community cancer education program: the Forsythe County, North Carolina cervical cancer prevention project. *Public Health Rep.* 1989;104:542–551.

18. *Healthy Communities 2000: Model Standards. Guidelines for Community Attainment of the Year 2000 National Health Objectives.* Washington, DC: American Public Health Association; 1991.

19. *APEX/PH Assessment Protocol for Excellence in Public Health.* Washington, DC: National Association of County Health Officials; 1991.

20. Farquhar J, Maccoby N, Wood P. Education and communication studies. In: Holland W, Detels R, Knox G, eds. *Oxford Textbook of Public Health.* New York, NY: Oxford University Press; 1985.

21. Farquhar JW, Fortmann ST, Wood PD, Haskell WL. Community studies of cardiovascular disease prevention. In: Kaplan NM, Stamler J, eds. *Prevention of Coronary Disease: Practical Management of Risk Factors.* Philadelphia, Pa: Saunders; 1983.

22. Kreuter MW. Health promotion: the role of public health in the community of free exchange. *Health Promotion Monographs* 1984:4 Center for Health Promotion, Columbia University.

23. Green LW, Kreuter MW. *Health Promotion Planning: An Educational and Diagnostic Approach.* Mountain View, CA: Mayfield Publishing; 1991.

24. Minkler M. Citizen participation in health of the Republic of Cuba. *Int Q Comm Health Ed.* 1980–81;1:56–78.

25. Green, LW. The theory of participation: a quantitative analysis of its expression in national and international health policies. In: Ward W, ed. *Advances in Health Education and Health Promotion.* Part A. New York: Columbia University Press; 1986.

26. Bracht N, Tsouros A. Principles and strategies of effective community participation. *Health Prom Int.* 1990;5(3):199–208.

27. *Model Standards: A Guide for Community Preventive Health Services.* 2nd ed. Washington, DC: American Public Health Association; 1985.

28. *Planned Approach to Community Health (PATCH).* Washington, DC: US Dept of Health and Human Services; November 1993.

29. *Promoting Health in the Urban Context, Five Year Planning Framework, A Guide to Assessing Healthy Cities.* Copenhagen, Denmark: World Health Organization regional office for Europe; 1988.

30. *Global Strategy of Health for All by the Year 2000.* Geneva, Switzerland: World Health Organization; 1981.

31. *World Health Organization, Five Year Planning Project.* Fadl, Copenhagen: World Health Organization Healthy Cities Project; 1988. WHO Healthy Cities Papers no. 2.

32. Ashton J. *Healthy Cities.* Philadelphia, Pa: Open University Press; 1992.

CHAPTER

Health Data Management for Public Health

Carl W. Tyler, Jr., M.D.
Richard C. Dicker, M.D., M.Sc.

The practice of public health influences the lifestyle and well-being not only of communities, counties, cities, and countries, but also of individuals, businesses, industries, and organizations. For example, in order to stop an illness from spreading among those who live in the community, a public health official may be called on to close a restaurant. Unfortunately, this action taken for the public's benefit also results in the elimination of income for the owner, his family, and his employees.

On a larger scale, a public health official may campaign against tobacco use and take on a nationwide industry. Public health practitioners may also be opposed by strong advocacy groups, such as the National Rifle Association, whose actions may aggravate community health problems, such as violence.

The need for current, accurate data and careful analysis on which to base health policy and public health practice decisions is obvious in scenarios like these. Epidemiology is the basic science of public health and the foundation of public health practice. Although effective management and policy decisions are made not solely on the basis of epidemiological information, a health agency that administers important public health programs and deals with public health crises still needs to have staff members with a sound understanding of the science and practice of epidemiology.

This chapter provides a synoptic snapshot of the following:

- the fundamental tasks of epidemiologic practice
- the measures used by the practicing epidemiologist
- required reporting of data used in public health practice
- major data sources used by public health practitioners
- uses of public health data by epidemiologists and other public health officials

PRINCIPLES OF THE PRACTICE OF EPIDEMIOLOGY

In this section, a definition of epidemiology is elaborated upon. This is followed by a description of the tasks of the epidemiologist. Finally, the relationship of the epidemiologist to other health practitioners is specified.

Defining Epidemiology

The definition of epidemiology has two dimensions; one is scientific, the other is related to public health practice. The most widely accepted definition is given in *The Dictionary of Epidemiology,*[1] which was developed and reviewed by an international panel of experts. According to this definition, "epidemiology is the study of the distribution and determinants of health-related states and events in specified populations and the application of this study to the control of health problems."

The phrase **health problem** is used in this definition in place of the word disease because epidemiologists and public health agencies now find themselves responsible for a wide range of health problems. In addition to infectious diseases such as tuberculosis, noninfectious health problems, such as automobile crash injuries in children, exposure of miners to coal dust in mines, and unintended pregnancies to teenagers, are also high priority public health problems.

The term **distribution** in the definition addresses the relationship of health events to person, place, and time, in other words, the relationship between the health problem and the population in which it exists. The characteristics of the population are usually given in terms of age, sex, and the places where people live and the health event occurs.

The word **determinants** refers to both the direct causes of the health problem and the factors that determine the risk for the problem. These factors are often classified into three groups:

1. host factors
2. agent factors
3. environmental factors

Host factors are those that characterize the people afflicted with the health problem and their susceptibility to it. **Agent factors** are those that characterize the agent that causes the disease. **Environmental factors** are those that determine the exposure of the host group to the agent.

In an epidemic of food poisoning, for example, the host group includes the people who ate the food and became ill. The agent factors are those related to the cause of the problem, such as the salmonella bacillus, which may infect turkey or egg dishes. The environmental factors are those that provide suitable circumstances for the agent to survive, such as improper handling of food, and those that determine the exposure of the host group.

The Tasks of Epidemiologic Practice

Even though epidemiology is thought of as the basic science of public health, a science is often best defined by what the scientist does. Langmuir, the renowned CDC epidemiologist who established the Epidemic Intelligence Service, stated that, "the basic operation of the epidemiologist is to count cases and measure the population in which they arise," so that rates can be calculated and the occurrence of a health problem can be compared in different groups of people.[2]

The contemporary epidemiologist has unique responsibilities that can be stated in more detail. These basic responsibilities are

• surveillance
• investigation
• analysis
• evaluation

In addition, the epidemiologist needs to assume other responsibilities, such as clear communication, effective management, consultation, group or public presentation, and human relations skills.

Surveillance

Surveillance is "the ongoing systematic collection, analysis and interpretation of health data essential to the planning, implementation and evaluation of public health practice, closely integrated with the timely dissemination of these data to those who need to know. The final link in the surveillance chain is the application of these data to prevention and control."[3] This definition is taken from the plan proposed by the Centers for Disease Control and Prevention for public health surveillance, which is also discussed in Chapters 16 and 20.

Investigation

The epidemiological investigation of health problems may be precipitated by a host of factors. Surveillance reports frequently initiate an investigation, for example, but phone calls to health agencies, as well as reports from other health departments, colleagues in epidemiology, or other health professionals or news reports may also play a role.

An epidemiologic investigation may focus on an epidemic, such as an outbreak of infection, a cluster of events, such as injuries or leukemia, or the presence of risk factors for disease, such as tobacco use or an occupational exposure. The basic steps in such an investigation are detailed later in the chapter.

Analysis

The analysis of epidemiologic data proceeds through an orderly series of steps that transform numbers into information that can lead to the control or prevention of a health problem.

Evaluation

Evaluation is the assessment of a specific public health action intended to deal with a clearly defined problem. Measuring vaccine effectiveness is one example of an evaluation that is generally the responsibility of epidemiologists.

Additional Essential Tasks

Dealing with health data and management requires a public health practitioner to be able to do more than those tasks that are uniquely epidemiologic. Clearly *communicating* the findings from epidemiologic studies to the public and to health professionals is needed if community cooperation with control and prevention measures is to be effective.

Management of the people who are needed to conduct epidemiologic studies and carry out control and prevention programs makes it essential for public health practitioners to be skilled in this area. Because practitioners skilled in working with health data and management problems are often called on for advice, competence in *consultation* is also important. Proficiency in *human relations* is required of every public health practitioner who deals with colleagues in carrying out tasks dealing with health data and the management of community health problems.

Relationships with Other Health Practitioners

Health data and its management are important for many public health practitioners with a wide range of special competences. *Statisticians* play a special role in accessing and managing data sources and evaluating and interpreting results. *Laboratory staff* have an important part to play in carrying out tests that identify the exact cause of a health problem and confirm the presence of the problem in those people who show symptoms and signs of the condition.

Health policy makers need to understand health data if effective strategies are to be designed to control and prevent a community health problem. *Health service and program managers* need to understand the findings of studies and policy analyses if they are to be persuaded to provide services and conduct effective programs.

Summary

In summary, public health practitioners who deal with health data and apply these data to the management of health problems must be part of a team that serves the health needs of a community. They need to be skilled with data, and they must be able to communicate their findings clearly and persuasively.

SURVEILLANCE SYSTEMS: THEIR ESTABLISHMENT AND USE

In this section, the role of surveillance in public health practice is outlined.

What Is Public Health Surveillance?

Public health surveillance is essential to making competent, well-informed public health policy decisions that are based on quantitative data. As a public health activity, surveillance was conceptualized by practicing epidemiologists as follows:

> Surveillance is the ongoing systematic collection, analysis, and interpretation of health data essential to the planning, implementation, and evaluation of public health practice, closely integrated with the timely dissemination of these data to those who need to know. The final link in the surveillance chain is the application of these data to prevention and control.[3]

Surveillance Versus Research

Surveillance must be defined in terms of what it is *not* as well as what it is. Public health surveillance is not research. The need for timeliness and for rapid dissemination is essential for effective public health surveillance. This attribute is not as important for research whose findings must be subject to careful and deliberate contemplation by scientists rather than by public health decision makers.

Surveillance data must be disseminated quickly to public health practitioners, including those who originally gathered the data, as well as to decision makers throughout the public health organization and, depending on the character of the information, to other public service agencies and the community. Surveillance data are more often related to identifying a public health problem than to problem solving. The dissemination of surveillance data frequently stimulates the search for additional data that may come from other sources.

Surveillance Systems Versus Health Information Systems

Surveillance systems are also different from health information systems. Health information systems span a broad range of health data, which may include interviews, abstracted hospital records, birth certificates, death certificates, physician office visit abstracts, and medical prescriptions. Data from a health information system may be used for surveillance, just as death certificates may be an indispensable component of a cancer surveillance system, but surveillance systems differ from health information systems in at least three ways:

1. Surveillance systems must be ongoing; health information systems may not be.
2. Surveillance systems must be integrated with timely dissemination.
3. Surveillance systems must be applicable to public health actions, such as control and prevention.

The Purpose of Public Health Surveillance

Public health surveillance has specific purposes that are fundamental to decision making, policy development, program implementation, and sometimes crisis management. The following are the key purposes of a surveillance system:

- describing trends and the natural history of health problems
- detecting epidemics
- providing details about patterns of disease
- monitoring changes in disease agents through laboratory testing
- planning and setting health program priorities
- evaluating the effects of control and prevention measures
- detecting critical changes in health practice
- evaluating hypotheses about the cause of health problems
- detecting rare but important cases of disease, such as botulism

To be certain that a surveillance system meets the needs of public health decision makers and their communities, the objectives of the system must be specified in detail. Everyone who might make decisions based on the surveillance data needs to be involved in the process.

The Surveillance Cycle

Public health surveillance is conducted in a systematic cycle that has four major steps. These steps and their most important characteristics are as follows:

1. *collection of data* (pertinent, regular, frequent, prompt, timely)
2. *consolidation and interpretation of data* (orderly, descriptive, evaluative, prompt, timely)
3. *dissemination of information* (prompt, timely; disseminated to all who need to know, such as data providers, for confirmation and support, policy makers, action takers)
4. action to control and prevent problems

The surveillance cycle is a concept that may be used for the entire spectrum of public health problems. Originally applied to infectious diseases, the surveillance cycle is now used in prevention and control programs for injury, cancer, certain cardiovascular diseases, and high-risk and unintended pregnancies. Understanding this cycle, especially the need for promptness in data collection and timely, accurate reporting, is essential for public health policy makers and action-oriented health program managers.

Specifically, the surveillance cycle highlights three important points for policy makers and program managers:

1. Promptness is important at every step of the cycle and is given priority over meticulousness. As a result, changes may occur in surveillance data that do not occur in vital statistics or in most health survey data.
2. Reports based on surveillance data are highly descriptive, that is, for the most part surveillance data provide the numerator numbers for estimated rates of disease occurrence. Surveillance reports generate hypotheses and suggest causes of health problems rather than confirm or establish them.
3. Under rare circumstances surveillance systems may be brought to an end. When smallpox was eradicated, for example, surveillance was terminated because the smallpox virus was no longer a public health threat.

Characteristics of a Surveillance System

A public health surveillance system has the following seven characteristics:

1. simplicity
2. sensitivity
3. flexibility
4. acceptability
5. timeliness
6. representativeness
7. high positive predictive value

In many ways, these characteristics are interdependent. *Simplicity* is essential if data quality is to be maintained and if consolidation, interpretation, and dissemination are to be carried out promptly. *Acceptability* is required because voluntary cooperation from busy public health practitioners is usually the cornerstone of data collection. *Sensitivity* and a *high positive predictive value* are important because surveillance is one approach to screening for the health problems of a community, especially for epidemic diseases and clusters of health events, such as injuries.

Flexibility is critical because surveillance systems often prove to be the only mechanisms for detecting new public health problems. This was the case in detecting the AIDS epidemic and in finding penicillinase-producing *Neisseria gonorrhoeae*. *Representativeness* is necessary if the system is to reflect accurately the occurrence of health problems in all sectors of a geographic area. Finally, *timeliness* must be an integral part of any surveillance system that is expected to detect health problems and to lead to the institution of effective control and prevention measures.[4]

The Problem of a Uniform Data Set

The desirability of a uniform set of basic data items has been recognized for decades. As data-based decision making has become more realistic, greater efforts have been made to construct such a set of basic data items. The rapidly changing health care environment has increased the number of these efforts.

The CDC's Surveillance Coordinating Group has addressed this problem, as has a group formed in connection with the issuance of national health objectives based on *Healthy People 2000.*[5] More recently the Public Health Foundation published *Data for the Year 2000 National Health Objectives: The ASTHO Reporting System's New Core Data Set.*[6] Anticipating the growing role of health maintenance organizations (HMOs),

the National Committee for Quality Assurance has issued a 156-page document titled *Health Plan Employer
Data and Information Set and User's Manual.*[7] The
last publication goes beyond the development of a basic data set to propose performance indicators for
HMOs in terms of access to health care, satisfaction of
those receiving care, health plan stability, and financial
performance.

The groups that developed these proposals all recognize the importance of data for decision making and the
proliferation of data systems and their attendant burden.
However, the overlapping interests of these diverse groups
do not appear to be considered. Although all of them
share a serious interest in health, many bring their own
perspective (for example, clinical, community-oriented,
research, or public health) and do not take account of
other views. For this reason, it is difficult to be optimistic
about the development within the next decade of a uniform set of core data for decision making about health.

SOURCES OF DATA

There are a diversity of sources of health data, including vital certificates, notifiable diseases surveillance systems, other communicable disease surveillance systems,
the National Health Survey, and other national data systems. Each of these sources of data are described next.

Vital Certificates

Vital statistics are significant in every way for a public health practitioner. They document vital events,
specifically births and deaths, and they have special
characteristics that make them vital for decision makers.
Most important, birth and death certificates are public
documents. In addition, they are widely accepted as accurate for health, medical, and legal purposes, because
vital event reporting is as nearly complete as any life
event can be, even though it is not perfect. The reporting of births is more complete than that of deaths.

Data Characteristics

Birth and death data have important detailed characteristics that help public health decision making.

Each certificate has an individual identifier, geographic
location, date of event, and certain important personal
characteristics. Of most use are gender, race, and marital status. Birth data include length of pregnancy, birth
weight, and exact time and place of birth. Death certificates generally report age, usual occupation, and
cause of death.

Drawbacks

As useful as they are, vital certificates pose several
problems for public health decision makers. They often
are not edited, aggregated, or made accessible in a
timely manner. The time lag is almost always greater
than three months and is sometimes measured in years.
In addition, not all items are reported with the same accuracy so critical variables may need verification.

Geographic information needs to be read with care
so that a decision maker knows whether the place reported is the individual's place of residence or the place
where the vital event occurred, for example, in a hospital rather than at home. Geographic information is also
often not as detailed as a public health practitioner
would like. In national or state reports, vital events are
often reported just for counties or cities, even though
data for the area served by public health nurses or
schools—the neighborhood or block are essential for
making decisions about health services in a community.
Locating births and deaths by census tract or, under
very special circumstances, by city block, can sometimes
be done with the help of local planning officials.

Causes of death have been carefully classified for
years, but if a specific cause of death is important to a
health decision, vital data may be of most use in developing preliminary hypotheses. The source document,
such as a hospital, medical, or autopsy record, may ultimately be required.

Other Public Records

Other public records, such as fetal death certificates,
marriage records, automobile driver licenses, or court
or other legal documents, may also be essential to health
decisions for communities. As the span of concern of
public health professionals and agencies increases, other

sources of public information are used for new approaches to improving health, such as injury control programs or family violence prevention.

Uses of Vital Data

Ultimately, a decision maker needs to know what and how vital data might be used. In most cases vital events provide the numerator for event rates in a community. Census data or local population estimates are usually the best denominator data, but this depends on the specific decision that is being considered and how it must be measured. These issues are addressed below.

Notifiable Diseases Surveillance Systems

A surveillance system includes the functional capacity for data collection and analysis, as well as the timely dissemination of these data to persons responsible for prevention and control activities. One mechanism for data collection is the system of legally required reporting of specified diseases. This system, dating back to the late 1800s, requires that health care providers and others report any case of a *reportable,* or *notifiable,* disease to the appropriate public health authorities. Although a few diseases are reportable under federal law, most are determined to be reportable at the state level.

Reporting from Individual to Local Health Department to State Health Department

Each state's morbidity reporting system is based on state laws and regulations adopted by the state board or department of health, which derives its authority to issue regulations from acts of the state legislature. In most states, state health authorities are empowered to establish and modify the morbidity reporting requirements. In a few states, the legislature keeps that authority.

Typically, the regulations specify not only which diseases or conditions are reportable, but also who is responsible for reporting, what information is required for each case of disease reported, how to report and to whom, and how quickly the information is to be reported. The regulations may also specify control measures to be taken in the event that certain diseases occur.

These case reports are usually considered confidential and are not available for public inspection.

Deciding What Is Reportable. The list of notifiable diseases differs for each state, reflecting the public health priorities and concerns of the state. In general, a disease is included on the list if it causes serious morbidity or death, has the potential to affect larger numbers of people, and can be controlled or prevented with proper intervention. In most states the list includes from 35 to over 100 conditions, mostly but not exclusively infectious diseases.

In addition to specific diseases or conditions that have been established as reportable within a given state, health department regulations commonly specify two other circumstances that require reporting: the occurrence of any outbreak or unusually high incidence of any disease and the occurrence of any unusual disease of public health importance. Some states also provide for the immediate addition to the list of any disease that becomes important from a public health standpoint. States can also modify the specific information required for each case of a reportable disease.

Who Must Report. In most states, reporting known or suspected cases of a reportable disease is generally considered to be an obligation of the following individuals:

- physicians, dentists, nurses, other health practitioners, and medical examiners
- laboratory directors
- administrators of hospitals, clinics, nursing homes, schools, and day care centers

In some states, responsibility for reporting also includes any other individuals who know of or suspect the existence of a reportable disease.

How Cases Are Reported. Usually, a case report is sent to the local health department, which has primary responsibility for taking appropriate action. In most states, reportable diseases are required to be reported within a week of diagnosis, but selected diseases and conditions that pose special threats to the public, such as botulism, quarantinable diseases, and epidemics, are required to be reported immediately by telephone.

The local health department then forwards a copy of the report to the state health department. In a few states case reports are sent directly to the state health department, either because there is no local health department in the reporting physician's area or because the local health department, for whatever reason, cannot effectively respond to the reports. In some cases, the state has determined that it will be primarily responsible for responding to the reports.

Passive Versus Active Surveillance. This form of data collection, in which health care providers send reports to a health department based on a known set of rules and regulations, is called *passive,* or *provider-initiated, surveillance.* Less commonly, health department staff may call or visit health care providers to solicit reports. This is called *active,* or *health-department-initiated, surveillance.* It is usually limited to specific diseases over a limited period of time, such as following a community exposure or during an epidemic.

Reporting Forms. In most states, health department regulations require that case reports be submitted on a standard form that the health department provides. However, some states allow reporting by telephone in lieu of written reports. In addition, some states are now experimenting with submission of reports by electronic telecommunication.

At a minimum, most case report forms ask for the patient's name, age, sex, race, address, and telephone number; the name of the patient's head-of-household; the date of onset of illness; the name and telephone number of the person reporting; and the date of the report. The place and date of hospitalization, if applicable, are also commonly requested. For many diseases, additional information is also collected about the diagnosis, manifestations, and epidemiologic features.

Failure to Report. Although it is the intention of the laws and regulations of each state that every case of a reportable disease be reported, the reality is otherwise. For rare, serious diseases of public health importance such as rabies, bubonic plague, or botulism, the cases actually reported may approach 100 percent. For some other diseases, however, such as aseptic meningitis, reporting has been found to be as low as 6 percent.[8]

The laws and regulations often include penalties for failure to report a notifiable condition, such as a fine or suspension of a license to practice, but these penalties are rarely enforced. Incomplete reporting of some diseases can be attributed to lack of knowledge about what is reportable, lack of knowledge about how to report, and the perception that reporting is not important.

Reporting from the State Health Department to CDC

The Council of State and Territorial Epidemiologists (CSTE) determines which diseases must be reported by states to CDC. Table 12.1 lists the nationally notifiable diseases for 1990.

The list of nationally notifiable diseases is a dynamic one. In 1961, the list included the six quarantinable diseases (cholera, plague, louse-borne relapsing fever, smallpox, epidemic typhus fever, and yellow fever), sixteen additional infectious diseases of humans, and one infectious disease of animals (rabies). Since then, the list has been revised several times, adding newly recognized diseases (toxic shock syndrome, legionellosis, AIDS), adding categories of disease (for example, hepatitis A, hepatitis B, hepatitis non-A non-B, and hepatitis, unspecified), and dropping some diseases from the weekly list (streptococcal sore throat, scarlet fever, chicken pox). The notifiable disease list in each state is longer than the nationally notifiable list, reflecting state surveillance of diseases and conditions of local importance.

In general, each week each state health department provides to CDC, by electronic telecommunication, a line listing of all case reports of nationally reportable diseases that were reported in the state during the preceding seven days. These reports represent provisional data because the diagnosis may not be confirmed and other data items may be incomplete. The actual disease report forms, which contain much more detailed information, follow by mail, though increasing use is being made of telecommunications. Usually, these reports are stripped of names and other personal identifiers by the state before being sent to CDC.

Within two days of receipt of the weekly reports from the states, CDC compiles, publishes, and distributes the

TABLE 12.1   Notifiable Diseases, United States, 1990

Diseases Reportable in Most States

*	Acquired immunodeficiency syndrome	*	Measles (rubeola)
*	Amebiasis	*	Meningitis, aseptic
*	Anthrax		Meningitis, bacterial
*	Botulism (foodborne, wound, and unspecified)	*	Meningococcal disease
*	Brucellosis	*	Mumps
	Campylobacteriosis		Outbreaks
*	Chancroid	*	Pertussis
*†	Cholera	*†	Plague
*	Diphtheria	*	Poliomyelitis, paralytic
*	Encephalitis	*	Psittacosis
	Giardiasis	*	Rabies, human
*	Gonorrhea / gonococcal disease		Reye syndrome
*	Granuloma inguinale	*	Rocky Mountain spotted fever
*	Hansen disease (leprosy)	*	Rubella
*	*Hemophilus influenzae*, invasive	*	Rubella, congenital
*	Hepatitis A	*	Salmonellosis
*	Hepatitis B	*	Shigellosis
*	Hepatitis Non-A, Non-B	*	Syphilis, primary & secondary
	HIV infection		Syphilis, congenital
	Influenza outbreak	*	Tetanus
	Kawasaki syndrome	*	Toxic shock syndrome
*	Legionellosis	*	Trichinosis
*	Leptospirosis	*	Tuberculosis
*	Lyme disease	*	Typhoid fever
*	Lymphogranuloma venereum	*	Typhus
*	Malaria	*†	Yellow fever

Diseases / Conditions Reportable in Some States

	Abortion		Nonspecific urethritis
	Adverse drug reaction		Nosocomial outbreak
	Animal bite		Occupational disease, any
	Asbestosis		Ophthalmia neonatorum
	Blastomycosis		Pesticide poisoning
*	Botulism, infant		Pneumoconiosis
*	Chicken pox (varicella)		Q fever
	Congenital defect		Rabies, animal
	Coccidioidomycosis		Relapsing fever
	Dengue fever	*	Rheumatic fever, acute
	Diarrhea caused by E. coli		Scarlet fever
	Guillain-Barre syndrome		Silicosis
	Herpes simplex		Smallpox
	Histoplasmosis		Staphylococcal disease
	Impetigo outbreak		Streptococcal disease
	Lead poisoning		Toxoplasmosis
	Listeriosis		Trachoma
	Mycobacterial infection, atypical		Yersiniosis

* Nationally notifiable disease
† Disease covered by International Quarantine Agreement
SOURCE: Centers for Disease Control. *Summary of Notifiable Diseases, United States, 1990.* MMWR. 1990; 39:53 (Modified by the authors)

data in the *Morbidity and Mortality Weekly Report.* CDC also prepares and distributes detailed surveillance reports on various diseases from the case report forms and other reports of cases, laboratory isolates, epidemics, and investigations.

Reporting by CDC to the World Health Organization

By international agreement, CDC promptly reports to the World Health Organization any reported cases of the internationally quarantinable diseases—plague, cholera, and yellow fever. CDC also reports influenza virus isolates and sends an annual summary of the disease reports received during the previous year.

Summary

The practice of reporting morbidity data to successively higher levels of government not only keeps each level informed of the current incidence in its jurisdiction but also makes possible the compilation of data for successively larger areas. These compilations provide opportunities for identifying common factors not discernible at lower levels, especially when the incidence of a disease is low in most local areas.

Other Communicable Disease Surveillance Systems

Most communicable diseases of interest to public health authorities are included in the notifiable disease surveillance system. However, a few diseases are detected through alternative mechanisms, such as laboratory reporting, sentinel surveillance, and specialized, often locally adapted or customized, systems.

Laboratory Reporting

Laboratory reporting is generally used for diseases such as salmonellosis and shigellosis, which require laboratory confirmation of a clinical diagnosis. State health laboratories may perform confirmatory testing, subtyping, or other specialized studies. These results and isolates of the organisms themselves may then be forwarded to CDC. The emphasis of the laboratory surveillance system is on the agent, in contrast to the emphasis of the nationally notifiable disease surveillance system, which is on the host.

Sentinel Surveillance

While the notifiable disease reporting system is intended to capture every recognized case of a notifiable disease, it is well known that underreporting is widespread. This underreporting creates problems in interpretation, because health officials generally do not know which cases are reported and which are not. An alternative to the traditional all-inclusive but passive system is a **sentinel** system. A sentinel surveillance system relies on a pre-arranged sample of reporting sources who agree to report all cases of one or more notifiable conditions. Usually the sample is not random but is comprised of sources, such as physicians, clinics, and hospitals, that are likely to see cases of the notifiable conditions and are willing to report them.

National population-based surveillance for HIV infection is not feasible in many developing countries. Sentinel surveillance, based on serial serosurveys conducted at selected sites with homogeneous, well-defined population subgroups, provides a practical alternative. Under this strategy, health officials define the population subgroups and regions to study, then identify institutions that are capable and willing and that serve the population subgroups of interest. Serosurveys are then conducted at least annually, using standard survey techniques, to provide statistically valid estimates of HIV prevalence.

Customized Systems

Another category of communicable diseases that are often missed by the notifiable disease surveillance systems are those which public health authorities want to know about when they occur in outbreak or epidemic proportions, but not necessarily when they occur as sporadic cases. Chicken pox and influenza are two such diseases.

Influenza: An Example. Because influenza can affect so many people and can cause considerable mortality, several customized surveillance systems have been developed that provide an assessment of influenza's incidence and impact without requiring that health care providers report every case of influenza-like illness. For example, at the local and state level, public health authorities assess influenza activity through reports of outbreaks of influenza-like illness, laboratory identification of influenza virus from nasopharyngeal swabs, and reports from schools with excess absenteeism (for example, more than 10 percent of the student body). Other, more localized, systems include monitoring of pneumonia and influenza mortality from local death certificates; reporting by cooperating (sentinel) physicians of the number of patients seen with influenza-like illness each week; and reports of excess employee absenteeism. At least one county health department monitors the number of chest X-rays done on nursing home patients by a mobile radiology group; when chest X-rays exceed 50 percent of the total X-rays ordered, an influenza epidemic is usually in progress.

At the national level, the CDC uses four different surveillance systems during the influenza season from October through May. Each week:

1. The laboratory-based system receives reports of influenza virus isolates from about 60 state, city, and university hospital laboratories.
2. The 121-city mortality reporting system receives data from 121 jurisdictions that include the total number of deaths by age and the proportion attributed to pneumonia or influenza.
3. The sentinel physician system receives reports of the number of patients seen with influenza-like illness from a network of about 150 family practice physicians.
4. Each state epidemiologist provides a summary assessment of influenza activity in his state, selecting from *no report, no activity, sporadic, regional,* or *widespread.*

Data from these four surveillance systems are combined to provide a reliable assessment of influenza activity throughout the United States that does not require all health care providers to report every case they see.

The National Health Survey

In the United States the National Center for Health Statistics (NCHS) conducts a series of national sample surveys, some of which began as early as 1957. The series includes both population-based and provider-based surveys. Computer-assisted telephone interviewing (CATI) now makes the use of community surveys more flexible, so they are a more important source of health data than ever before. Collectively, these data systems, which are also discussed in Chapter 16, are the foundation of health survey information in the United States.[9]

The National Health Interview Survey

The National Health Interview Survey (NHIS) is an annual survey of a stratified nationwide probability sample of the civilian population who are interviewed as household members (as distinct from members of residential institutions). A core of information is gathered each year on the characteristics of respondents' health problems, the disability associated with them, and the care sought and received by the respondents. In addition, each survey inquires in detail about health problems related to a specific system of the body (such as the cardiovascular system), a special group of diseases (for example, infections), or personal health practices. Reports of NHIS findings are published as part of the NCHS series, *Vital and Health Statistics.*

The National Health and Examination Survey

The National Health and Examination Survey (NHANES) was first conducted in 1959. It extended the NHIS by including selected physical and biological measurements of each respondent. Height, weight, blood pressure, hemoglobin, visual acuity, and other more specialized tests were carried out in mobile examination facilities. In 1970, a nutrition examination was added to the survey on a regular basis. Now this survey has the capacity to sample special population groups, such as Hispanics living in the United States.

The National Hospital Discharge Survey

The National Hospital Discharge Survey (NHDS) surveys a stratified probability sample of hospital record discharge sheets. The sample includes short-stay, non-federal hospitals and is stratified by size of hospital, as measured by the number of beds in the institution. Large hospitals (1,000 beds or more) are highly likely to be included in the sample.

Data from hospitals are useful for assessing the need for care in hospitals, the kinds of procedures performed in hospitals, and the characteristics of illnesses severe enough to require hospital care. The data are limited by the number of diagnoses and procedures that can be abstracted. Because hospitalized individuals may have complicated health problems, the limited number of data items that can be recorded may limit the usefulness of information collected. Nonetheless, the general quality of the NHDS data and its use of probability sampling makes it uniquely valuable for national and regional decisions and comparisons.

The National Ambulatory Medical Care Survey

The National Ambulatory Medical Care Survey (NAMCS) is a probability sample of patient visits to physician offices. Based on reports from a panel of clinical practitioners, this survey includes information on patients' symptoms, physicians' diagnoses, medications prescribed, and referrals.

NAMCS began in 1974 and was carried out annually until 1981. Then, the annual cycle was interrupted, and surveys were conducted only in 1985 and 1989, but not in the intervening years. The most recent cycle of NAMCS data, in 1991, was the National Hospital Ambulatory Medical Care Survey.

Detailed descriptions of the data systems of the NCHS are published in *Vital and Health Statistics, Series 1*, which gives information about the programs and collection procedures. Number 23 in this series is the most recent comprehensive characterization of these systems. The most current results of these systems appear in *Advance Data from Vital and Health Statistics* as well as in the *Monthly Vital Statistics Report*.

Other National Data Systems

There are several other national health data systems. Three of them are described next.

Surveillance, Epidemiology, and End Results (SEER) Program

The Surveillance, Epidemiology, and End Results, or SEER, program of the National Cancer Institute has collected cancer data from population-based cancer registries scattered throughout the country since 1973. The SEER program currently enrolls roughly 120,000 new cases of cancer each year from nine geographic areas containing about 10 percent of the United States population. For each type of cancer, data are collected on patient demographics, tumor site, morphology, confirmation of diagnosis, extent of disease, treatment, and survival. Though not part of the SEER program, many other states maintain similar cancer registries for parts or all of the state.

National Electronic Injury Surveillance System (NEISS)

The National Electronic Injury Surveillance System (NEISS), sponsored by the Consumer Product Safety Commission since 1972, collects emergency room data on injuries related to consumer products. National projections on injuries, poisonings, and burns related to consumer products other than automobiles are based on the small (currently 62) but representative sample of hospitals.

Medical Care Provider Analysis and Review (MEDPARS)

Medical Care Provider Analysis and Review (MEDPARS) files were created by the Health Care Financing Administration to monitor the quality of care provided through Medicare programs. The files link demographic information from eligibility files, diagnosis and treatment information from part A and part B of the Medicare claims files, and health care provider information from facilities files. Because about 96 percent of the population age 65 and over is enrolled in at least part A of the Medicare program, these files are useful for the epidemiologic study of problems of older Americans, as well as for their original purpose of examining the quality of health care.

EPIDEMIOLOGIC MEASURES

While effective public health practitioners do not need to be expert in all of the epidemiologic tasks described above, they do need to be knowledgable enough about basic epidemiologic measures to interpret data appropriately and make rational public health decisions.

Numbers and Rates

Counting the numbers of events—the number of new cases of hepatitis A reported this week, the number of infants who died this year, the number of doses of measles-mumps-rubella vaccine administered this month—is a common and essential activity of a health department. The numbers can be added or grouped by time, place, and person to provide an informative description of the magnitude and pattern of a health problem or service. The numbers can also be used to guide health policy and resource allocation—the number of hospital beds needed, the best location of a satellite clinic, or the dollar amount to request for HIV-related counseling in next year's budget.

The use of counts alone has limitations, however. Because counts do not take into account population size or dynamics, they are insufficient for assessing an individual's or a population's risk of some adverse health event. To characterize risk, *rates* rather than counts must be used. Calculating rates for different subgroups by age, sex, geographic location, exposure history, or other characteristics can identify groups at elevated risk of disease. Identification of these high-risk groups is vital to the development and targeting of effective control and prevention measures. Rates also are preferred over counts for comparing health conditions in a population over time or among different populations, because rates take into account the size of the population and the specific time period.

To calculate a rate, the count must be divided by an appropriate denominator. The denominator is usually an estimate of the population that gave rise to the counts in the numerator. For example, if the numerator is the number of women diagnosed with breast cancer as identified by a statewide cancer registry during the past year,

an appropriate denominator might be the estimated midyear female population of the state based on census figures. If the numerator is restricted to women above a certain age, the denominator should be similarly restricted. These rates provide an estimate of the one-year risk of breast cancer among women in that population.

As illustrated by this example, denominators for public health data are often population estimates from the United States Bureau of the Census. Based on the census conducted every 10 years, the bureau provides detailed breakdowns of the population by age, race or ethnic group, sex, and census track. Between census years, the bureau provides less detailed estimates. Many states develop more detailed estimates for use in their own jurisdictions for the years between the national censuses.

Common Measures

The most common health outcomes measured by health agencies are those related to natality (birth), morbidity (illness, injury, disability), and mortality (death). Morbidity measures include disease incidence and prevalence. Mortality measures include crude, specific, and standardized mortality rates as well as years of potential life lost. Some common measures of natality, morbidity, and mortality are listed in Table 12.2.

Morbidity Measures

Morbidity measures quantify a population's likelihood of developing or having an illness, injury, disability, or other adverse health condition.

Incidence Rate. An **incidence rate,** sometimes referred to simply as incidence, is the rate at which new events, such as a new case of illness, occur in a population in a stated period of time.[1]

Prevalence Rates. In contrast, the **prevalence rate,** often referred to simply as prevalence, is the proportion of persons in a population who have a particular disease or attribute at a specified point in time or over a specified period of time. Prevalence differs from incidence in that prevalence includes all cases, both new and old, in

TABLE 12.2. Commonly Used Epidemiologic Measures

Natality measure	Numerator	Denominator	Expressed per Number at Risk
Crude Birth Rate	# live births reported during a given time interval	estimated total population at midinterval	1,000
Crude Fertility Rate	# live births reported during a given time interval	estimated number of women age 15–44 years at midinterval	1,000
Morbidity Measure			
Incidence Rate	# new cases of a specified disease reported during a given time interval	average or midpoint population during time interval	variable: 10^x where $x = 2,3,4,5,6$
Attack Rate	# new cases of a specified disease reported during an epidemic period of time	population at start of the epidemic period	variable: 10^x where $x = 2,3,4,5,6$
Point Prevalence	# current cases, new and old, of a specified disease at a given point in time	estimated population at the same point in time	variable: 10^x where $x = 2,3,4,5,6$
Period Prevalence	# current cases, new and old, of a specified disease identified over a given time interval	estimated population at midinterval	variable: 10^x where $x = 2,3,4,5,6$
Mortality Measure			
Crude Death Rate	total number of deaths reported during a given time interval	estimated midinterval population	1,000 or 100,000
Cause-Specific Death Rate	# deaths assigned to a specific cause during a given time interval	estimated midinterval population	100,000
Death-To-Case Ratio (case-fatality rate, case-fatality ratio)	# deaths assigned to a specific disease during a given time interval	# new cases of that disease reported during the same time interval	100
Neonatal Mortality Rate	# deaths under 28 days of age during a given time interval	# live births during the same time interval	1,000
Infant Mortality Rate	# deaths under one year of age during a given time interval	# live births reported during the same time interval	1,000

SOURCE: *Self-Study Course 3030-G: Principles of Epidemiology.* 2nd ed. Atlanta, Ga: Centers for Disease Control; 1992.

the population at the specified time, whereas incidence is limited to new cases only.

Point prevalence refers to prevalence measured at a particular point in time, that is, the proportion of persons with a particular disease or attribute on a particular date. **Period prevalence** refers to prevalence measured over an interval of time, that is, the proportion of persons who had a particular disease or attribute at any time during the interval.

Mortality measures

The **mortality rate** is an estimate of the proportion of a defined population that dies during a specified time period.[1]

Crude Mortality Rate. The **crude mortality rate** (or crude death rate) is the mortality rate from all causes of death for an entire population. In the United States in 1990, 2,148,463 deaths occurred; the 1990 midyear population was 248,710,000. The crude mortality rate was, therefore, 863.8 per 100,000.

Specific Mortality Rates. To assess or compare the mortality experience of different subpopulations, mortality rates may be calculated for those subpopulations. An **age-specific mortality rate** is a mortality rate limited to a particular age group. Similarly, a **sex-specific** or **race-specific mortality rate** is limited to one sex or one racial group, respectively.

The **infant mortality rate,** a type of age-specific mortality rate, is used by all nations as an important public health indicator. The numerator is the number of deaths among children under one year of age reported during a given time period, usually a calendar year. The denominator is the number of live births reported during the same time period. The infant mortality rate is usually expressed per 1,000 live births. Other frequently used mortality rates are described in Table 12.2.

A **cause-specific mortality rate** is the mortality rate from a specified cause for a population. The numerator is the number of deaths attributed to a specific cause. The denominator is the midinterval size of the entire population. Cause-specific mortality rates are usually expressed per 100,000 population.

Age-Standardized Mortality Rates. Often, one wishes to compare the mortality experience of different populations. However, because mortality rates increase with age, a higher crude mortality rate in one population than another may simply reflect the fact that the first population is older, on average, than the second. When the underlying age distribution of two (or more) populations varies, one could either compare age-specific mortality rates or compute **age-standardized mortality rates**.

Age-standardized mortality rates are based on statistical techniques that eliminate the effects of different age distributions in different populations. Age standardization is used not only to compare mortality rates between nations with different underlying age distributions but also to compare mortality rates over time for a single nation, because the underlying age distribution has changed over time.

Years of Potential Life Lost. **Years of potential life lost (YPLL)** is a measure of the impact of premature mortality on a population.[10] For an individual who dies "prematurely" (usually defined as either before age 65 years or before the average life expectancy is reached), YPLL is calculated as the difference between that defined end point and the actual age of death. For an entire population, the YPLL is the sum of the individual YPLLs. **Cause-specific YPLL** can be calculated analogously for specific causes of death.

The **years-of-potential-life-lost rate** represents years of potential life lost per 1,000 population who are below the specified end point in age. YPLL rates are used to compare premature mortality in different populations, because YPLL alone does not take into account differences in population size. Furthermore, YPLL rates may be standardized by age to adjust for differences in the underlying age distribution of populations.

THE USES OF EPIDEMIOLOGY IN PUBLIC HEALTH MANAGEMENT AND PRACTICE

Epidemiology is not only "the study of the distribution and determinants of health-related events in populations," but it is also "the application of this study to control health problems." The applications of most importance to public health decision makers are community assessment, epidemic detection, public health policy development, and assurance of the provision of services. Ideally, the detection of epidemics should be integrated into community assessment. However, experience shows that public health emergencies are rarely anticipated, despite their frequent influence on the formulation of public health policy.

Community Analysis

Analyzing community health events and problems often follows five steps:

1. defining the problem
2. estimating the magnitude, characteristics, and occurrence of the problem

3. refining the definition of the problem
4. estimating the population needing health service
5. reevaluating the problem

Each of these five steps is applied to public health decision making. The first three are basic to assessing a community health problem. Step four is the quantitative basis for policy development because it determines the number, characteristics, and location of people in need of service. Assurance is provided by the reevaluation of the public health problem in step five.

Defining the Problem

This step poses both conceptual and measurement issues. The way in which a community analysis is done is influenced by the perceptions of health officials and community members. If a community experiences excessive injuries among young adults, for example, the analysis needs to examine measures appropriate to this concern. Potentially preventable cancer of the cervix, on the other hand, would require a different approach, as would sleep disorders in the elderly or unintended fertility among teenagers.

Measurement problems are often dealt with by using the most accessible data. Mortality measures are often used, as McGrady[11] did in his use of death certificates to examine cancer in the Fulton County portion of Atlanta, Georgia. The ready availability of death certificates, their validity for a cause of death such as cancer, and the characteristics of the information in these documents make them very useful for this purpose.

Fertility analysis using birth certificates has been applied to assessing the nature and extent of unintended pregnancy as a community health problem. One such approach analyzed teenage fertility, out-of-wedlock births, and marital births by birth order, but other measures could have been developed depending on the way in which health officials and community members perceived and conceptualized the problem in their locale.[12]

Medical care analysis often provides a community with the most vivid perception of a health problem. It may also be the best way to measure health events that do not lead to death or that have a long interval between the initiation of the condition and death. Hospital admission or discharge data, emergency room records, or clinical records in ambulatory care facilities may be important data sources in these cases.

Potential pitfalls in defining community health problems may seem obvious, but they can catch even those with the best of intentions off guard. Individual privacy, for example, even in the use of public documents, is a serious community problem that became obvious during the AIDS epidemic. Data quality is also variable, often to an unanticipated extent. This is true for medical care records and public documents. Data quality is influenced by data collection, transcription, and editing procedures. Analyses may produce results that are not expected, so the verification of those results is important before public statements are made based on them.

Defining community health problems is not easy or cheap. This step is often skipped, despite its obvious importance. Good examples of community health problem definitions are hard to find, and many writers use national or international data rather than that for a particular city or neighborhood. Publications by the National Center for Health Statistics in the *Health, United States* series, especially those that include a *Prevention Profile* or *Healthy People 2000 Review*,[13] are excellent sources of ideas and inspiration. The same is true of the books by Holland and his colleagues on avoidable mortality in the European community.[14] Defining a community's health problems requires good professional judgment and can benefit from including the perceptions of knowledgeable citizens in the community.

Estimating Health and Population Measures

Accurate measurement of community health problems will have an important influence on the community's perception of the problems and on the management of programs meant to solve them. The first step in doing this part of a community analysis is to scour the community for sources of data. Census data will be valuable. Health department vital statistics offices often have information with surprising detail. Local or state planning groups can be very helpful; they may have already done important portions of the analysis. University libraries, computer centers, market research groups, and economic analyses by financial institutions may also warrant consideration.

The analysis of health events and populations in small areas involves professional judgment and knowledge of the community. Independent estimates may differ. If this is the case, all of them must be examined to reconcile the differences and arrive at a judgment that is widely accepted by the community and its officials.

Refining the Problem Definition

Once a problem has been conceptualized and measured, experience shows that the initial definition must be refined for effective intervention. A community analysis of cancer, for example, may show areas where cancer deaths are excessive. Further analysis of the site of the cancer or of the potential risk factors may be needed to develop a program to control or prevent the problem.

Consider the following example. Suppose that a neighborhood or group of census tracts had an excessive number of cancer deaths. This was known from population estimates that permitted rates to be calculated. These confirmed the excessive occurrence of cancer. If the community had limited resources, what approach to cancer control would be most acceptable? This requires refining the definition of the problem. If an examination of death certificates showed that many of the cancers were cancers of the lung, for example, then tobacco control would be the program to initiate. If cancer of the cervix was frequent instead, screening women using cervical smears and cytology (Pap smears) would be a more relevant program.

As another example, if unintended pregnancy was determined to be a serious problem for a community, based on a fertility analysis, then a range of health program decisions might be considered. These could be narrowed down by refining the problem definition. A community with an abundance of women in their late childbearing years who were having larger families than they intended, for example, might need sterilization services. A community with frequent unintended teenage and/or out-of-wedlock pregnancies, on the other hand, might want to consider school-based birth control education and services.

Estimating the Population Needing Service

Once the highest priority problem for a community has been identified and community support and an effective intervention have been established, further analysis can characterize the population for which the intervention is needed. Typically, the analysis needs to identify the geographic distribution of the people; their age, gender, and special activities; and the most likely means by which they can access communications and receive (or be given) service.

The type of intervention that is selected will guide this phase of the analysis. Community-based programs, such as food sanitation and environmental cleanup, may be implemented without community members going to a special location. On the other hand, clinical preventive health services, such as vaccine administration, blood pressure measurement, and breast cancer screening, require technically skilled people and specialized equipment that are usually only available in a clinical setting.

Characterizing the population needing service, specifying the means of intervention, and determining how it will be delivered provide the basis for resource estimation. New, imaginative approaches to intervention, such as blood pressure screening in shopping malls rather than health department clinics or physician offices, may require pilot studies to evaluate usefulness and cost. Experience suggests that resource estimation often must allow for a limited amount of operational research if established interventions are to be used in a community with unique characteristics and requirements.

Reevaluating the Problem

Reevaluating the community's health problem should be integrated into the original plan aimed at its resolution. For some health issues, long-term, highly accurate measures that are the basis of the initial analysis may need to be reconsidered. Less accurate short-term measures might be useable if their results can be occasionally confirmed by measures that are better established. In addition, analysis of measures of intervention program performance often detect difficulties with program management. Identification of measures needs to be an integral part of initial program planning.

Summary

Community analysis is a process that is cyclic and needs to be repeated. Dealing with small areas and population groups requires a combination of careful analysis, detailed knowledge of community characteristics and dynamics, and sound intuitive judgment if the resultant health policy is to affect community health in a positive way.

Applying Community Analysis to a Community Mumps Epidemic

Community health problems may be acute or chronic, endemic or epidemic. They may include such conditions as infections, injuries, or infarctions of the heart. All are amenable to community analysis. A health department's response to a mumps epidemic illustrates the community analysis approach to using health data for managing a sudden, serious health problem.

Defining the Problem. Defining the problem in this instance began with the analysis of communicable disease surveillance data. These data showed officials in a southeastern state that, in the current year, an unexpected and large number of mumps cases were being reported. The unexpected cases were occurring primarily in people between the ages of 10 and 19 years, rather than in the usual age group of between 5 and 9 years.

Estimating the Magnitude, Characteristics, and Occurence of the Problem. Estimates of the magnitude, characteristics and occurrence of these cases focused especially on a metropolitan area in which 840 people with mumps had been reported to city/county health officials. The young people in whom this illness was concentrated were school age, and the illness struck both boys and girls.

Refining the Definition of the Problem. Refining the problem definition according to age and school attendance allowed the epidemiologists to pinpoint its location. Almost half the cases were students at a single high school. Further investigation indicated that a specific pep rally probably contributed to the initiation of widespread transmission. Studying the problem in even

more detail uncovered evidence that mumps afflicted an additional 126 middle school students and 28 elementary school students who attended feeder schools for this high school.

Estimating the Population Needing Health Service. Estimating the population needing health service had two dimensions in this instance. First, intervention was needed to halt the epidemic. Second, the prevention of future epidemics required a broader, statewide program.

Immunization against the mumps virus is clearly the best method of intervention. The key policy question is who should be immunized. The policy decision regarding control of the epidemic was conceptually straightforward. Everyone susceptible to mumps needed to be immunized. Because mumps vaccine carries no risk of side effects, there is no problem immunizing everyone exposed. In this instance, all students at the high school and its feeder schools as well as all family members of the ill children were targeted to receive vaccine.[15]

Mounting an effective program for the entire population at risk of mumps involved additional policy considerations as well as additional and difficult administrative action. The greater number of people (all children age one or older), the larger geographic area (the entire state), and the increasing number of cases showed that this epidemic heralded a long-term, statewide problem. It thus required a substantially greater investment of public resources for a longer period of time. In this instance, public officials added $300,000 to the health department budget for its immunization program.[16]

Reevaluating the Problem. Reevaluating the problem was done using the established surveillance system of infectious disease reporting, which in this state included mumps. In addition, detailed studies showed that the mumps vaccine was effective, confirming that the epidemic resulted from a failure to vaccinate and not from failure of the vaccine.

Following the increase in the budget for the state immunization program, no unexpected occurrences of mumps have been reported, and an effective surveillance system remains in place as a basic part of the public health infrastructure. Continued public health surveillance provides the people of this state assurance of immunization services and the capacity to detect new epidemics should immunization levels decline in the future.

Outbreak Detection And Investigation

One of the primary reasons for conducting surveillance of communicable diseases is to detect outbreaks so that prompt and appropriate public health action can be taken.

An *outbreak* or an *epidemic* is the occurrence of more cases of a disease than expected in a given area or among a specific group of people over a particular period of time.

Detecting Outbreaks

In order to detect an outbreak, it is essential that case reports and summary tabulations be reviewed by public health authorities on a regular basis, such as weekly. Regular review provides the staff with a sense of the *usual* numbers and patterns of disease, and this knowledge allows them to determine numbers or patterns that are *unusual* and worthy of further investigation.

For a disease that occurs infrequently in a jurisdiction, health department staff usually look at the number and contents of the individual case reports. If only one or two cases of a disease are expected all year, every case report represents an unusual event, and two or more in a short period of time represent a cluster worthy of explanation. For such diseases, more can be learned by looking at detailed information on the case report than by summarizing the reports by abstracting information for basic descriptive variables. For example, if a health department were to receive a case report of malaria, for which the expected number of cases is zero per week in most health departments in the United States, a member of the health department staff would likely review the case report closely, focusing particular attention on the section describing where the patient may have acquired the infection.

Many notifiable diseases are more common than can be analyzed practically by reviewing individual case reports. Therefore, many health departments enter key information from case reports into a computer database and run a computer program each week to perform descriptive epidemiology—grouping numbers of cases by time, place, and person. The most common methods for displaying the data are simple cross-tabulations and graphs. The usefulness of more sophisticated techniques, such as analysis of time-space clustering, time-series analysis, and computer-mapping techniques, is currently being explored.

Nonetheless, even for more common diseases, important information may be gleaned by looking at the case reports themselves. For example, state health department staff in one state were able to detect an outbreak of hepatitis B that was transmitted by a dentist because they regularly reviewed and compared the dental exposures reported for hepatitis B cases.[17]

Analysis of surveillance data primarily involves comparing current numbers and patterns of cases with some usual or expected value, identifying differences between them, and assessing the importance of those differences. Usually, the expected values are based on numbers for recent reporting periods or for the corresponding week of previous years. In addition, current data from one reporting area (for example, a county) can be compared with data from neighboring areas or with data for the larger area to which it belongs (for example, comparing county data with state data).

Despite this emphasis on data collection and analysis, many outbreaks come to the attention of public health officials by telephone, long before the case report forms are filled out. Alert health care providers—physicians and nurses in particular—frequently piece together information based on their contacts with patients and notify the health department of suspicious clusterings of disease. In addition, members of affected groups may call the health department to report or express concern about unusual occurrences of disease.

To illustrate, in late October 1989, two physicians from Bogalusa, Louisiana telephoned the epidemiology office in the Louisiana State Health Department to report that over 50 cases of pneumonia had occurred among persons in and around that community since early October, of whom six had died.[18] Although the clinical histories and presentations of many patients were consistent with legionellosis, the hospital laboratory was not equipped to test sputum for *Legionella pneumophila*, so no specimens were collected. In addition, insufficient time had elapsed to compare titers in acute and convalescent sera. Therefore, no cases could be reported through the traditional case–reporting system because the specific disease was unidentified. The physicians were nonetheless concerned, and they prompted public health officials to initiate a more detailed investigation of these cases of pneumonia.

Investigating Outbreaks

Some outbreaks are over by the time the health authorities learn of them. Others may be handled over the telephone. However, for ongoing outbreaks that require field investigation, working quickly is essential. Getting the right answer is essential, too. Under such circumstances, epidemiologists find it useful to have a systematic approach to follow, such as the sequence of steps listed in Table 12.3. This approach assures that the investigation proceeds without missing important steps along the way.

The steps described in Table 12.3 are listed in conceptual order. In practice, however, several steps may be done at the same time, or the circumstances of the outbreak may dictate that a different order be followed. For example, control measures should be implemented as

TABLE 12.3   Steps of an Outbreak Investigation

1. Prepare for field work
2. Establish the existence of an outbreak
3. Verify the diagnosis
4. Define and identify cases
   a. Establish a case definition
   b. Identify and count cases
5. Perform descriptive epidemiology
6. Develop hypotheses
7. Evaluate hypotheses
8. As necessary, reconsider / refine hypotheses and execute additional studies
   a. Additional epidemiologic studies
   b. Other types of studies—laboratory, environmental
9. Implement control and prevention measures
10. Communicate findings

soon as the source and mode of transmission are known, which may be early or late in any particular outbreak investigation.

Preparing for Fieldwork. Anyone about to embark on an outbreak investigation should be well prepared before leaving for the field. Preparations fall into three categories: scientific, administrative, and consultative. The investigator first must have the requisite scientific knowledge, supplies, and equipment to carry out the investigation. Second, because most investigators work for an agency with bureaucratic requirements, the investigator must follow administrative travel and related procedures. Third, because most field investigations are collaborative, the investigator must know who the local contacts are, as well as the role the investigator is expected to play in the field, for example, leader versus consultant.

Before departing for Bogalusa, the team from the state health department updated their knowledge of the clinical, epidemiologic, and laboratory aspects of Legionnaires' disease. Then they gathered the appropriate supplies. They also discussed the role and responsibilities of each member of the team, including an epidemiologist and laboratorian called in from the CDC to assist.

Establishing the Existence of an Outbreak. One of the first tasks of a field investigator is to verify that a purported outbreak is indeed an outbreak. In an outbreak, the investigator usually presumes that the cases are related to one another or that they have a common cause. Some purported outbreaks turn out to be true outbreaks with a common cause, some turn out to be sporadic and unrelated cases of the same disease, and others turn out to be unrelated cases of similar but unrelated diseases.

Often, the investigator must first determine the expected number of cases before deciding whether the observed number exceeds the expected number. Even if the current number of reported cases exceeds the expected number, the excess may not necessarily indicate an outbreak. Reporting may rise even without any increase in disease for several reasons, including changes in local reporting procedures, changes in the case definition, increased interest because of local or national awareness, or improvements in diagnostic procedures. A new physician, infection control nurse, or health care facility, for example, may see referred cases and more consistently report cases, when in fact there has been no change in the actual occurrence of the disease. In areas with sudden changes in population size, such as resort areas, college towns, and migrant farming areas, changes in the numerator (number of reported cases) may simply reflect changes in the denominator (size of the population).

Whether an apparent problem is worth investigating further is not strictly tied to verifying that it is a true outbreak. The severity of the illness, the potential for spread, political considerations, public relations, available resources, and other factors all influence the decision to launch a field investigation.

The decision to conduct the field investigation in Bogalusa was made even before accurate background data were available. The physicians estimated that the number of patients with pneumonia seen in October was at least five times higher than usual, and six deaths were highly unusual. By reviewing hospital discharge data, the investigators determined that the number of patients discharged with a diagnosis of pneumonia in October of the previous three years were 15, 8, and 10, with a mean of 11, as compared to 70 patients in 1989.

Verifying the Diagnosis. Closely linked to verifying the existence of an outbreak is establishing what disease is occurring. In fact, the investigator frequently can address these two steps at the same time. The goals in verifying the diagnosis are to assure that the problem has been properly diagnosed and to rule out laboratory error as the basis for the increase in diagnosed cases. In Bogalusa, the investigators had to wait for a comparison of acute and convalescent sera to eventually confirm that the outbreak had been caused by *Legionella*. Later, lung tissue from two autopsied patients grew *Legionella* of the same subtype.

Establishing a Case Definition. A *case definition* is a standard set of criteria for deciding whether an individual should be classified as having the health condition of interest. A case definition includes clinical criteria and—particularly in the setting of an outbreak investigation—restrictions by time, place, and person.

The clinical criteria should be based on simple and objective measures, such as elevated antibody titers, fever greater than 101°F, three or more loose bowel movements per day, or myalgia (muscle pain) severe enough to restrict the patient's usual activities. A good case definition will include most if not all of the actual cases, but very few or none of the *false-positive* cases, persons who meet the case definition but do not have the disease in question. Recognizing the uncertainty of some diagnoses, investigators often classify cases as confirmed (usually with definitive laboratory findings), probable (meeting most of the criteria), or possible (meeting some of the criteria).

In Bogalusa, the investigators defined a possible case of Legionnaires' disease as illness in a resident or visitor of Washington Parish, about 20 years of age or older, admitted to one of the five local hospitals after October 1, 1989, with an infiltrate on chest radiograph. A confirmed case had to meet the criteria for a possible case, plus have lab evidence of legionellosis (four-fold rise in antibody titer, a single convalescent antibody titer $\geq$1:256, positive urine antigen test, positive sputum culture, or positive biopsy).

Identifying and Counting Cases. The cases which led to the recognition of an outbreak are often only a small and nonrepresentative fraction of the total number of cases. The next step is to determine the geographic extent of the problem and the populations affected by it.

Regardless of the disease under investigation, the information shown in Table 12.4 should be collected for every case.

Usually, the information listed in the table is collected on a standard case report form, questionnaire, or data abstraction form. Critical data items may be extracted onto a form called a **line listing**. A line listing resembles a spreadsheet, with each column representing an important variable, such as name or identification number, age, sex, case classification, and so on. Each row represents a different case, and new cases are added to a line listing as they are identified. Thus, a line listing contains key information on every case and can be scanned and updated as necessary. Even in the era of microcomputers, many epidemiologists still maintain a hand-written line listing of key data items and turn to

TABLE 12.4   Information Collected on a Standard Case Report Form

Type	Specifics/Examples	Use to the Investigator
Identifying information	name, address, and telephone number	allows the investigator to contact patients for additional questions, notify them of laboratory results and the outcome of the investigation, check for duplicate records, and map the geographic extent of the problem
Demographic information	age, sex, race, and occupation	provides the "person" characteristics of descriptive epidemiology needed to characterize the populations at risk
Clinical information	symptoms, physical examination findings, laboratory and x-ray results	allows the investigator to verify that the case definition has been met, plot dates of onset, and describe the spectrum of illness
Risk-factor information		tailored to the specific disease in question, may be used for both hypothesis generation and hypothesis testing
Reporter		enables investigator to seek additional clinical information and report back the results of the investigation

their computers for more complex manipulations, cross-tabulations, and the like.

The Bogalusa investigators set up active surveillance for case finding at all five local hospitals. In addition, they used a standard questionnaire to abstract information from the medical records of all persons admitted or discharged with a diagnosis of pneumonia, respiratory distress, or possible Legionnaires' disease since October 1, 1989. These data were maintained in an *Epi Info* file on a portable computer.

Performing Descriptive Epidemiology. Descriptive epidemiology means characterizing the outbreak by time, place, and person. This step is critical for several reasons. First, by looking at the data carefully, the investigator gets a sense of which information is reliable and informative (for example, many cases reporting the same unusual exposure) and which may be less reliable (for example, many missing or "don't know" responses to a particular question). Second, descriptive epidemiology provides a comprehensive description of the outbreak by portraying its time course, its geographic extent (place), and the populations (persons) affected by the disease. By assessing the descriptive epidemiology in light of what is known about the disease (usual source, mode of transmission, risk factors, and populations affected, among others), the investigator can develop rational causal hypotheses to evaluate.

By November 19, the Bogalusa team had identified 79 patients who met the definition of possible Legionnaires' disease. Fourteen of these patients had died without *Legionella* testing. Of the 79, 64 percent were female and 31 percent were African-American. Over half the patients were residents of Bogalusa. Of the Bogalusa residents, 67 percent lived on the east side of town. Most patients had been admitted in mid-October, with few if any new cases occurring in mid-November, as shown in Figure 12.1. To date, no sputum culture had shown growth for *Legionella* or other pathogens.

Developing Hypotheses. While developing hypotheses may be the next conceptual step, hypothesis generation may actually begin with the first phone call. Hypotheses may be generated by scientific knowledge (What are the usual vehicles or risk factors for this disease), discussions with affected patients and local health staff, descriptive epidemiology (What are the common features of the cases?), and outliers (What did the one person from out of town have in common with the affected residents?). The hypotheses should address the source of the agent, the mode and vehicle or vector of transmission, and the exposures that caused the disease. Also, the hypotheses should be testable, because evaluating hypotheses is one of the goals of the next step in an investigation.

At this point in the Bogalusa investigation, the leading hypothesis was that the outbreak was caused by

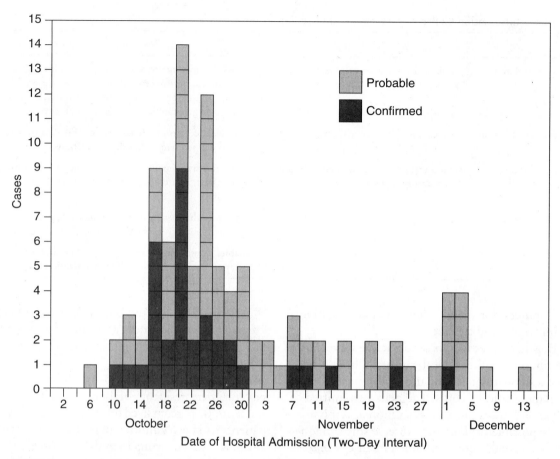

FIGURE 12.1 Probable* and confirmed cases of Legionnaires' disease by date of hospital admission, Bogalusa, Louisiana, October 1 to December 15, 1989.

*Pneumonia without laboratory-confirmed *Legionella pneumophila*.

outdoor exposure to cooling towers, a cause of several previous Legionnaires' disease outbreaks. After talking to a few of the patients, investigators also began to compile a list of retail stores and other commercial establishments that were frequently mentioned. In addition, investigators noted the unusual preponderance of females and the locus on the east side of town.

Evaluating Hypotheses. In field investigations, hypotheses can be evaluated in one of two ways: either by comparing the hypotheses with the established facts or by using analytic epidemiology to quantify relationships and assess the role of chance. The first method

would be used when the clinical, laboratory, environmental, and/or epidemiologic evidence so obviously supports the hypotheses that formal hypothesis testing is unnecessary.

In many other settings, however, the circumstances are not as straightforward, and even very careful analysis of the series of cases is insufficient to determine if the hypotheses are supported. In such circumstances, **analytic epidemiology,** characterized by the presence of a comparison group, is required to test hypotheses. A comparison group enables the investigator to quantify relationships between exposures and disease and to test hypotheses about causal relationships. The investigator usually chooses between a case-control study and a retrospective cohort study design, depending on the type of health outcome under study, the population affected, and the resources available.

The Bogalusa investigators decided to conduct a case-control study to test their hypotheses. Two controls per case would be selected from office records of physicians who admitted the cases. A total of 28 cases and 56 controls were enrolled. Cases and controls were asked about exposures to cooling towers and nearby buildings. Exposure to area cooling towers and to nearby buildings was not substantially different for cases and controls. However, 93 percent of the cases, but only 52 percent of the controls, frequently visited a particular grocery store.

Refining Hypotheses and Executing Additional Studies. If the original study was unrevealing or pointed in a general direction without sufficient specificity, the investigator needs to reconsider the hypotheses. Perhaps the investigator needs to return to the hypothesis generation stage, or perhaps a different comparison group is needed to test a more specific hypothesis.

In the Bogalusa investigation, additional epidemiologic analysis demonstrated a dose-response relationship between time spent in the grocery store and risk of disease. The investigators visited the grocery store and looked for potential sources of aerosolized water. An ultrasonic mist machine was operating over one section of the produce display. No one at the grocery store was familiar with the maintenance or operation of this machine. Permission was obtained to culture a specimen of water from the reservoir of the misting device. The culture from the misting device contained *Legionella pneumophilia* serotype 1 (LP-1). Cultures from various cooling towers around town also contained LP-1, but of different subtypes.

Four additional activities were undertaken. A serosurvey was conducted among all grocery store employees in Bogalusa to determine antibody status against LP-1. A second case-control study was undertaken to determine if exposure to the misting device was associated with developing Legionnaire's disease. Ten similar misting devices from other parts of the country were

cultured. The investigators asked for permission to perform autopsies on two patients who had died of pneumonia early in the epidemic.

Employees at the suspected grocery store were more likely to have elevated antibody titers to *Legionella* than employees at the other grocery stores included in the study. Analysis of the second case-control revealed a significant association between disease and purchasing produce, which was nearest to the mister. Of the ten mist machines from other parts of the country, six grew *Legionella*. The subtype of *Legionella* found in the grocery store misting device was also isolated in a small cooling tower, which was far from public access and not in proximity to the grocery store in question. Lung tissue from the two autopsied patients revealed *Legionella* of the same subtype as that found in the grocery store.

Implementing Control and Prevention Measures. In most outbreak investigations, the primary goal is control and prevention. Although control and prevention are conceptually step nine, health authorities should, in fact, implement control measures as soon as possible. Control measures can usually be implemented early if the source of the outbreak is known.

In general, control measures are aimed at the weak links in the chain of infection. Control measures can be aimed at eliminating the agent/source/reservoir, such as destroying mosquito breeding sites; interrupting transmission/exposure, such as instructing people to avoid wooded areas or wear protective clothing to reduce the risk of acquiring Lyme disease; or reducing susceptibility of the host, such as giving immune globulin to travelers.

Communicating the Findings. The final task is to communicate the findings. This communication usually takes two forms, an oral briefing and a written report. The oral briefing should be directed to local health authorities and persons responsible for implementing control and prevention measures. The findings must be presented in clear and convincing fashion with appropriate and justifiable recommendations for action. The written report serves as a record of performance, a blueprint for action, and a document for potential legal issues. It also serves as a reference if the health department encounters a similar situation in the future. Finally, a report that finds its way into the public health literature serves the broader purpose of contributing to the knowledge base of epidemiology and public health.

The Bogalusa investigators concluded that the misting device was the source of aerosols that caused the outbreak. They were reluctant to publish the results until the laboratory was able to demonstrate that viable *Legionella* could be isolated from aerosols produced by the machine. This was expected to take several weeks. In mid-December, the machine was removed from the grocery store and sent to the CDC for further study. Because it seemed likely that other mist machines could harbor *Legionella,* the Food and Drug Administration (FDA) was notified. The FDA quickly developed guidelines for maintaining the mist machines.

The Louisiana State Health Department issued a press release and an electronic mail message describing the mist machine findings. Grocery industry officials were notified about the potential problem in trade newspapers and at meetings. The press release was widely quoted in newspaper articles. Additional findings were published in the *MMWR* after laboratory staff were able to isolate *Legionella* organisms from aerosols produced by the machine.[19]

CONCLUSION

Epidemiology and health data play a central role in public health practice. Whether the data come from long-established surveillance systems, vital records, periodic or special surveys, registries, or special studies, judicious use of quantitative information should lead to better planning, program administration, and policy development in the public health arena.

REFERENCES

1. Last JM, ed. *A Dictionary of Epidemiology. 2nd ed.* New York, NY: Oxford University Press; 1988.

2. Langmuir AD. The territory of epidemiology; pedimento. *J Infect Dis.* 1987;155:3.

3. *Comprehensive Plan for Epidemiologic Surveillance.* Atlanta, Ga: Centers for Disease Control; 1986.

4. Centers for Disease Control. Guidelines for evaluating surveillance systems. *MMWR.* 1988;3(suppl S–5).

5. *Healthy People 2000; National Health Promotion and Disease Prevention Objectives.* Washington DC: US Dept of Health and Human Services; 1991. PHS publication 91-50213.

6. *Data for the Year 2000 National Health Objectives: The ASTHO Reporting System's New Core Data Set.* Washington, DC: Public Health Foundation; 1990.

7. *Health Plan Employer Data and Information Set and User's Manual.* version 2.0. Washington, DC: National Committee on Quality Assurance; 1993.

8. Vogt RL, Clark SW, Kappel S. Evaluation of the state surveillance system using hospital discharge diagnoses, 1982–1983. *Am J Epidemiol.* 1986;123:197–198.

9. Kovar MG. *Data Systems of the National Center for Health Statistics.* National Center for Health Statistics, Vital and Health Statistics; 1989. Series 1(23).

10. Wise RP, Livengood JR, Berkelman RL, Goodman RA. Methodologic alternatives for measuring premature mortality. *Am J Prev Med.* 1988;4:268–273.

11. McGrady E. *Community Atlas of Cancer Mortality, Fulton County, Georgia, 1989–1991.* Atlanta, Ga: Centers for Disease Control; 1993. Report to the Association of Minority Health Professions Schools Foundation.

12. *Training for Family Planning Program Evaluators; Course Manager's Manual.* Atlanta, Ga: Centers for Disease Control; 1978.

13. *Health, United States, 1992 and Healthy People 2000 Review.* Hyattsville, Md: National Center for Health Statistics, US Dept of Health and Human Services; 1993. PHS publication 93-1232.

14. Holland WW, ed. *European Community Atlas of Avoidable Death.* New York, NY: Oxford University Press; 1988.

15. Wharton M, et al. A large outbreak of mumps in the postvaccine era. *J Infect Dis.* 1988;158:6.

16. Milner L. Prevention's the cure officials should seek. *Sunday Tennessean.* January 17, 1988.

17. Rimland D, Parkin WE, Miller GB, Schrack WD. Hepatitis B outbreak traced to an oral surgeon. *N Engl J Med.* 1977; 296:953–958.

18. Mahoney FJ, Hoge C, Farley TF, et al. Legionnaires' disease associated with a grocery store mist machine. *J Infect Dis.* 1992;165:736–739.

19. Centers for Disease Control. Legionnaires' disease outbreak associated with a grocery store mist machine—Louisiana, 1989. *MMWR.* 1990;39:108–110.

CHAPTER

Communications and Public Health

Larry Wallack, Dr.P.H.

Lori Dorfman, Dr.P.H.

Katie Woodruff, M.P.H.

For advocates, the press is a grand piano waiting for a player. Strike the chords through a news story, a guest column, or an editorial and thousands will hear. Working in concert, unbiased reporters and smart advocates can make music together.

Susan Wilson
New Jersey Network for Family Life

The practice of public health means regularly confronting significant problems that often seem intractable. Cancer, alcohol and other drug problems, homelessness, HIV/AIDS, and violence are just some of the problems that public health professionals face on a daily basis. Given the enormous task at hand, it is essential to use all available resources as efficiently as possible. The mass media constitute a powerful resource that typically has not been well used. Too often the media have been used only to address changes in individual behavior. The "new public health" requires that

consideration of the social, economic, and physical environment, as well as the individual person, be included in problem definitions and solutions.

This chapter shows how public health advocates can make better use of the mass media to address significant public health problems. First, a thumbnail sketch of how the media have traditionally been used in public health is provided. Then, the basic foundation for a new approach, called **media advocacy,** is reviewed. Finally, a 10-step guide to using media advocacy is presented.

TRADITIONAL MEDIA APPROACHES AND PUBLIC HEALTH

The most common use of the mass media to promote health has been to communicate specific health information to large audiences.[1] More recently, a social market approach has been developed.

Public Information Approach

The public information approach is based on the assumption that if people know the facts, they will change their health habits and consequently improve their health. For example, if people understand that smoking cigarettes can lead to health problems, they will never start smoking, or, if already smokers, they will quit immediately.

Although this approach sounds rational and makes a great deal of sense, in most cases it simply does not work. Despite the best health information, children and adults seem to be motivated by something other than facts, general knowledge, and attitudes. There is virtually no research evidence to show that public information campaigns or public service advertising are successful methods for changing health behavior and improving health.[2]

Most public service advertising focuses on individual choice as the crux of public health problems. This approach presumes that individuals' health decisions result from rational considerations of self–interest. Therefore, so–called behavioral problems, such as drinking and driving, tobacco or drug use, poor diet, or lack of exercise, are interpreted at best as health professionals' failure to present the right information in the right way to the right people. At worst, such problems are blamed directly on individuals' laziness, fatalism, or lack of motivation. In a very specific way, such public service campaigns represent propaganda of the status quo: by placing responsibility for health on the actions of individuals, they exonerate the political and economic system from significant responsibility for addressing the problem.[2,3]

Social Marketing Approach

In recent years, a somewhat more sophisticated approach to using the mass media for changing health behavior has emerged called **social marketing**. Social marketing has evolved as a popular approach that attempts to apply advertising and marketing principles to the "selling" of positive health behaviors. Social marketing has become a key concept in addressing some of the shortcomings of previous public communication campaigns. In general, social marketing provides a framework in which marketing principles are integrated with social–psychological theories to develop programs better able to change behavior. It takes the planning variables from marketing—product, price, promotion, and place—and reinterprets them for particular health issues.[2]

Social marketing has gained visibility through its careful application by community heart disease prevention programs in the United States[4] and Finland.[5] Social marketers have also claimed success in promoting contraceptive use and oral rehydration therapy in developing countries.[6] However, the positive health effects of these efforts have yet to be demonstrated convincingly.

Social marketing attempts to make it as easy and attractive as possible for the consumer to act in compliance with the message. This is achieved by creating the ideal marketing mix of product, price, promotion, and place. The *product* is the behavior or idea that the consumer needs to accept. In some cases it is a literal product, such as a condom; in other cases, it is a behavior, such as not drinking and driving. *Price* can refer to psychological, social, economic, or convenience costs associated with message compliance. For example, the act of not drinking in a group can have psychological costs of anxiety and social costs of reduced status. *Promotion* refers to how the behavior is packaged to compensate for the costs. It answers the questions: What are the benefits? What is the best way to communicate this message? Benefits could include health, increased status, self–esteem, or freedom from criticism. Finally, *place* refers to the availability of the product or behavior. If the intervention is promoting condom use, for example, then it is essential that condoms be widely available—both physically and socially. Condoms are more likely to be used when their use is supported and reinforced by peer groups and the community at large.[7]

The most significant contribution of social marketing has been the strong focus on consumer needs. Consumer orientation[8] means identifying and responding to the needs of the target audience. This is a departure from many past campaigns (and many current ones) where professionals developed messages and strategies with little input from those whom the message was designed to reach.[9]

Formative Research

To help tailor public communication efforts to specific audiences, formative research is used.[10] Formative research provides information and viewpoints to improve communication messages before they are finalized. At all stages of intervention design and implementation, such research provides important feedback to the planners. For example, small groups representing the target audience might convene to give their ideas about program strategy and their reactions to specific messages. Strategy and content can be modified based on the results of these focus groups.

Other kinds of formative research might include analyzing the audience in order to segment it into homogeneous groups; monitoring the target population's media habits so messages can be placed in the proper channels at the optimal time; and assessing preexisting knowledge and attitudes in the target population. Formative research, when done correctly, serves to reduce some of the uncertainty associated with campaigns. Testing possible campaign slogans, for example, can assure that such slogans are culturally sensitive and likely to be interpreted in a way that is consistent with campaign goals.

The Exchange Process

Special attention to the process of *exchange* is critical to the efficacy of social marketing approaches. The concept of exchange means that people are willing to give up some resource, such as time or money, for a benefit, perhaps a product or positive attribute. The marketing process attempts to facilitate a voluntary exchange that provides the consumer with tangible benefits at minimal costs in terms of money, physical or emotional effort, or group support. If, in the end, the intervention is not successful in facilitating this voluntary exchange, it is not likely to be effective.[8]

Limitations of Social Marketing

Social marketing has a number of limitations that inhibit its usefulness. It has been criticized as being manipulative and ethically suspect.[11] This is not surprising given social marketing's close correspondence to more general advertising and marketing practices. It has also been criticized for promoting single solutions to complex health problems and ignoring the conditions that give rise to and sustain disease. For example, in developing countries social marketing focuses on changing individual health habits rather than addressing environmental problems such as assuring a clean water supply.[6]

Social marketing is also limited by the difficulty of motivating the consumer to exchange immediate gratification for long–term benefit. Typical health promotion programs promise increased health status, positive image, and presumed peer approval in exchange for delayed gratification (for example, diet, smoking cessation), increased physical effort (for example, exercise), risk of social rejection (for example, abstinence from drugs), or physical discomfort (for example, withdrawal from nicotine). The limited success of these programs is not encouraging.

Another notable limitation is the relatively narrow, reductionist approach of social marketing. It tends to reduce serious health problems to individual risk factors and to ignore the proven role of the social and economic environments as major determinants of health. In the long run, this risk factor approach may contribute relatively little to reducing the incidence of disease in a population.

Summary

In sum, typical public service campaigns can raise awareness about public health problems and contribute to attitude change but generally do little to modify behavior. Indeed, these campaigns may serve the political function of maintaining a narrow definition of the problem and deflecting concerns about environmental factors that contribute to it, including production and marketing practices. Finally, these campaigns may also serve to minimize government responsibility for addressing the broader social and economic conditions that contribute to the problem.[3]

MEDIA ADVOCACY

In recent years, a "new public health" has emerged. This new approach to public health practice is based largely on a set of principles that stress broad–based participation, multisectoral planning, and the development of healthy public policy. Traditionally, public health professionals have not used the mass media to advance policy but rather to provide information about personal behavioral habits. For example, the media focused on messages telling people not to drink and drive and not to smoke. In recent years this focus has shifted, and the media are now being used to promote policies that would limit the availability of alcohol and tobacco products.

Recognizing the power of the media and the need for policy level interventions to improve health, advocates around the country have developed a new approach to using the media called **media advocacy**. Media advocacy is the strategic use of mass media to advance healthy public policy by applying pressure to policy makers. It focuses attention on those who have the power to change policy. This can occur when a news story draws attention to the actions of a specific individual (such as a mayor) or group (such as a planning commission). This can also occur when the news story alerts people to an issue or an action and mobilizes community support.

Media advocacy aims to have the news story told from a public health perspective. This means emphasizing the public policy dimensions of prevention, and shifting the focus from individual health behavior to the social, cultural, economic, and political context of health problems. Media advocacy also aims at making the problem visible so it can be put on the public agenda. Once a problem is on the agenda, media advocacy helps advance policy by drawing public attention to the actions of those responsible for enacting or opposing the policy.

Setting the Agenda: Framing for Access

A primary task of media advocacy is to direct the media spotlight to a particular issue and hold it there. In the early to mid–1980s, when AIDS was not covered by the *New York Times*, the issue did not make it to the nation's policy agenda either. As Daniel Schorr, National Public Radio commentator and longtime journalist, says, "If you don't exist in the media, for all practical purposes, you don't exist."[12] If the news media do not cover a demonstration highlighting a contradiction in health policy, for example, the event might as well not have taken place as far as the broader community—and probably the person with the power to make the desired change—is concerned.

Gaining access to the media is the first step for media advocates who want to set the agenda. Media access is important for two reasons. First, the public agenda-setting process is linked to the level of media coverage and thus the broad visibility of an issue. The media tell people what to think about: the more coverage a topic receives in the media, the more likely it is to be a concern of the general public.[13–16] Second, the media provide a vehicle for gaining access to specific opinion leaders. Politicians, government regulators, community leaders, and corporate executives are some of the specific people that it might be useful to reach.

In successful media advocacy, both objectives will be met. For example, alcohol advocates who wanted to remove PowerMaster malt liquor from the market were able to get the problem covered in the media, which helped to make it a public issue.[17] At the same time, specific politicians and government regulators at the Bureau of Alcohol, Tobacco and Firearms were exposed to media reports, which heightened their sensitivity to the issue and their belief that others around them were aware of the issue as well. Journalists put pressure on bureaucrats just by reporting the story, apart from what happened with public opinion after the story was broadcast. With tape rolling, officials had to answer for their actions. Consequently, advocates were able to muster enough public and regulatory pressure to remove PowerMaster from the market.

Newsworthiness

Journalists and editors are interested in stories that sell newspapers and attract viewers. In a variety of ways, media advocates take advantage of how news is constructed and what its objectives are. An issue will be covered only to the extent that it is timely, is relevant, is defined to be in the public's interest, and/or meets a number of other criteria of newsworthiness. Convincing journalists to cover a story often involves calling attention to the aspects of the story that meet these criteria.

Factors that determine newsworthiness include controversy, conflict, injustice, irony, celebrity, deviance, tragedy, uniqueness, and proximity.[17,18] Other important factors include the "breaking" quality of a news issue and the human interest element, which focuses on people overcoming difficult odds or helping others.[19]

Shaping the Debate: Framing for Content

Gaining access to the media is an important first step, but it is only a first step in influencing the public policy agenda. Once advocates have media attention, the challenge is to reframe the dominant view of health problems from individual matters to public issues. As Henrik Blum, a well–known health planner, notes, "There is little doubt that how a society views major problems . . . will be critical in how it acts on the problems."[20] Problem definition is a battle to determine which group and which perspective will gain primary "ownership" of the solution to the problem.

Clear and concise definitions of problems are appealing in that they facilitate concrete, commonsense solutions. Often, however, problems of health and social well–being are difficult to define, much less solve. The tendency is to simplify problems by breaking them down into basic elements that are easier to manage. Most public health problems are broken down into biological elements if the solution is medical treatment or informational elements if the solution is education.

This misguided pragmatism about problem solving reduces society's drug problem, an enormously complex issue, to a matter of individual failure to "just say no." Similarly, public and private institutions focus on identifying the gene for alcoholism while leaving the activities of the alcoholic beverage industry largely unexamined. Even though 30 percent of all cancer deaths and 87 percent of lung cancer deaths are attributed to tobacco use,[21] the main focus of cancer research is not on the behavior of the tobacco industry but on the biochemical and genetic interactions of cells.

The alternative is to see problems as part of a larger context. Tobacco use, for example, can be seen as a function of a corporate enterprise that actively promotes the use of a health–compromising product. Individual decisions about whether to smoke can be seen as inextricably linked to the decisions of relatively few people at the corporate level regarding production, marketing, and widespread promotion. Smoking, in this larger context, can be seen as a property of a larger system in which a smoker or potential smoker is only one part. The same approach can be applied to automobile safety, nutrition, alcohol, and many other issues.

Research and historical experience have established that the major determinants of health are not located as much in individual behavior as in the individual's social and physical environment. Therefore, public health professionals are charged with shifting the focus of the news media and the public from individual–oriented perspectives to policy approaches that aim to make the environment healthier.

Shifting the focus is a formidable challenge, because the tendency to define problems in terms of individual responsibility is deeply ingrained in our culture. For example, when a female jogger was brutally beaten by a group of "wilding" youths in Central Park in 1989, the first question in everyone's mind was, "What was she doing jogging alone in Central Park at 9:00 at night?" The media coverage of the tragedy focused on the personalities of the attackers and the defenselessness of the victim. No one asked, "Why isn't Central Park safe?" Thus, environmental factors such as lighting and patrols in the park, alternatives to crime for youth, and the broader issue of violence against women were not highlighted on the public agenda.

Many traditional public health media campaigns are guilty of a similar focus on individual responsibility to the exclusion of communal concerns. For example, a prominent nutrition campaign in California urges people to eat "five a day" in a promotion of the benefits of fresh fruits and vegetables. However, many Californians live in neighborhoods where there are no supermarkets or produce stands, only liquor stores and convenience stores. For those without access to fresh, affordable produce, the five–a–day campaign is worse than useless, because it may lead policy makers to the complacent belief that something is being done about the problem of inadequate nutrition.

DEVELOPING A MEDIA ADVOCACY PLAN

Successful media advocacy assures that the story is told from a public health perspective. This means maintaining a focus on the public policy dimensions of prevention; emphasizing the social, cultural, economic, and political context of health problems; and stressing participation in decision making. Media advocacy uses a range of media and advocacy strategies to define and stimulate broad–based coverage of health and social issues in order to advance healthy public policies.

The success of media advocacy may well depend on how well the advocacy is rooted in the community. As Tuchman notes, " . . . the more members, the more legitimate their spokesperson."[22] Media advocacy is not a strategy used alone but a tool that combines the separate functions of mass communication and community advocacy.

Groups and organizations seldom have a commitment to making good use of mass media. Often they fear talking with the media, or they respond to the media only when they absolutely must. It is also common for organizations to think simply of public affairs approaches to the media and thus focus their efforts on the least effective mechanisms.

Successful media advocacy is integrated throughout the organization's work. This requires a great deal of planning, creativity, and energy. To be effective, media advocacy must be an organizational commitment. Organizations must dedicate resources to making sure everyone in the organization understands the media advocacy approach and can apply it to various policy issues.

Steps to Follow

Media advocacy efforts will be most productive if the following steps are taken: monitor the media, develop a media list, cultivate relationships, carefully review policy objectives, set specific media objectives to pursue policy goals, identify targets, develop the message, specify the outlets for delivering the message, and carry out the plan. Note that the first three steps are basic to any

media advocacy efforts. They are conducted continuously regardless of which policy issues are currently of interest. Steps four through ten help plan for specific policy objectives.

Step One: Monitor the Media

The purpose of monitoring the media is to understand if and how the issue is being presented. For example, the issue of youth violence is often presented as a problem due to gangs or "bad" youth. This frame runs counter to the public health understanding of violence as a systems issue rather than as a personal problem. Importantly, the usual media frame reinforces a law—enforcement and punitive response that attempts to punish and remove bad youth. Instead it should suggest and reinforce prevention measures.

In order to work well with journalists, it is necessary to understand how they define and report news. This can be done by carefully watching television news, reading newspapers, and listening to the radio. This will identify the underlying text that is the "formula" that shapes most stories and usually must be changed to portray the issue more accurately. The formula generally emphasizes the typical elements of newsworthiness—tragedy, deviance, celebrity, and the others listed above—and neglects the social accountability aspects of the story.

The media outlets that serve the community in question are the outlets to monitor. They should be monitored for how often they cover the issues that are of concern and what they say about the issues. Do they tell the whole story? What parts of the story do they tell well? What parts have they left out?

Through careful attention to news stories about issues of interest, one can determine which journalists are most interested in the topic and which aspects of the topic interest them most. The different symbols and journalistic conventions that are used to tell the stories should be noted. This is the foundation from which journalists can be approached about aspects of the story that are not receiving attention.

Step Two: Develop a Media List

The purpose of developing a media list is to know where to send news releases, to whom to pitch stories, and to whom to provide ongoing background on the issues. The media list can evolve directly from monitoring by using as sources the names of reporters who attend to the issues. Other sources of reporters' names for the media list include previous contacts, reporters known by colleagues and friends, and media guidebooks, which are available in libraries and stores.

The objective is to keep a list of media people who can be contacted in the future—to invite to an event or to pitch a story. It can also be used to keep notes on journalists in order to keep current on their work. Media lists are living documents, constantly changing because people in the industry change jobs frequently. Thus, keeping an updated media list can be a big job, so agencies often share a single list.

Step Three: Cultivate Relationships

As the media are monitored and names of reporters, producers, and editors are collected for the media list, frequent contact should be made with journalists. Even the most casual contact is important, because it allows the development of relationships that can increase the media accessibility and credibility of public health projects.

A journalist's rolodex is an essential tool. When journalists are given a story assignment, their first step is to pick up the phone to gather information. Media advocates need to get into the journalist's rolodex. This can happen when a journalist calls and the advocate responds quickly with good information. It can also happen when the journalist knows the advocate is well connected to the community.

Another way to build relationships with journalists is to contact them directly. This can be done to pitch a story they may be interested in or to comment on a story they already did. For example, they should be told when they have done an important story. Public health practitioners also have a valuable commodity to offer to journalists; health issues are legitimate news, and journalists need expertise. Practitioners should let journalists know they are interested in their stories and have information that may make their next story more complete.

Step Four: Carefully Review Policy Objectives

Not every policy objective requires a media advocacy initiative to see it through. For example, if an organization wants to change a local school policy, and the school board agrees with the proposed change, there may be no need for media coverage. However, if there are school board members who do not think the proposal is important, media coverage may convince them otherwise or at least get their attention.

Both policy and media advocacy goals and objectives should be reviewed and revised if necessary. In fact, in the process of developing the target and message in the next two steps, policy advocacy goals may be clarified and revised or changed.

The organization's policy objectives should be examined to identify which ones would benefit from media coverage. This process can be done as policy objectives are prioritized. It may make sense to group together those objectives that will have media advocacy, or they may be prioritized based on community or political contingencies. The point is that policy objectives should drive the media advocacy plan, not the other way around.

After the decision is made regarding which policy objectives to pursue with media advocacy, the necessary background information to educate policy makers and the news media must be collected. Accuracy is extremely important and requires meticulous work when gathering and sharing information. An advocate who becomes a reliable source of useful, accurate information on an important social issue will be recontacted by journalists. On the other hand, an advocate who gives exaggerated or false information will lose credibility as a source and may never be recontacted by journalists. Moreover, an opportunity to educate the community will be lost.

Step Five: Set Specific Media Objectives to Pursue Policy Goals

Specific media objectives usually fall into two general categories: getting media attention and advancing the policy. Setting specific media objectives in those two areas can help narrow the focus of the work to a manageable plan.

The short–term question is: What needs to be done to get journalists' attention? It may be that local media are already interested in the issue in question, in which case getting their attention may mean a phone call to the reporters working on that beat to let them know of information or a side of the story that can help them with their work. If the issue is not already on the agenda, it must be put there. Sometimes a news release or a cold call will be enough to get a journalist's attention. At other times a more visible news event is necessary. As the issue is framed, potentially newsworthy elements, such as the controversy a policy is likely to generate, should be identified.

One example of creating news is the work of the Dangerous Promises Campaign, a coalition of alcohol policy and domestic violence advocates in California. Concerned about the ways in which sexist alcohol advertising reinforces attitudes of violence against women, the Dangerous Promises Campaign asked the Beer Institute, the Wine Institute, and the Distilled Spirits Council of the United States to adopt a code of ethics about portrayals of women and violence in alcohol advertising. To turn up the heat on the alcohol trade associations, the coalition developed a pair of counteradvertisements: one showed three serious women with the slogan, "Hey Bud—Stop using our cans to sell yours," and the other, playing directly on the Budweiser logo, had the slogan "Bloodweiser, King of Tears—Selling Violence against Women."

Billboard companies in both Los Angeles and San Francisco rejected the counterads, despite the fact that the coalition was not asking for public service spots but paid advertising space. The controversial content of the counterads, and the fact that a group of nonprofit agencies was denied the right to buy space for two small antiviolence advertisements, whereas alcohol companies spend over $2 billion a year to promote their deadly products, created controversy and irony that helped make the story newsworthy.

Besides controversy and irony, other conventions of newsworthiness can be attached to an issue. Is there a compelling injustice that can be highlighted? Does the issue relate to other news events locally? In making a national story local, reporters ask: Do the conditions that made this happen there also exist here? Is there a celebrity willing to endorse the policy or a "victim" who

will speak out who also knows how to link personal tragedy to social policy? Does the issue relate to a local or national anniversary or a seasonal event? For example, the news media routinely do stories about youth and drinking during prom week and the six-month or one-year anniversary of a tragic shooting is a reason to do stories on shootings that try to answer the question: Do the conditions that made the violence possible the first time still exist today? The reporter's job is to localize and personalize the story. To the extent that advocates can do that for journalists with their issues, the greater the likelihood that the advocate's perspective will be incorporated in the story or report.

The long–term question for planning specific media objectives is: What must be done to advance the policy? Getting the media's attention may prove to be much easier than influencing the interpretation of the problem and its solution to reflect policy goals. One strategy is to provide an "authentic voice," a person who has been affected personally by the issue and who can also promote policy goals. For example, if the issue is alcohol availability, the teenage victim of a drinking and driving crash might well attract a reporter's attention. However, rather than talking about her personal feelings about nearly being killed, the teen might talk about the need for stricter local enforcement of laws against merchants selling alcohol to youth.

Long–term goals involve strategizing about the message and the recipient, as discussed in steps six and seven below. Long–term goals also aim to build the capacity of the organization to anticipate journalists' needs and questions and attract their attention when necessary. Long–term objectives may involve organizational objectives, such as developing a media list and cultivating relationships with journalists.

Step Six: Identify Target(s)

Mass media messages are always more effective when they are specifically defined for certain recipients. The general public often gets information as a result of media advocacy initiatives, but they are not usually the primary target. Sometimes the recipient of media advocacy may be a single individual. The power to influence that individual comes from his knowing that everyone in the community is in on the conversation.

When the target is just one key person, paid media can be useful in reaching her. For example, at a critical stage in the legislative process of the Tobacco Products Control Act, the Canadian Non-Smokers' Rights Association took out a full-page ad in a Toronto newspaper. The ad showed a picture of the prime minister with the president of the Canadian Tobacco Manufacturers Council. The headline read, "How many thousands of Canadians will die from tobacco industry products may be in the hands of these two men." The text of the ad appealed to the prime minister to act in the interests of future generations by supporting the tobacco control legislation. By suggesting that the prime minister might be influenced more by the tobacco industry than by concern for the public's health, the ad used controversy to publicly shame its target. The legislation passed, and the prime minister supported it.

There are two key questions to help determine who should be receiving the message. Which person or group has the power to make the desired policy change? Who in the community can be mobilized to draw attention to the policy? These two questions guide the next two steps.

Step Seven: Develop the Message

It is very important to have a consistent, direct, and clear message that will minimize confusion and create a common bond among all those who speak with the news media. The sometimes objectionable reality is that the media rely on sound bites of sometimes fewer than 10 seconds to make a point. Quotations may be longer in print than on television but not always. The sound bite reality requires that the message be concise.

Framing the message is an important part of media advocacy strategizing. Media advocates take advantage of the conventions of newsworthiness to frame the message to get media attention. Too often news stories focus on personal tragedy rather than social action and policy solutions. After getting media attention, media advocates must frame the message to emphasize specific aspects of the story that help journalists move from the person to the policy, from feeling to action.

This can be difficult, because journalists feel it is their job to make stories meaningful by personalizing them. One of the authors of this chapter, Larry Wallack, was once interviewed on The Today Show for his thoughts on the efficacy of the scare tactics commonly used to keep teens from drinking and driving. In this case, youths who had been brain-damaged in drunk-driving crashes spoke to high school audiences before prom night. While Wallack proposed more effective, environmental interventions, such as limiting alcohol's availability and raising its price, the interviewer repeatedly asked individual-oriented questions, such as, "Can't these programs change *some* kids' behavior?" and, "What can parents do to keep their kids from drinking and driving?" The result was a thematic tug-of-war throughout the interview. Ultimately, Wallack was able to expand the journalist's frame to include the activities of the alcoholic beverage industry—in this case, its marketing to youth. By the end of the interview, the problem of teen drinking was addressed as a social issue as well as an individual issue.

Whatever the issue, journalists will want to know some version of the following: What is the problem here? What do you think the solution is? If each of those questions can be answered in just a few sentences, then it is time to make contact with the news media. The objective is advancing the policy, so the answer to the solution question should include some aspect of the policy that is being advanced.

Step Eight: Specify the Outlets for Delivering the Message

Nearly every city or town in the United States has a variety of print and electronic media outlets attended to by a variety of audiences. The outlet for the message is determined by whom it should reach.

Newspapers are read by policy makers everywhere. They pay attention to hard news, editorials, letters to the editor, and op-ed pieces (editorials and guest editorials). There are other parts of the paper that may be just as valuable depending on the policy objective, target, and message. A community group seeking to ban tobacco and alcohol sponsorship in their local sports arena may benefit from a story on the sports pages, for example.

Television news can bring visibility to an issue. Television generally takes its cues from local newspapers, but each medium can influence the other. Public affairs and talk shows offer space for more in-depth views and community perspectives. Though seen by fewer people, those who do watch public affairs shows are more likely to be interested or involved in policy.

Radio news and talk shows provide opportunities to speak relatively longer than on television. There are also usually far more radio stations than television stations or newspapers, and radio is often precisely targeted to specific audiences. For those reasons radio can be useful for reaching policy makers as well as for mobilizing community members to become active in policy advocacy.

Paid advertising in newspapers, on billboards, or on radio can be very effective outlets for a message for two reasons. First, the ad can deliver the message directly in an outlet the target is likely to see. It functions like news in that the recipients of the message know they were not the only ones to see the message. They know others also saw the ad and now know who is responsible for doing something, and can hold the responsible party accountable. Second, when an ad is controversial, as with the Canadian Non-Smokers' Rights Association advertisement described earlier, it can generate news coverage on its own.

Outlets should be chosen based on which media the target pays attention to. For example, during the confirmation hearings of William Bennett, tobacco advocates wanted to call the Senate nominating committee's attention to the irony of an active tobacco addict being nominated as the first national drug czar. They purchased a full-page ad in the *Washington Times* to issue a drug-free challenge to Bennett, a two-pack-a-day smoker. The controversial ad campaign generated news coverage in the *Washington Post* as well as other papers. Advocates knew their campaign had reached its target when congressional committee members questioned Bennett about tobacco issues during his confirmation hearings.

It is necessary to find out which papers the targets read and which news they listen to—that is where the message should be placed. If one of the objectives is to influ-ence the mayor, for example, the message should appear on the editorial pages of one of the local papers. If one of the objectives is to mobilize community support for a particular policy, the media channels that are most likely to reach community members should be used.

Step Nine: Carry Out the Plan

Implementation activities may not become clear until the organization has determined which policy objectives it wants to focus on and the targets and messages that will be developed. In general, the activities will include getting journalists' attention and having background materials ready for them. This means developing accurate and comprehensive yet concise background materials, planning events such as demonstrations, pitching stories, and meeting with members of the news media. A general rule for implementation is to question each activity in terms of overall goals and objectives. Ask whether the activities lead to the accomplishment of specific objectives.

Step Ten: Rethink and Assess Steps One to Nine

Periodically, the media advocacy plan should be assessed and revised to assure that activities are on target. It is critical to evaluate both the process and the outcome of the initiative.

Media advocacy depends upon the policy being advanced. Policy change work, like other political activity, can evolve from the planning stage through implementation. Therefore, to be sure a media advocacy plan is responsive to current circumstances, it should be reviewed periodically. This evaluation of process objectives builds on experience to date and makes adjustments for the future. In particular, it is important to consider whether policy goals have changed. The following questions should also be asked:

- Based on the media coverage, does the media advocacy plan need revision?
- Is the target still appropriate?
- Is the message still what is intended?
- Is monitoring capturing what is needed?
- Is the media list complete and current?

Answering these questions will help in making appropriate adjustments during the media advocacy initiative. For example, if a policy board takes an action that advances a policy, rather than using media messages to put pressure on them, one might use a news conference to congratulate their sense of responsibility and wise action.

Evaluation. No two media advocacy initiatives will be the same. Each initiative will reveal itself in particular community and policy circumstances, yet there is much that can be learned about media advocacy from others. Most evaluations of media advocacy have been in the form of case studies.[17,23] Case studies are an effective way to evaluate media advocacy because they can capture the nuances that each initiative exhibits.

The following outcome evaluation measures can help assess the effectiveness of a media advocacy initiative:

- Placement: Where did the message appear? Did it appear where it was meant to?
- Message: Was the story told with the desired emphasis?
- Outcome: What was the reaction to the message? Did the target respond? Were there phone calls from community members, other media or anyone else?
- Impact: What happened as a result of the coverage? Was there movement on the policy? Were others brought into the effort?

Summary

In summary, media advocacy planning can be thought of as occurring in three stages: self-defense, reflection, and action. Self-defense refers to understanding the forces that shape the mass media and knowing how the issue is being portrayed. This allows reframing of the overall presentation to reflect policy goals. Reflection involves blending knowledge of the issue with knowledge of how the news media work in order to develop an overall media strategy. Reflection helps formulate the overall goal, the target to address through the media, and the outcome that is desired. Finally, action entails building the capacity to work with the news media, implementing the plan, and maintaining the power of media in the organization's efforts.

CONCLUSION

The media are too powerful a resource to be squandered on disappointing, individual-focused public health campaigns. Public health issues are also too important to be hidden away in public service corners. Media advocacy is a promising tool for combining the power of the media with the legitimacy of community advocacy to promote healthy, responsible public policy.

The tightening economy is affecting the newsroom as much as it is affecting every other sector of the world. There are fewer journalists to cover more stories. Although that is bad news for journalists, it can be good news for media advocates. As media resources shrink, opportunities for advocates grow because they can take up the slack. By establishing relationships with reporters and providing them with solid information on important health issues, media advocates can help reporters do their job. By developing a savvy understanding of the media's conventions and needs, advocates can also help place their issues and perspectives on the public agenda more easily.

Health professionals are valuable, credible resources with legitimate news stories to promote. By combining the leadership of the profession with the reach and impact of the news media, public health professionals can be powerful advocates for healthy public policy.

REFERENCES

1. Rice R, Atkin C, eds. *Public Communication Campaigns.* Newbury Park, Ca: Sage Publications; 1990.

2. Wallack L. Two approaches to health promotion in the mass media. *World Health Forum.* 1990;11:143–154.

3. Dorfman L, Wallack L. Advertising health: the case for counter-ads. *Public Health Rep.* 1993;108:716–726.

4. Farquhar J, et al. Community applications of behavioral medicine. In: Gentry W, ed. *Handbook of Behavioral Medicine.* New York, NY: Guilford Press; 1984.

5. Puska P, Wiio J, McAlister A, et al. Planned use of mass media in national health promotion: the "Keys to Health" TV program in 1982 in Finland. *Can J Public Health.* 1985;76: 336–342.

6. Aufderheide P. Hucksting health. *Channels.* 1985;5:51–52.

7. Kashima Y, Gallois C, McCamish M. Predicting the use of condoms: past behavior, norms, and the sexual partner. In:

Edgar T, Fitzpatrick M, Freimuth V, eds. *AIDS: A Communication Perspective*. Hillsdale, NJ: Lawrence Erlbaum Associates; 1992.

8. Lefebvre C, Flora J. Social marketing and public health intervention. *Health Educ Q*. 1988;15:299–315.

9. Dervin B. Audience as listener and learner, teacher and confidante: the sense making approach. In: Rice R, Atkin C, eds. *Public Communication Campaigns*. Newbury Park, Ca: Sage Publications; 1990.

10. Atkin CK, Freimuth V. Formative evaluation _____ _____ _____-paign design. In: Rice R, Atkin C, eds. *Publi_____ Campaigns*. Newbury Park, Ca: Sage Publica_____

11. Buchanan D, Reddi S, Hossain Z. Social n_____ appraisal. *Health Prom Int*. 1994;9:1–9.

12. Communications Consortium Media C_____ *_____munications for Nonprofits: Strategic Med_____ lic Interest Campaign*. Washington, DC_____ and the Center for Strategic Communi_____

13. Cohen B. *The Press and Foreign Polic_____ ton University Press; 1963.

14. Iyengar S, Kinder DR. *News That_____ versity of Chicago Press; 1987.

15. McCombs M, Shaw D. The ager_____ media. *Public Opinion Q*. 1972;3_____

16. Rogers E, Dearing J. Agenda setting research: where has it been and where is it going? In: Anderson JA, ed. *Communication Yearbook*. Beverly Hills, Ca: Sage Publications; 1988.

17. Wallack L, Dorfman L, Jernigan D, Themba M. *Media Advocacy and Public Health: Power for Prevention*. Newbury Park, Ca: Sage Publications; 1993.

18. Shoemaker P, Mayfield E. Building a theory of news content: a syntheses of current approaches. *Journalism Monographs*. 1987;103:1–36.

19. Dearing J, Rogers E. AIDS and the media agenda. In: Edgar T, Fitzpatrick M, Freimuth V, eds. *AIDS: A Communication* _____ Hillsdale, NJ: Lawrence Erlbaum Associates;

_____ _____uction. *Fam and Commu-*

_____ and dietary patterns among _____tes, 1991. MMWRR. 1992

_____ *Study in the Construction of Re-* _____ Press; 1978:92.

_____. Making news, changing policy: _____acy on alcohol and tobacco issues. _____ for Substance Abuse Prevention;

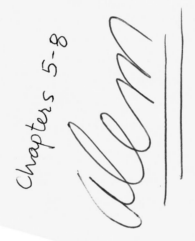

CHAPTER

14

The Management of Public Health Services

Gregory A. Ervin, M.P.H.
Dominic Frissora, M.P.A.

For many people, the area of budgeting and fiscal management signifies mystery, uncertainty, and perhaps uneasiness. In reality, budgeting should be viewed in a very positive light. It is a basic part of the overall planning process for public health. Good planning for the future requires both an understanding of community needs and an awareness of available resources. Budgeting is an important part of planning for the utilization of personnel, supplies, materials and equipment in the most efficient and effective manner to accomplish a specific set of goals and objectives.

The objective of this chapter is to help the reader gain a better understanding of the budget process in order to effectively manage the resources available to address public health issues. A public health officer must be aware of the fiscal status of his program or department in order to be an effective manager. She must meet payroll and pay vendors or service objectives will not be met.

The more leaders know about budgeting, the more effectively they will be able to communicate with those who help establish the budget, whether they are finance director, mayor, county commission, city council, financial/budget committee, or the voters.

BUDGETS

The word **budget** is derived from the French word *bougette* that means a leather bag, pouch, or purse and its contents. According to Webster, the word budget is both a noun and a verb. As a noun, budget is defined as, "a plan for the coordination of resources and expenditures; the amount of money that is available for, required for, or assigned to a particular purpose." As a verb, budget is defined as, "to plan expenditures for a budget."[1]

The National Committee on Governmental Accounting defined a budget as "a plan of financial operation that includes an estimate of proposed expenditures for a given period of time and the proposed means of financing them."[2]

Most definitions of budget contain the word *plan*. In this chapter we will try to emphasize budgeting as a dynamic planning function and not "number crunching" or "bean counting," a perception held by many. Developing a budget is a process for prioritizing resources and activities, a mechanism for managers to control spending and operational procedures, and it can serve as a basis for program evaluation. In essence, a budget is a mechanism to assist management in operating an organization more effectively and to put the scarce resources of qualified personnel and funds to the best possible uses. Because public health agencies operate day-to-day in a dynamic environment, a budget must be flexible in order to be effective.

The budget can be thought of as a road map showing how to get from point A to point B. In addition to providing a plan that shows how resources will be utilized to accomplish agency goals and objectives, an accurate budget is required by various funding sources in order to properly account for the expenditure of public funds.

A budget is a financial plan specifying how much money or revenue a department expects to receive during a given period and how that projected revenue will be expended for the provision of goods and services. Budgets must be developed, reviewed, and approved by appropriate authorities, and they must remain flexible to account for various economic and work load changes. Specific objectives of the budget may have to be revised during the budgeting period to match changing needs for services with available revenue.

BUDGETING

Many people have an innate fear of budgeting. The process, the magnitude of the numbers, and the need for control overwhelm them. However, budgeting can be one of the most exciting, innovative, and creative areas of public health administration. Every phase of management is influenced by the budget. Budgeting provides the opportunity to envision and examine problems and to creatively develop alternatives for addressing problems and controlling operations. It allows

one to be involved in one of the most important planning and operating processes of a public health agency.

In budgeting, goals and objectives must be defined and their costs identified. The cost of providing services must be compared with the benefits expected to determine whether the cost justifies the benefit to be gained. Should $50,000 be expended to provide a popular program that has little tangible impact on the health of the community, or should that popular program be deleted in favor of a new program almost certain to improve health status? The cost of providing service includes, but is not limited to, salaries, employee fringe benefits, travel costs, administrative support, supervision, supplies, materials, equipment, and additional overhead costs.

Budgets must remain flexible to accommodate an agency's needs and be responsive to a changing environment. Budgeting is not an end in itself; rather, it is the identification of needs and resources and a guide for the prudent expenditure of those resources during the budget period in order to accomplish a specific set of objectives.

There are a variety of effective ways to develop a budget. A public health manager should be familiar with each of them so the most appropriate can be chosen to fit the circumstances at hand. Each job may require a different budgeting tool or perhaps a combination of budgeting tools. Making the correct choice(s) is an important element of the success of a program or agency.

Common Budgeting Tools and Concepts

Budgeting concepts have evolved over time from basic input-oriented models to sophisticated models that focus on public impacts. In this section, the basics of four budgeting frameworks are presented: line-item budgeting, performance budgeting, program budgeting, and zero–base budgeting. Variations and combinations of these frameworks are utilized in practice.

Line-Item Budgeting

Perhaps the most basic form of budgeting is the **line-item budget**. The focus of this form of budgeting is on inputs, such as the amount of money to be spent on line items and objects of expenditures (for example, personnel, equipment, and supplies). It does not focus on outputs, such as number of people to be served, cost per unit of service, or quality of service.

In order to achieve a balanced budget, anticipated revenues are **allotted,** or distributed, among various categories, such as departments, objects of expenditures, or functions. This type of budgeting is relatively easy to employ and expends minimal resources of staff time for budgeting, accounting, and evaluation.

Fund accounting is used to provide technical control. Fund accounting controls and accounts for each line-item in checkbook–like fashion. Expenditures and obligations are compared to appropriations for each line item, thereby providing the amount of the appropriation still available for spending. Success is based on not exceeding the budget spending limits.

Drawbacks. A disadvantage of line-item budgeting is that it is based on prior funding levels and provides for incremental funding. Competition among agencies and departments is encouraged, and cooperation among them is discouraged. There is no incentive for analysis and creativity.

Are there public needs that are not being met? Are there alternative ways for addressing the public needs that will provide higher-quality service at a comparable or lower cost? Are duplicate services provided in multiple departments? These are questions that are not answered when a line-item budget is utilized. By focusing on the inputs instead of the outputs, it becomes difficult to use the budgeting process for planning purposes.

Example. Consider the following example. The manager of a small local health department uses a line–item budget to help manage the department. Two operating divisions are created: The Environmental Services Division and the Personal Health Services Division. The manager allocates resources between the two divisions.

All activities related to the environment, such as well water monitoring, sewage disposal, solid waste management, food service operations, vector control, litter control, and nuisance abatement, are addressed by the Environmental Services Division. All activities related to individual or personal health, such as child and family health services, disease control and investigation, clinical services, and home health services, are addressed by the Personal Health Services Division.

Both environmental services and personal health services are essential programs. Both divisions must function at the highest level in order to assure that all health needs of the community are fully addressed. Each division has a budget that provides for a specific number of staff members as well as the supplies, materials, and equipment needed to provide services to the community.

With a line-item budget, the individual division managers are responsible for assuring that the environmental services and personal health needs of the community are met and that their budgets are not exceeded. The total budgeted amount for the department and each division is dependent solely upon available revenue, and only broad, general funding categories appear in such a budget.

If there are no major problems, the primary control of services provided are the funds made available for division managers. As department head, the manager has no means of knowing whether available resources are being maximized, whether services are being provided in an efficient manner, whether needed services are being provided, or whether services are being duplicated. The manager does, however, have a clear budget plan allocating available resources between the Environmental Services Division and the Personal Health Services Division. Table 14.1 shows a sample line-item budget for this example.

TABLE 14.1 Line-Item Budget

Environmental health services	$ 500,000.00
Personal health services	700,000.00
	$1,200,000.00

Environmental health services include personnel conducting environmental inspections and direct program support, such as registered sanitarians, supervisors, clerical support; and supplies, material, and travel.

The personal health services include public health nurses, clerical support, travel expenses, medical/clinic supplies, and materials.

The only detail provided in this line-item budget is the allocation of funds between the two divisions.

Broad discretion remains in this type of budget, allowing the movement of funds among various programs within the divisions. No feedback regarding performance is provided.

Performance Budgeting

Performance budgeting focuses on activities pursued by establishing standards for measuring success. It provides for managerial control to improve the quality of services at the same or lower cost. Cost accounting and operations research are the methods used to measure success. The act of establishing good, reasonable standards is critical for performance budgeting to be successful.

Drawbacks. Unlike line-item budgeting, performance budgeting addresses output, but it still shares many of the disadvantages of line-item budgeting described above. For example, it does not identify unmet public needs and unnecessary services, and it does not address services that are duplicated. Whereas feedback to monitor and control a line-item budget is readily available through the fund–accounting system, feedback for a performance budget requires gathering information that may not have been available before and analyzing it. Thus, more resources are required to implement and maintain a performance budget than a line-item budget.

Example. Using the same example as earlier, implementing a performance budget to manage a small local health department with two major operating divisions, the Environmental Services Division and the Personal Health Services Division, requires the establishment of standards for all activities of the health department. These standards define desired levels of performance, and data collection procedures must be in place in order to collect information for performance analysis.

Assume the Personal Health Services Division is responsible for improving the immunization status of children in the community, and it has a goal of immunizing 9,000 of 12,000 preschoolers in the community at a cost not to exceed $9.50 per child immunized. Data collected to determine the success of this activity include the number of preschool–age children seen; the number of immunizations given; and the cost of vaccines, personnel, supplies, space, waste disposal, and equipment. A sample performance budget for this example is shown in Table 14.2.

TABLE 14.2   Performance Budget

Performance Statistics—Childhood Immunization Program	
Staffing for 52 weeks (2 RNs)	$60,000.00
Contract office assistant	15,000.00
Vaccine, supplies, and infectious waste disposal	8,000.00
Clinic rental	1,300.00
Replacement equipment (typewriter)	500.00
	$84,800.00

Children immunized = 9,000

Cost per child − $84,800/9,000 = $9.42 per child immunized

The performance budget can determine the cost of a unit of service and allows cost benefit analysis to be conducted. The budget is set up to address a specific service area need. Feedback is provided to evaluate the impact of the program and its contribution to the mission of the agency.

Note that this performance budget can only provide services if children find their way to the clinic. There is no connection to an outreach service if children fail to come for services.

Program Budgeting

Program budgeting's primary focus is on goals. Line-item and performance budgets are usually passed by legislative bodies to initiate programs, often in a nonintegrated manner that results in duplication. Program budgeting, by contrast, is frequently used by public administrators to make goal–oriented proposals for funding approval. The public administrator thus guides the programs to attain the goals set forth in the budget.

Goals are developed through **strategic planning,** which develops budget policy by:

- identifying necessary goals and services that are not provided by the private sector
- establishing goals and objectives for providing such services
- identifying alternative ways to meet goals and objectives
- identifying resources available and needed for each alternative
- selecting the best possible alternative
- determining how to measure program successes and failures, that is, program evaluation

Cost–Benefit Analysis. **Cost-benefit analysis,** a commonly used evaluative method, analyzes the price of program success. Cost-benefit analysis allows for comparison of the services provided by the various programs with their costs in order to maximize the benefits of available resources.

Drawbacks. There is often legislative resistance to program budgeting because it is perceived to reduce legislative authority. Another disadvantage of program budgeting is that it requires a commitment of human resources to perform the cost–benefit analysis of the many alternatives. In addition, program budgeting does not always fit in the public budgeting process because it requires strategic planning that often extends beyond the budget period.

Planning Programming Budgeting System (PPBS). An advanced program budget model is the **Planning Programming Budgeting System.** This model incorporates scientific management and priority setting to maximize resource utilization and allocation. PPBS examines what needs to be done, establishes objectives, develops alternative means for meeting the established objectives, determines what resources are needed for each alternative, and prioritizes the use of available resources. PPBS gained considerable attention in the early 1960s during the Kennedy administration when it was utilized by the Department of Defense under Secretary Robert McNamara.

Example. Using the earlier example, a program budget requires that goals be established for all activities of the Environmental Services and Personal Health Services divisions of the department. For example, one goal might be to inspect all restaurants and bring them into compliance with all food service regulations so that foodborne disease is reduced by a certain percentage. Another goal might be to immunize fully all children prior to entering the first grade of school so that no child is allowed to go unprotected from a disease for which a vaccine is available.

In line-item budgeting there are no definitions of desired outcomes, only the allocation of resources for general program activities. In performance budgeting a specific amount of staff time and resources is budgeted to address specific activities, such as restaurant inspections and immunization clinics. With program budgeting, by contrast, a managerial decision is required to assure that inspections are provided as needed to gain compliance and that educational activities are provided to help eliminate foodborne diseases. In the program budget process, the cost of increased inspection and educational activities may exceed the benefits of reducing foodborne diseases by a set percentage, and the activities may be discontinued or done less frequently by changing the predetermined level of foodborne disease cases that may be deemed acceptable. A sample program budget for this example is shown in Table 14.3.

TABLE 14.3 Program Budget

Goal I—Inspect all restaurants in the health district twice a year.

Field sanitarians/inspectors/ support persons	$40,000.00
Supplies and materials	500.00
Transportation	1,000.00
	$41,500.00

The program manager may opt to increase or decrease the level of inspections based on the quality of the restaurants and the number of suspected cases of foodborne illness reported. Poor restaurant quality and increased cases would justify increased inspection activities. A high level of compliance with standards and minimal suspected cases of foodborne illness would allow resources to be redirected to other activities.

Goal II—Investigate all rodent complaints within 24 hours and place bait when appropriate

Rodent abatement staff	$10,000.00
Supplies	500.00
Transportation	500.00
	$11,000.00

Should complaints decrease, personnel could be reassigned to other activities such as food service/restaurant inspections. Should complaints increase, additional personnel could be assigned or the goal of making inspections within 24 hours could be increased to match needs and resources.

In both the restaurant inspection program and the rodent abatement program, the manager would utilize data to adjust personnel as needed to meet program needs.

Zero-Base Budgeting

Zero-base budgeting (ZBB) was developed in 1969 by Peter Pyhrr for private sector application and adopted for government use in 1973 in the Georgia state budget.[3] With ZBB, all management levels participate in setting the organization's objectives and developing the budget.

The ZBB model in its pure form breaks down programs into smaller decision packages and ranks the decision packages based on need. More managers and more management time are utilized in the ZBB approach because *all* programs are broken down, evaluated, and systematically compared to determine their effectiveness and efficiency. Unmet needs are analyzed, alternatives for meeting these needs are developed, and decision packages are created. As many decision packages are prioritized as funding permits. All, part, or none of a current program may be funded along with new initiatives. In this manner, ZBB not only determines whether things are being done right, but also whether the right things are being done.

ZBB in its purest form is not commonly used, however, because of the resources needed to manage it. Nonetheless it is a useful tool for developing large agency or programmatic budgets or for long–term planning. It is also useful when there is a significant change in available funds to be budgeted.

Variations of the ZBB model are also used. The Ohio state budget, for example, has used a 90 percent base budget—each state agency had a base equivalent to 90 percent of its current budget. The agencies then developed and prioritized decision packages for the remaining 10 percent of their current budget and any new initiatives they wished to address. The primary focus of the state budget process was then on all costs above the 90 percent base.[4]

Example. Returning to the earlier example, ZBB requires development and ranking of decision packages that encompass current activities of the Environmental Services and Personal Health Services Divisions. Restaurant inspections or immunization activities might each be broken into two decision packages.

One inspection per year might satisfy minimum state requirements. Semiannual inspections might gain 90 percent compliance with food service laws, whereas three or more inspections might be required to reach 100 percent compliance. Weekly immunization clinics might be sufficient to immunize 75 percent of the children prior to school. Outreach to alternative sites and home visits might be required to approach 100 percent immunization levels.

The four decision packages might be ranked as follows:

1. one basic required restaurant inspection at a cost of $41,500
2. semiannual inspections at a cost of $83,000
3. immunization clinic at a cost of $84,800
4. alternative clinic sites and home visits to reach additional children at a cost of $41,400

If these are the only activities performed by the two divisions in the example and there is only $126,300 available, packages one and three could be included in the budget. If $167,700 is available, packages one, three, and four could be included. The Personal Health Services Division would thus be fully funded and the Environmental Services Division would receive a budget reduction that would fund only the basic state–required activities.

The decision packages are actually microbudgets, and alternative means of accomplishing the objectives are encouraged. For example, the Environmental Services Division might explore alternative, lower–cost ways of improving the quality of food service operations and reducing foodborne diseases. It might propose a training program for food service operators in the health department to reduce the number of rechecks and thus decrease travel and staff time. This could significantly lower costs and might change budget priorities. A sample zero–based budget for this example is shown in Table 14.4.

Budgeting Tool and Concept Summary

Budgeting has evolved from a focus on inputs and processes to a focus on outputs and outcomes. It provides an exciting and creative process for managing a government agency, department, or program while maximizing the use of limited resources.

TABLE 14.4 Zero-Base Budget

A true zero-based budget requires each program or division to start at zero and build a case for funding. Variations of zero-based budgeting are more common in public funding. A 75 percent or 90 percent base of previous funding may be provided, and additional funds are added based on a manager's ability to describe services that will be provided.

	Modified Zero-Base Budget		
	90%	10% continuation	Total
Environmental health	$1,800,000	$200,000	$2,000,000
Nursing services	1,800,000	200,000	2,000,000
Administration	900,000	100,000	1,000,000
Laboratory	315,000	35,000	350,000
	$4,815,000	$535,000	$5,350,000

Examples of Justifications for Full Continuation Funding

A $200,000 funding level above the 90 percent base would allow the Environmental Health Division to continue rodent abatement activities through the continued employment of four field staff and one supervisor and the purchase of rodent bait.

A $200,000 funding level above the 90 percent base level would allow the Nursing Services Division to continue weekly child health clinics at two sites that see 5,000 children annually.

A $100,000 funding level above the 90 percent base level in the Administration Division would allow the department to retain one grant writer and two accountants that are responsible for $3,000,000 in grant funds.

A $35,000 funding level above the 90 percent base level would allow the laboratory to keep a microbiologist who is currently conducting a childhood blood lead program analyzing 5,000 blood samples annually.

The four programs could be compared and contrasted by the authority approving the budget. Environmental health, nursing, administration, and the laboratory would each be evaluated on its own merits for full or partial funding. The impact of both full and reduced funding would be made clear for all programs.

The **rainmaker theory** presented by Joseph Peters at the Delbert Pugh Health Planning Conference demonstrates the need for this evolution of the budget process.[4]

- The rainmaker gets so involved with the rain dance, that he forgets the goal is to make rain.
(The focus is on process, not goals.)
- "I know I didn't make rain, but wasn't the dance beautiful?"
(The desired outcome is missed, but the process is good.)
- The science of rainmaking turns into the science of rainmaking dancing.
(The process replaces the desired outcome as the end goal.)

When public administrators are responsible for the financial management of a health agency, they cannot afford to make the rainmaker's error and allow the beautiful dance that has no positive outcome to replace the purpose of budgeting. The outcome of the process must be to provide for the public good, and financial management tools are the vehicles to assure that the community receives the maximum benefit from use of its resources.

Real–Life Budgeting and Public Health

In the past, a public administrator might demonstrate with medical research and pilot programs that an immunization program could prevent diseases and improve the health of specific populations. In response, a convinced legislative body might earmark a specific amount of resources for this purpose. Documentation of a successful program would come from the accounting records that showed spending within the budgeted amount and from programmatic information that documented the number of people immunized and protected from a specific disease. The focus was on input.

Today, that proposed immunization program has become harder to sell. Questions likely to be asked now include: How much of an impact does the immunization program have in preventing diseases compared to a scaled-down program or no program at all? How does the impact of the immunization program compare to that of other programs utilizing the same resources? What is the political climate at this time? Is there a search for funds to support another initiative? How does that initiative (for example, health care reform or a special maternal and child health program) interrelate with the proposed immunization program?

Resources are needed to develop a public health agency's budget proposal. An information base is also required to develop issue papers for budget proposals. This information base might include the agency's accounting and program data, vital statistics, and the results of studies and surveys. In addition, human resources are needed for developing the budget document and shepherding it through the budget process. Staff need training and experience in budget theory, the agency's budget process, public health, accounting, statistics, and organizational management, as well as partisan and nonpartisan political awareness and communication skills.

The Budget Process

A typical public health agency's budget process might proceed according to the following seven steps. Note that the first four steps are internal to the agency, and the last three are external.

1. The director solicits new initiatives from the agency's administrators, board members, constituents, elected officials, and/or concerned citizens.
2. After an analysis of existing programs and new initiatives, meetings with agency administrators and forums with constituents are held.
3. Priorities are established by the director, and the budget document is prepared.
4. The budget is presented to the central governmental body (for example, the mayor, governor, or county administrator), along with other agencies' budgets.
5. From this information, the governmental budget is prepared and submitted to the legislative authority (for example, city council, state legislature, or county commissioners) for approval.
6. Hearings are held at which the submitting agencies, proponents, opponents, and expert witnesses testify.
7. The legislative authority usually modifies and then passes the budget. This is probably the single most important legislative action affecting the public health agency.

The budget process does not begin and end with the budget being prepared and approved. In reality, the process is an ongoing cycle, as illustrated in Figure 14.1. Once the budget is approved, it is implemented and managed as information is continually provided. Program results and outcomes are evaluated, and the evaluations serve as a basis for developing the next budget.

PUBLIC FUNDING: A PUBLIC TRUST

A public health official has the important responsibility of faithful stewardship of public funds. Decisions regarding expenditures must be prudent and in the best interests of the public. Public perception is an important consideration. Should the confidence of the public be lost due to poor financial management or the perception of poor financial management, it is very difficult for a public agency to regain it. Regardless of the quality of services, a lack of public confidence due to poor financial management can render an agency ineffective in addressing community needs.

Maintaining Accountability

Local health agencies must establish and follow basic financial management standards. Many state and local government units have adopted such standards to help assure accountability. They include the formal adoption of an annual budget document by the board or governing body, the connection of the budget to specific program objectives to be accomplished with

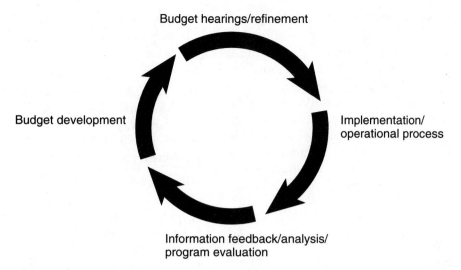

Budget hearings/refinement

Budget development

Implementation/
operational process

Information feedback/analysis/
program evaluation

FIGURE 14.1 Budget Cycle

the funds appropriated in the budget, and the development of a system to review the extent to which the objectives are met.

Generally accepted accounting and auditing procedures and policies should also be adopted to assure the proper expenditure of public funds through a system of checks and balances. Appropriate journals, ledgers, registers, and financial reports should be developed and maintained. The financial management system must identify and track both the receipt and expenditure of funds. As part of the system of checks and balances, there should be a separation of powers: personnel responsible for the receipt of funds should not also be responsible for the final expenditure of funds or for inventory control. Such checks and balances are essential for maintaining credibility and accountability in any agency.

Internal Controls and the Control Environment

A series of internal controls are needed to assure that public funds and property are safeguarded from exploitation. Basic internal controls should include, as part of the accounting system, a voucher system and

control procedures that allow all invoices to be checked for accuracy prior to the release of payment. A receiving report verifying the receipt of goods or services should also be generated prior to the release of payment. In addition, an inventory system that tracks ascending and descending totals of goods and supplies should be tied into the receiving report and voucher system.

A good system of internal controls that tracks the receipt of goods, inventories goods, and issues appropriate payments upon receipt and verification of stated quantities helps protect public funds and agency credibility. An additional benefit of such internal controls is the ability to take advantage of discounts for prompt payments. This type of system also assures that invoices are not lost and allowed to go unpaid, perhaps accruing late payment charges. Errors in noting the quantity of goods received and/or dispersed may be a major problem that can drain an agency of needed resources. A good inventory system with trigger reorder points helps keep an agency from running out of essential supplies, such as vaccine or mosquito insecticide.

Whenever possible, different persons should handle each area of the control environment. The segregation of duties can greatly improve accountability. As noted earlier, the person receiving goods should complete the receiving report but not issue the payment. The person conducting inventories should not be allowed to write off lost or damaged goods independently, but with the approval of a superior outside the immediate unit. This helps maintain the credibility of the system.

In general, control efforts do not add to the productivity of an agency, but they are essential to protect the agency and the public from loss. They are not infallible, but they do make it more difficult to misappropriate goods or services. Thus, they make it less likely that an incident of misuse or misconduct will occur that could erode public confidence and waste public funds.

Assessing Effectiveness of Internal Controls

The following questions can help public administrators assess the effectiveness of internal controls and help them adjust internal controls to meet agency needs.

- Is a chart of accounts used?
- Does the accounting system monitor both the encumbrance and expenditure of funds?
- Does the accounting system provide current and accurate information?
- Does the accountant/bookkeeper provide monthly updates of revenues, encumbrances, and expenditures?
- Are cash receipts supported by prenumbered, multipart receipt forms that can be reviewed by a different party during a daily reconciliation?
- Are revenue deposits collected and deposited daily?
- Does a system exist to address cash overage and/or underage, that is, cash in excess of receipts or cash less than receipts.
- Are all receipts and disbursements tracked in appropriate journals?
- Is there an appropriate petty cash policy in effect?
- Is someone other than the bookkeeper responsible for the inventory functions?
- Are periodic physical inventories taken to verify quantities of goods?
- Are accurate inventory records maintained?
- Is access to supplies and materials limited to appropriate personnel?
- Are purchase requisitions or purchase orders used to authorize purchases?
- Are purchase requisitions/orders tied into the accounting system with appropriate personnel responsible for the authorization of purchases?

In most public agencies, the greatest proportion of the budget goes towards salary and related costs for employees. Time and attendance thus represent significant potential for errors or misconduct on the part of public officials. The following additional questions are therefore especially important:

- Is there an accurate system to record time and attendance and make appropriate entries on payroll records?
- Are attendance and time worked verified for all employees?
- Are employees' balances charged for their annual leave, sick leave, and/or compensatory time?

CONCLUSION

This chapter has illustrated the basic concepts of budgeting and financial management. A budget is nothing more than a plan to help utilize financial resources in the most effective manner to accomplish a specific set of goals or objectives. It is a basic road map that shows how to get from point A to point B. Obstacles (changing needs, changing resources) present detours that require adjustments. The budget process must therefore remain flexible enough to adjust to real–world situations and allow responses to an ever changing environment. At the same time, safeguards must be in place to ensure accountability so that public funds are guarded and public confidence is maintained. Budgeting is not an end in itself but only one of many management tools to help meet the objectives of the agency.

REFERENCES

1. *Webster's Seventh New Collegiate Dictionary*. Springfield, Ma: G & C Merriam Company; 1963.

2. National Committee on Governmental Accounting, Municipal Financial Officers Association of the United States and Canada. *Governmental Accounting, Auditing, and Financial Reporting*. Ann Arbor, Mi: Coshing-Melloy Inc; 1968.

3. Pattillo JW. *Zero-Base Budgeting: A Planning, Resource Allocation and Control Tool.* New York, NY: National Association of Accountants; 1977.

4. Stoltz R, Ervin G, Frissora D. Budgeting, A tool of public health nursing services. Columbus, Oh: Ohio Department of Health; Spring 1991.

SUGGESTED READINGS

Babunakis M. *Budgets: An Analytical and Procedural Handbook for Government and Non Profit Organizations.* Westport, Ct: Greenwood Press; 1976.

Butt HA, Palmer DR. *Value for Money in the Public Sector: The Decision Maker's Guide.* New York, NY: Basil Blackwell; 1985.

Dillon RD. *Zero-Base Budgeting for Health Care Institutions.* Germantown, Md.: Aspen Systems Corp; 1979.

Griesemer JR. *Accountants' and Administrators' Guide: Budgeting for Results in Government.* New York, NY: John Wiley & Sons; 1983.

Hanlon JJ. *Public Health Administration and Practice.* St. Louis, Mo: The CV Mosby Company; 1974.

Haveman RH, Margolis J. *Public Expenditures and Policy Analysis.* Chicago, Il: Markham Publishing Company; 1970.

Hoffman FM. *Financial Management for Nurse Managers.* Norwalk, Ct: Appleton-Century-Crofts; 1984.

Jancura EG. City of Akron Internal Control Training Program. Akron, Oh: City of Akron; December 2, 1993.

Osborne D, Gaebler T. *Reinventing Government.* Reading, Ma: Addison Wesley Publishing Company Inc; 1992.

Premchand A. *Government Budgeting and Expenditure Controls: Theory and Practice.* Washington, DC: International Monetary Fund; 1993.

Premchand A. *Public Expenditure Management.* Washington, DC: International Monetary Fund; 1993.

Pyhrr PA. *Zero-Base Budgeting: A Practical Management Tool for Evaluating Expenses.* New York, NY: John Wiley & Sons; 1973.

Raftery WJ. *Government Accounting and Financial Reporting Manual.* Boston, Ma: Warren Gorham Lamont; 1993.

Rubin J, Hildreth WB, Miller GJ. *Public Budget Laboratory Workbook.* Athens, Ga: the University of Georgia Carl Vinson Institute of Government; 1983.

State of Ohio. Local Health Department, Self-Study Guide/Report in Preparation for Peer Review. Columbus, Oh: Ohio Department of Health; 1989.

Steiner PO. *Public Expenditure Budgeting.* Washington, DC: The Brookings Institution; 1969.

Steiss AW. *Public Budgeting and Management.* Lexington, Ma: Lexington Books; 1972.

Wholey JS. *Zero-Base Budgeting and Program Evaluation.* Lexington, Ma: Lexington Books; 1978.

CHAPTER

Teaching and Research

F. Douglas Scutchfield, M.D.
C. William Keck, M.D., M.P.H.

This chapter is designed to illustrate the linkage of public health practice to education and research in public health. It discusses the public health workforce, its composition, and its education and training needs. It describes educational programs for public health professionals. It describes current research focused on public health and links that research to the role of public health agencies.

It might seem inappropriate to some that a text dedicated to the practice of public health should include a chapter on teaching and research. It is appropriate when one considers that the effective public health practice site is dependent for its success upon well-trained practitioners who can draw upon an expanding knowledge base about effective public health strategies. Indeed, public health practice settings have a responsibility to support and participate in both teaching and research activities. "Real–world" practice opportunities for students and community-based, practice-oriented

research projects are otherwise very difficult, if not impossible, to arrange.

THE PUBLIC HEALTH WORKFORCE

In order to be able to make accurate decisions about the supply, demand, and need for public health personnel, a complete and accurate data base about the public health workforce should be available for analysis. Unfortunately, that kind of information does not yet exist. Collecting workforce data has been difficult because so many different professions are active in public health, and a substantial portion of the workforce does not have formal public health training. Recently, the Health Services and Resources Administration organized a consortium of federal agencies and professional organizations to address the need for workforce data to guide planning for professional public health education.

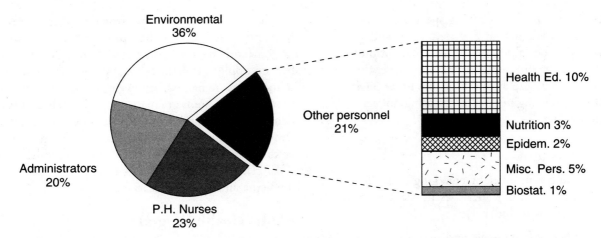

FIGURE 15.1 Public Health Personnel in 1989. SOURCE: *Health Personnel in the United States, Eighth Report to Congress 1991.* Washington, DC: US Dept of Health and Human Services, Health Resources and Services Agency and Public Health Service; 1992.

Nonetheless, it is possible to provide a general description of the public health workforce. It has been estimated that there are approximately 500,000 individuals working in public health in the United States. Of those, 220,000 have formal public health training, whereas the remaining 280,000 received their education in other settings. The latter include individuals with technical or professional education, such as engineers, chemists, physicians, and dentists. Figure 15.1 shows the percentages of the types of individuals who comprise the public health workforce.

Data are not available from federal government agencies about personnel currently employed or positions now vacant at the federal level, but they are for the local and state levels.

Local Health Department Personnel

The National Association of County and City Health Officials surveyed the nation's 2,888 local health departments in 1992 to 1993. The 2,091 departments that responded to the survey reported approximately 192,000 employees, of whom about 145,000 were employed full–time.[1] Because of concerns about reliability, data obtained about numbers of people employed by professional category were not published. However those departments responding to questions about personnel reported nurses to be the largest number of employed professionals (over 28,000 budgeted positions, of which 7 percent were vacant). Sanitarians and environmentalists were the next largest professional groups employed (with almost 10,000 budgeted positions, of which 4.5 percent were vacant. (Nancy Rawding, NACCHO, oral communication).

State Health Agencies

Some data are also available for state health agencies. In 1989, state health agencies reported that they had a total of 63,200 professional and technical staff who were not working in an institution. The largest proportion, 18.4 percent, or 11,650, were public health nurses. The next largest group were sanitarians who comprised 4,790 individuals, or 7.8 percent of the total employed. Public health physicians and epidemiologists had the greatest vacancy rate, but the largest group represented was public health nurses, who had 38 percent of the total vacancies. These data, along with others, have led the Department of Health and Human Services to conclude again in its eighth report to Congress on health personnel in the United States that, "Shortages of public and community health personnel currently exist in the following specialties: epidemiology, biostatistics, several environmental and occupational health specialties, public health nutrition, public health nursing, and public health and preventive medicine."[2] There is also a consensus that fewer physicians, scientists, and engineers are choosing to get public health training.

Future Outlook

Addressing a number of emerging issues in public health will also require increases in the public health workforce. They include:

- achievement of the goals and objectives in *Healthy People 2000*[3]
- an evolving health system that focuses increasingly on community-based preventive services
- a growing awareness of the need to focus on the problems of environmental hazards and degradation
- the growing epidemic of HIV disease
- the re-emergence of tuberculosis with its multiple drug–resistant strains
- the newer epidemics of drug abuse and violence

These and other issues make it clear that attention must be devoted to the appropriate training of public health workers in sufficient numbers and disciplines to adequately respond to the evolving public health problems of our society.

GRADUATE EDUCATION IN PUBLIC HEALTH

A substantial portion of the public health workforce, as pointed out above, does not have formal training in public health. Public health training is available in schools and graduate programs in public health and on-the-job at local health departments.

Schools of Public Health

A major source of public health professional education in the United States is the nation's 27 accredited schools of public health. Table 15.1 lists those institutions.

The schools are disproportionately located on the East and West Coasts of the nation. In fact, 32 states do not currently have schools of public health. The number of applicants, students, and graduates of these schools has remained relatively stable over the last decade. The schools graduate approximately 3,500 students per year, and they have a total enrollment of about 11,000 students. Schools of public health are accredited by the Council on Education for Public Health (CEPH), which also accredits programs in preventive medicine and health education.[4]

Public Health Programs

In addition to schools of public health there are a number of graduate programs in other institutions that provide professional public health education. In 1982, there were 317 graduate programs in public health disciplines outside of schools of public health.[5] These were predominately in health education, environmental health, nutrition, and health administration. Many of these programs are accredited: health education programs by CEPH, environmental health programs by the National Environmental Health Association, nutrition programs by the American Dietetics Association, and health administration programs by the Accrediting Commission on Education in Health Administration.

It is likely that these programs of public health, although smaller than schools of public health, produce as many or more graduates.[5] Clearly, the demand for public health professionals is such that academic institutions have responded. It is important to point out that schools of public health remain the predominant institutions in creating certain types of public health personnel, most notably epidemiologists and biostatisticians.

The Need for Linkages with Public Health Agencies

Schools of public health have come under criticism recently. The Institute of Medicine report, *The Future of Public Health*, made several observations about schools of public health and some recommendations for them to follow. Probably the most important recommendation was that schools (and presumably pro-

TABLE 15.1   Association of Schools of Public Health

University of Alabama-Birmingham 305 Tidwell Hall Birmingham, Alabama 35294	The Johns Hopkins University 615 North Wolfe Street Baltimore, Maryland 21205-2179	San Diego State University College and Montezuma San Diego, California 92182-0405
University of Albany SUNY Executive Park South Albany, New York 12203-3727	Loma Linda University 1708 Nichol Hall—Hill Street Loma Linda, California 92350	University of South Carolina Sumter and Greene Columbia, South Carolina 29208
Boston University 80 East Concord Street, A-407 Boston, Massachusetts 02118-2394	University of Massachusetts 108 Arnold House Amherst, Massachusetts 01003-0037	University of South Florida 13201 Bruce B. Downs Blvd. (MHH-104) Tampa, Florida 33612-3899
University of California at Berkeley 19 Earl Warren Hall Berkeley, California 94720	University of Michigan 109 South Observatory Street Ann Arbor, Michigan 48109-2029	University of Texas Health Science Center at Houston Reuel A. Stallones Building 1200 Hermann Pressler Houston, Texas 77225
University of California at Los Angeles Center for Health Sciences 10833 Le Conte Avenue (Rm. 16-035) Los Angeles, California 90024-1772	University of Minnesota A-304, Box 197, Mayo Memorial Bldg. 420 Delaware Street, SE Minneapolis, Minnesota 55455-0381	Tulane University Medical Center 1430 Tulane Avenue New Orleans, Louisiana 70112
Columbia University 617 West 168th Street (Rm. 319) New York, New York 10032	University of North Carolina S. Columbia Street (Rm. 169) Campus Box 7400 Rosenau Hall Chapel Hill, North Carolina 27599	University of Washington 1959 N.E. Pacific (SC-30) Seattle, Washington 98185
Emory University 1599 Clifton Road, NE Atlanta, Georgia 30329	University of Oklahoma Health Sciences Center 801 Northeast 13th Street Oklahoma City, Oklahoma 73104-5072	Yale University School of Medicine P. O. Box 3333 60 College Street New Haven, Connecticut 06510
Harvard University 677 Huntington Avenue Boston, Massachusetts 02115	University of Pittsburgh 111 Parran Hall Pittsburgh, Pennsylvania 15261	St. Louis University 3663 Lindell Boulevard (Rm. 380) O'Donnell Hall St. Louis, Missouri 63108
University of Hawaii 1960 East-West Road Honolulu, Hawaii 96822	University of Puerto Rico Main Building—Medical Center G.P.O. Box 5067 San Juan, Puerto Rico 00936	
University of Illinois at Chicago Health Sciences Center 2121 W. Taylor Street (Rm. 113) Chicago, Illinois 60612		

grams) of public health should establish closer linkages with public health agencies.[6] This point has been elaborated further by the Public Health Faculty/Agency Forum, a group funded by the Centers for Disease Control and Prevention, to bring practitioners and academics together to develop recommendations for improving linkages between academia and practice.[7] The Council on Linkages Between Academia and Public Health Practice, which includes representatives of national public health practice organizations and the national public health educational establishment, is now working to implement the recommendations of the forum.[8]

Continuing Education

The fact that so many individuals working in public health do not have formal public health education also concerned the Institute of Medicine. In its report, it calls on schools of public health to take the lead in making continuing education opportunities available to practicing public health professionals in order to maximize their public health competence.[6] The need for continuing education is also a concern for those who received formal public health education earlier in their careers but want their public health knowledge and skills to remain current.

In response to these continuing education needs, a number of schools of public health have begun to offer distance learning opportunities, either to earn a public health degree or to continue the education of those currently employed full-time in public health. Schools of public health have been more aggressive in their efforts to provide other kinds of continuing education opportunities for practicing professionals as well. For example, a number of schools (and some state health departments) have developed public health leadership workshops and institutes, and the Centers for Disease Control and Prevention has supported a national Public Health Leadership Institute, administered by three schools of public health, in order to improve leadership skills in state and local health departments. It is likely that opportunities such as these will continue to develop, as a wide array of continuing education opportunities becomes available to practicing public health professionals.

The Role of the Community Agency

The major responsibility for teaching public health professionals lies with academic institutions, but effective public health training cannot take place without opportunities for students to have "real-world" experiences. State and local health departments should provide student slots. They should also work closely with referring academic institutions to assure that goals and objectives for student performance meet the needs of students as well as the needs or problems of the host agency.

The Institute of Medicine noted in its report that training involves substantial experience and development in one or more specific aspects of public health (including, but not limited to, epidemiology, biostatistics, environmental health science, health education, and administration), but it also entails an understanding of how a particular discipline relates to the whole of

public health, and how public health relates to social endeavor as a whole. Thus, the effective public health professional is well-grounded in the values of public health, that is, has a commitment to the social good; has an ability to analyze public health problems from a pragmatic perspective; and understands the political process.[6(p157)] These values and skills will be reinforced in the student who has a capstone—practical experience that requires integration in the field of material taught at the academic institution.

Not all health departments have the opportunity to incorporate students into their activities. There may be no academic institution nearby training public health professionals, for example. All health departments should remain open to the possibility, however, because local individuals away at school may wish to return home for practical rotations. Where the presence of an academic institution makes regular access to students a possibility, efforts should be made to hire their faculty for part-time work in the health department and to procure faculty appointments for appropriate health department employees.

Benefits of Linkages Between Education and Practice

The association of practice settings with academic institutions brings the potential for a variety of benefits to both. Student placements for practical experience in community health settings provide students with opportunities to synthesize classroom theory with real—world issues. They also provide agencies with "extra hands," supported by faculty, to address pragmatic problems. A side benefit is the special opportunity agencies have to observe and recruit talented students. Access to data and programs in local agencies can provide faculty with almost unlimited community research opportunities, and faculty involvement with students and research provides agencies with faculty expertise (on such subjects as tobacco, substance abuse, and lead poisoning, among others) that can be applied to program development and evaluation.

There are a variety of academic resources, in addition to faculty, that can be tapped by local health agencies with linkages to academic institutions. These include:

- physical facilities and technical capacity for analyzing data
- physical facilities to support meetings, seminars, workshops, and the like
- capacity to foster continuing education credits for public health professionals by providing both qualified teachers and the accreditation mechanism
- access to survey research centers for the design and execution of community surveys
- capacity to underwrite expensive consulting costs

Close linkages between academic institutions and practice agencies can lead to important outcomes. For example, expanded local health department technical capacity should produce better public health "products." Awareness and specification of local community health problems and issues should also be enhanced. Importantly, the capacity to compete for outside funding of research projects that require both scientific and practitioner involvement is dramatically improved. The synergism that emerges when education and practice meet allows ideas to develop and play off one another to the significant advantage of both.

RESEARCH

The research base of public health has expanded rapidly over the last several decades. Advances in epidemiology and in the social and behavioral sciences that apply to contemporary public health problems have allowed health workers to be more aggressive in their personal and community-based public health interventions. The vast majority of this research information comes as the result of the work of faculty in the nation's schools of public health and medicine, highlighting the dual role that institutions of higher education play—teaching and research.

The Role of NIH

The majority of research efforts have been funded by National Institutes of Health (NIH) extramural funding programs. The systems of peer–reviewed grants and the legacy of the rapid growth in research funding that occurred after World War II are the envy of other countries and are largely responsible for our success in

biomedical research. Unfortunately, a comparable program specifically aimed at prevention research has not developed as rapidly as the biomedical program. NIH only recently has begun to focus on prevention research. Hopefully, the appointment at NIH of an associate director for prevention will raise awareness of the importance of funding prevention research.

Role of CDC

A major source of research on prevention has been the Centers for Disease Control and Prevention. Much of the nation's prevention research has been performed at this institution, which has been a major supporter of public health–related research since its founding in the 1930s. Unfortunately, CDC has not been as well endowed as its counterpart, NIH, so it has not been a major source of extramural research support for academic institutions.

Not surprisingly, CDC has had a strong sense of service to practicing public health programs, but not a strong sense of commitment or ties to academia. Fortunately, the creation of cooperative agreements between the CDC and both the Association of Schools of Public Health and the Association of Teachers of Preventive Medicine has increased research efforts of mutual interest to the CDC, faculty members of schools of medicine and public health, and practitioners who will use the new knowledge that is gained.

The Role of Community Agencies

State and local health departments should become important partners with academic institutions as research in public health expands. Academic institutions should be doing not only basic research in fields related to public health, but they should also increasingly engage in research that is relevant to real-world public health problems, such as applied research and development and program evaluation and implementation research. The best settings for such research are state and local health departments and other community agencies.

The relationships established between local public health agencies and academic institutions for the purpose of providing students with necessary practical experience are also key for increasing the amount and quality of pragmatic research done. Teaching and research are both integral to academicians, and they should also be, to a lesser extent, to public health practitioners. Relationships developed to facilitate the interaction of academics and practitioners for the sake of students are the same relationships that can stimulate collaboration on research to answer public health priority and service questions. Success in these endeavors requires the faculty of academic institutions to value applied research and service agencies to facilitate and support their research efforts.

The blend of skills and interests when academics and practitioners interact should lead to an enhanced capacity of the local agency to respond to community health needs. It should also lead to an improved capacity for policy development as research further defines local needs and involves academics in the policy-making process. Academic institutions should benefit from a realistic public health experience for students and a broad array of opportunities for faculty scholarly endeavors. The greatest benefits, of course, are reaped by the community, which should be rewarded with enhanced health status as a result of its investment in both government and education.

TEACHING HEALTH DEPARTMENTS

One way to achieve strong linkages between education and practice is to develop the concept of *teaching health departments,* parallel to the teaching hospitals associated with schools of medicine. This concept was first implemented in 1977 by Weiler and Clawson of the Lexington-Fayette County Health Department and the University of Kentucky College of Medicine.[9] They describe an affiliation agreement between the health department and the college of medicine that recognized the mutual interdependence of the health department and the college's Department of Community Medicine. The agreement was crafted to facilitate joint effort and action by each party for the achievement of common objectives in the broad areas of public health, education, research, patient care, and community service, while also allowing emphasis on separate goals. This arrangement formalized the types of academic and practice linkages that are described in this chapter and created a real partnership in the pursuit of improved public health. It is a concept that deserves attention throughout the United States.

CONCLUSION

Education and research are vital to maintaining and improving our ability to provide needed public health services. Linkage between community health agencies, schools of public health, medicine, and other education and research programs assure the capacity to provide high quality public health services. Efforts to enhance the education of our nation's public health workforce and to provide new tools through research need the support of the entire public health community if we are to achieve the best health status for our communities.

REFERENCES

1. *1992–1993 Profile of Local Health Departments.* Washington, DC: National Association of County and City Health Officials; 1995.

2. *Health Personnel in the United States, Eighth Report to Congress 1991.* Washington, DC: US Dept of Health and Human Services, Health Resources and Services Agency and Public Health Service; 1992.

3. *Healthy People 2000: National Health Promotion and Disease Prevention Objectives.* Washington, DC: US Dept of Health and Human Services, Public Health Service; 1990.

4. Fact sheet. Washington, DC: Association of Schools of Public Health; 1994.

5. Conrad CC. *Proceedings of Conference on the Education, Training, and the Future of Public Health.* Yordy KD, ed. Washington, DC: Institute of Medicine; 1991.

6. Institute of Medicine, Committee for the Study of the Future of Public Health. *The Future of Public Health.* Washington, DC: National Academy Press; 1988.

7. Sorensen AA, Bialek RG. *The Public Health Faculty/Agency Forum: Linking Graduate Education and Practice.* Gainesville, Fl: University of Florida Press; 1993.

8. Council on Linkages Between Academia and Public Health Practice. *The Link.* Winter 1995:7.

9. Weiler PG, Clawson DK. Medical schools and public health departments: a new alliance for progress. *J Med Ed.* March 1979; 54:217–223.

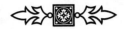

PART FOUR

THE PROVISION OF PUBLIC HEALTH SERVICES

CHAPTER

Chronic Disease Control

Jeffrey R. Harris, M.D., M.P.H.
David V. McQueen, Sc.D.
Jeffrey P. Koplan, M.D., M.P.H.

Chronic diseases account for about 75 percent of all deaths in the United States.[1] Every year, nearly 40 percent of deaths in the United States can be attributed to smoking, physical inactivity, poor diet, and alcohol misuse—all modifiable risk factors for chronic diseases.[2] Tobacco use alone has been described as the largest single factor resulting in early and unnecessary deaths in most of the developed world.[3] The contribution of these risk factors to mortality is profound.

The certainty that everyone must die eventually should not deter us from seeking to improve Americans' quality of life in order to prevent unnecessarily early deaths and morbidity. Many health experts and policy planners have argued that a significant reduction in these modifiable risk factors would result in fewer premature deaths and a compressed period of morbidity during a lifetime, leading to a healthier life.[4,5]

While recognizing the extraordinary breadth of topics related to chronic disease prevention and control, this chapter focuses on three basic areas: surveillance, intervention design, and programs. In doing so, the aim is to present the broad consensus relating to these topics.

BACKGROUND

Chronic diseases pose complicated challenges for public health professionals in the United States, as they continue to claim a significant number of lives each year.[6] Although deaths from cardiovascular disease in the United States have declined steadily since the 1960s, cardiovascular disease has remained the leading chronic disease in terms of mortality and its overall economic impact on society.[7,8] About one-fourth of Americans now have cardiovascular disease, and 43 percent of all deaths in the United States are related to cardiovascular disease.[9] In addition, cancer—the nation's second leading cause of death—accounts for about one-fourth of all United States deaths. Although cancer survival rates have improved since the early part of the century, many cancers still have low survival rates. For example, lung cancer currently has a survival rate of about one in ten.[10]

SURVEILLANCE

Surveillance has long played a critical role in chronic disease prevention and control because it allows public health professionals to monitor disease changes and trends over time and in various populations.[11–14] (A more detailed discussion of surveillance is presented in Chapter 20.) Together, epidemiology and surveillance provide the background information and knowledge on which to base public health interventions and programs to prevent and control chronic diseases.[15] From the above, it is clear that chronic diseases are important to monitor because they take a tremendous toll in lives and in the quality of life.

In the United States, there are numerous sources of chronic disease data, including:

- mortality data from vital statistics
- hospital discharge information
- health care claims and data collected by the Health Care Financing Administration
- periodic national health surveys, such as the National Health and Nutrition Examination Survey and the National Health Interview Survey, both performed by the Centers for Disease Control and Prevention
- state and local surveys, such as those conducted as part of the state–based Behavioral Risk Factor Surveillance System, supported by CDC
- individual targeted studies

The most effective surveillance systems are those that are driven by epidemiologic principles and follow a systematic approach to data collection, so the data are high quality, representative, sensitive, specific, and timely.[16] These surveillance systems not only collect data, but they also analyze, interpret, and disseminate information.[17] Thus, surveillance is more than mere data collection. It also involves a system of related actions, ranging from recognizing epidemiologic parameters to taking public health actions on the basis of analysis and interpretation of the collected data.

Its systematic approach and the dynamic nature of its data collection distinguish surveillance from the collection of vital statistics and records. Data collection relates less powerfully to the role of modern epidemiology, with its focus on the reasons *why* disease patterns change in a population. The long-term goal of chronic disease surveillance is to help monitor changes in risk factors that can be modified to prevent disease and promote health.

The breadth of chronic disease surveillance is great, and several detailed summaries provide good overviews of this public health endeavor.[18,19] Here the focus is on four primary types of surveillance: vital statistics and record systems, surveys on behavioral risk factors, assessments of multiple risk factors, and linked data systems.

Vital Statistics and Record Systems

In the past, chronic disease surveillance has relied on such data sources as disease notification systems, registries, medical records, and death certificates. Each of these sources has well–documented strengths and limitations that are familiar to every public health scientist. Unfortunately, few of these systems provide data that are timely enough to be useful for surveillance. Instead, from public health and prevention perspectives, these systems are largely a record of the failure of prevention activities; they chronicle the later and end states of chronic disease. Thus, although these systems are effective at establishing the magnitude of the problem and highlighting the overall importance of chronic disease in the population, the data arrive too late to be useful for early intervention.

Behavioral Risk Factor Surveys

Many chronic diseases, from the highly prevalent to the less common, are caused by risk factors that can be modified at both individual and social levels, as shown in Table 16.1.[2] The role of surveillance is to track these reputed causes as they occur in the population. The tracking of behavioral risk factors at the population level relies principally on population-based surveys. When such surveys are performed in a continuous series of surveys over time, such as the Behavioral Risk

TABLE 16.1 Major External (Nongenetic) Factors that Contributed to Death in the United States, 1990

	Deaths	
Cause*	Estimated no.†	Percentage of total deaths
Tobacco use	400,000	19
Diet/activity patterns	300,000	14
Alcohol use	100,000	5
Microbial agents	90,000	4
Toxic agents	60,000	3
Firearms use	35,000	2
Sexual behavior	30,000	1
Motor vehicle crashes	25,000	1
Illicit use of drugs	20,000	≤1
Total	1,060,000	50

Italic type denotes risk factors related to chronic disease.
†Composite approximation drawn from studies that used different approaches to derive estimates, ranging from actual counts (for example, firearms use) to population-attributable risk calculations (for example, tobacco use). Numbers over 50,000 are rounded to the nearest 10,000 and those below 50,000 are rounded to the nearest 5,000.
SOURCE: McGinnis JM, Foege WH. Actual causes of death in the United States. *JAMA.* 1993; 270:2207–2212.

Factor Surveillance System, they are considered a basic surveillance system. In conducting survey-based surveillance, epidemiologic methods and approaches need to be significantly enhanced by statistics and the social and behavioral sciences. Whereas vital statistics and record keeping have a long and distinguished history in public health in Europe and North America, survey research is a relatively new phenomenon linked to the advent of modern high-speed computers.

Furthermore, the art of asking questions about behavior is a highly synthetic task that requires a deep understanding of the cognitive processes of participants in the survey. As a result, current public health surveillance systems of this type are subject to considerable scrutiny and challenge. The result of this scrutiny has been a voluminous record of concern with technical detail. Much of the criticism focuses on the fact that survey data are self-reported by survey participants. The alternatives to self-reported data collected by surveys are fraught with their own methodological inadequacies but suffer chiefly from exorbitant costs for collecting population-based data. Increasingly, some areas of behavior surveillance—for example, the reporting of personal sexual practices—must rely solely on self-reported responses from survey participants. However, behavioral surveillance system administrators acknowledge the limitations of survey-based systems and that risk-related behaviors of hard-to-reach segments of the population are not well assessed by surveys.

Assessments of Multiple Risk Factors

Behind most surveillance systems, notably those that are survey based, is the notion that individual risk factors cause disease. This has been both a strength and a limitation of surveillance in public health. Much research in chronic disease now stresses the idea of multiple causation in the etiology of chronic disease. Yet surveillance systems still tend to treat risk factors as single entities. An extreme case of this limitation is seen in surveillance systems that are developed to assess changes and trends in a single risk factor or disease outcome. Data collection techniques now allow for more complicated data sets requiring the use of analytic techniques that take multiple risk factors into account. The future for chronic disease surveillance undoubtedly will lie in the assessment of patterns of risk in populations.

Linked Data Systems

Many areas of chronic disease surveillance cut across different data collection systems. For example, assessments of how well screening and medical services provide early detection of chronic diseases require data from a number of sources, including clinical records and self-reported survey data. Thus, surveillance for chronic disease should rely on linkages of data systems whenever possible.

Linking data systems was once a tedious, time-consuming, and expensive task. However, the future for data linkage in surveillance appears promising. Although most examples of linked data systems are currently found outside the United States, for example, in Sweden[20] and Canada,[21] the practice is beginning to emerge in the United States as well. With the permission of the individuals involved, some health maintenance organizations are linking clinical records with survey-based data, such as information on behavioral risk factors.

Criteria for Effective Surveillance

To be effective, surveillance systems must meet the usual criteria for public health surveillance, which include the following seven essential attributes:[16]

1. simplicity
2. sensitivity
3. specificity
4. flexibility
5. acceptability
6. timeliness
7. representativeness

The major surveillance systems now in use in the United States, which are shown in Table 16.2, share these seven essential attributes. They also have the following four characteristics in common:

1. a systematic approach to data collection
2. modern methods of data collection
3. the potential to analyze multiple risk factors for chronic disease
4. availability for public use

INTERVENTION DESIGN

Interventions for chronic diseases and their risk factors have been well studied and form the basis of much of what we know about health-related behavior change. The literature contains numerous reports of local interventions that have reduced risky behaviors and produced mass behavior changes.[22–26] The most impressive evidence of mass behavior change has been the reduction in cigarette smoking in the United States. Between 1965 and 1990, smoking rates fell from 50 percent to 28 percent for men and from 32 percent to 23 percent for women.[27]

Levels of Intervention

Efforts to change human behavior dominate most if not all interventions against chronic disease. This be-

TABLE 16.2 Three Major Survey-Based Chronic Disease Surveillance Systems

	BRFSS*	NHIS†	NHANES§
Date established	1982	1957	1960
Outcome	risk factor data for individual states	data on health status and risk factors in the United States	risk factor and disease data in the United States; focus on diet
Scope	nationwide, state by state; adults >17 years of age	national sample; primarily adults >17 years of age	noninstitutionalized national sample; primarily adults >17 years of age
Method	random-digit-dial household computer-assisted telephone interviews	household survey	household interview plus medical exam and lab work
Strengths	timely, state-level data; monthly data points	depth of question areas; supplemental surveys	very comprehensive; objective lab work
Weaknesses	lack of depth; data not local	self-reported data; analytical	complicated challenges; not timely
Comments	highly flexible system that allows states to add questions on numerous health topics	the standard for health status data in the United States	extensive information on chronic diseases

*Behavioral Risk Factor Surveillance System.
†National Health Interview Survey.
§National Health and Nutrition Examination Survey.

havioral component is obvious for primary prevention efforts, such as those aimed at reducing smoking. However, behavior change is also essential in more clinically oriented secondary and tertiary prevention efforts, such as screenings for breast cancer and diabetic retinopathy, in which both client and provider behaviors must be considered. Examples of primary, secondary, and tertiary prevention efforts are shown in Table 16.3.

Caveats

For a number of reasons, interpreting and using the literature on behavior change can be difficult. First, the literature's sheer size is overwhelming. Second, the terminology can be confusing because of numerous overlapping theories and perspectives. Third, although the science of behavior change is well developed, the precision, perceived or real, that dominates the medical literature is less appropriate for the behavioral literature. For the most part, behavioral interventions cannot be administered as reliably or precisely as surgery or drugs. Also, many behavioral interventions work at both individual and community levels, and their effects vary not only from individual to individual but also from community to community.

Practical Approach to Chronic Disease Intervention

With those caveats in mind, in this section a practical approach to changing human behaviors for preventing and controlling chronic disease is presented. The goal is not to review the literature in detail but to provide a referenced consensus on the principles and key issues involved in the design and evaluation of behavioral interventions. For the sake of clarity, many of the examples focus on efforts to reduce smoking.

Figure 16.1 provides a conceptual framework for thinking about the interrelated nature of three major components of interventions: the behaviors to be discouraged or promoted, the population for the interventions, and the site at which the interventions will take place. With that framework in mind, the design of an intervention can be divided into six steps:

1. selecting an approach
2. specifying objectives
3. identifying intervention populations
4. choosing intervention sites
5. selecting channels of communication
6. evaluating and modifying the intervention

Step One: Selecting an Approach

The first step in designing a behavioral intervention is selecting an appropriate intervention approach. A strong consensus suggests that theory is valuable in designing approaches to behavioral intervention.[28] As Hornik points out, all behavioral interventions are driven by a theory, even though that theory may be more implicit in some interventions than in others.[28] For example, implicit theoretical assumptions are made about the relationship between knowledge and behavior in an intervention in which people are educated about smoking as a risk factor for cancer and heart disease and then expected to simply stop smoking.

TABLE 16.3 Chronic Disease Intervention: Levels of Intervention

Prevention Behaviors		
Primary	Secondary	Tertiary
avoiding smoking eating a healthy diet undertaking physical activity controlling alcohol misuse	screening for breast, cervical, and colorectal cancers; hypertension; and hypercholesterolemia	conducting retinal examinations to detect diabetic retinopathy and controlling glycemia in diabetics

SOURCE: National Center for Health Statistics. *Annual Summary of Births, Marriages, Divorces, and Deaths: United States, 1992.* Hyattsville, MD: Public Health Service; 1993. Monthly Vital Statistics Report 41(13):1–9.

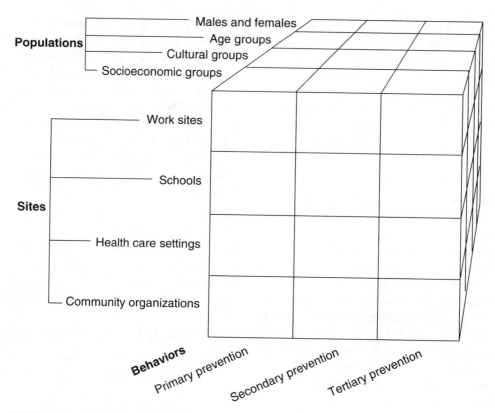

FIGURE 16.1 Cube of Chronic Disease Intervention: Interrelationships Among Populations, Sites, and Behaviors*
*Concept developed by Virginia S. Bales, M.P.H.,
Deputy Director, National Center for Chronic Disease Prevention and Health
Promotion, Centers for Disease Control and Prevention.

Of the numerous theories and models of human behavior change that have been employed, the following are used most often in health-related interventions:

- diffusion of innovations[29]
- health belief model[30]
- PRECEDE/PROCEED[24]
- social learning theory[31]
- social marketing[32]
- stages of change[33]
- theory of reasoned action[34]

Although all of these approaches provide valuable perspectives on intervention design, they may conflict with one another and leave the intervention designer confused. Liskin and colleagues have proposed an integrated approach that gleans key concepts from many of these models and theories. They propose five key elements of human behavior change and argue that all five elements are important for any full-scale intervention to change behavior.[35] The five elements are

1. *Rational element* (based on knowledge). People need to know what the disease is, which behaviors increase risk, what their risk level is, and what they can do to reduce risk.
2. *Emotional element* (based on attitudes). People need to feel vulnerable to the disease and have an emotional commitment to the behavior that reduces risk of the disease.

3. *Practical element* (based on skill). People need to be confident and competent in practicing the risk-reducing behavior.
4. *Interpersonal element* (based on social networks). People need to associate with and be supported by trusted others who reinforce risk-reducing behavior change.
5. *Structural element* (based on the social, economic, legal, and technological environment). People need to have easy access to necessary supplies and facilities for risk-reducing behaviors, and they also need barriers that hinder risky behaviors.

A further simplification of this approach divides behavioral interventions into those that operate at the individual level and those that operate at the environmental and policy levels. Both types of interventions play important roles in changing the behavior of individuals, and they should not be seen as mutually exclusive alternatives.

The individual level interventions are roughly analogous to the rational, emotional, practical, and interpersonal elements listed above. Environmental and policy level interventions are analogous to the structural element and include legislative strategies. Examples of the latter are cigarette excise taxes, minors' access laws to prevent teenagers from starting to smoke, and smoke-free workplace policies to encourage smoking cessation. Environmental and policy level interventions, such as Canada's high cigarette excise tax,[36] can be extremely effective and may even produce revenues rather than incur costs. However, these interventions often require a strong societal consensus that may not exist.

Step Two: Specifying Objectives

The second step in designing an effective intervention is specifying objectives that are specific, measurable, and time limited. For example, an objective may specify that "a smoking mass media campaign to be carried out in April and May in Cartersville seeks, by August 15, to promote a 10 percent increase over the March 15 baseline in awareness among teenaged boys (aged 13 to 19 years) of the lung cancer risk associated with smoking." The objective identifies a specific target, awareness, that is measurable. The objective also specifies dates for baseline measurement, intervention, and follow-up measurement.

Step Three: Identifying Intervention Populations

The third step in designing an intervention is to identify intervention populations. The teen smoking objective we just described identifies a fairly narrow intervention population, by age and sex, but even this population may be too diverse for the purposes of intervention. Key criteria for further segmentation include culture and socioeconomic status. An intervention that works in white culture may not work in African-American culture. Ideal language for college-educated adults may differ from that for blue-collar workers. Although the criteria may vary, the underlying principle is to divide the intervention population into subpopulations that are as homogeneous as possible and then to develop interventions specifically for each subpopulation.

Step Four: Choosing Sites

The fourth step in designing an intervention is choosing sites. The four principal sites for interventions are health care settings, schools, workplaces, and meeting sites of community organizations. Each setting has its own rationale and record of experience. More and more frequently, interventions in these sites are combined into community-wide interventions.

Health Care Settings. The rationale for using health care settings for chronic disease interventions is strong. Health care providers are generally respected advisors on health-related matters, and health care settings provide good access to patients, in whom risk-inducing behaviors tend to cluster. In addition, some screening services, such as Pap smears, can be provided only in health care settings.

Health care settings also have their negative aspects. For example, training busy health care providers to carry out the intervention and getting them to comply with training can be difficult, especially given their general lack of background in the principles of behavior change. Health care provider time is also expensive, and reimbursement is often difficult to obtain.

These limitations can be overcome by learning from the experiences of successful interventions.[37–40] For interventions that require clinical care, the systems that work best are those that facilitate care by reminding providers about the intervention and giving them easy access to the necessary supplies and equipment. For counseling interventions, multiple reinforcing messages from multiple sources—such as physicians, nurses, mailings, posters, pamphlets, and videos—over sustained periods of time are most effective. These messages are also more effective if they are individualized. Finally, health care settings do not exist in a vacuum, and providers should be knowledgeable about and refer patients to other community-based intervention programs.

Schools. School-based interventions against chronic disease can be highly effective for three primary reasons. First, schools are where the children are. Some 48 million children attend schools in the United States every day.[22] Second, many habits formed in adolescence, such as smoking and physical inactivity, have lifelong implications for the risk of chronic disease. For example, the vast majority of smoking initiation occurs before the end of adolescence; thus, deterring children from smoking until after adolescence may prevent them from ever smoking.[27] Third, schools are relatively controlled environments and are therefore excellent sites for environmental interventions such as the enforcement of no-smoking policies, the promotion of physical activity during physical education classes, and the availability of low-fat meals in school cafeterias.

Numerous curricula for school health education are available,[41,42] and those educating students against smoking have been the most heavily evaluated.[43,44] These evaluations show that changing knowledge is much easier than changing attitudes or behavior. They also show that theory-based approaches that go beyond increasing knowledge have more success in changing behavior.

Workplaces. Workplaces also serve as effective settings for chronic disease prevention interventions, be-cause they have large captive audiences and are some of the only sites readily available for reaching blue–collar workers.[45–48] Employers have financial incentives to improve their workers' health—to lower not only health insurance costs but also life and disability insurance costs and the costs of workers' compensation, absenteeism, low productivity, and high turnover. Workplaces also provide excellent opportunities for increasing social support for behavior change as well as for environmental interventions similar to school-based smoking, nutritional, and physical activity interventions.

For these reasons, workplace health promotion is increasingly common and growing in popularity. A majority of employers with more than 50 employees now offer health promotion activities.[49,50] Employee participation, however, remains quite low—usually at less than 20 percent. Unfortunately, rigorous evaluations of the effectiveness of workplace interventions are uncommon, and sound evaluations of their cost effectiveness are even less common.[45,51] The best studied and most cost-effective interventions are those providing work-based monitoring and treatment for hypertension. Workplace smoking cessation programs also appear to be cost effective.

Meeting Sites for Community Organizations. Community organizations include religious organizations such as churches; social organizations, such as men's and women's clubs; and voluntary health organizations. The rationale for selecting community organizations for intervention sites is that they provide access to specific populations, particularly minorities and the underserved. They also provide an opportunity for individuals within those intervention populations to help establish their own health priorities and agendas. In addition, health education and health messages are more likely to be effective if they are delivered by someone who is socially and culturally similar to recipients and who speaks their language. Like workplace intervention sites, community organizations provide the opportunity for social support for behavior change.

Community organizations have frequently been selected as sites for community–wide interventions.[48] These interventions have generally produced positive results. However, few interventions in community organizations have been evaluated.[52,53] Drawing from the experience to date, Sorenson and colleagues warn of six special barriers that health intervention planners may have to overcome when working with community organizations:[48]

1. concern about differential treatment and discrimination
2. concern about control and ownership of projects
3. lack of trust
4. apathy or lack of interest
5. economic costs of participation
6. cultural insensitivity and ignorance

Combined Sites for Community-wide Interventions. In recent years, a number of well–orchestrated, large–scale interventions have used principles of community organization to combine different types of intervention sites, along with generous use of the mass media.[54] The intent of these interventions has been to achieve more than the combined effects of interventions at individual sites. Instead, the intent has been a community–wide re-establishment of norms regarding health-related behaviors.

The best studied of these intervention projects included comparison communities and focused on preventing cardiovascular disease. The largest and most intensive began in North Karelia, Finland, in 1971. It resulted in significant reductions in risk behaviors, biological risk factors, and cardiovascular disease morbidity and mortality.[25] The National Heart, Lung, and Blood Institute funded the other four intervention projects—two in California, one in Minnesota, and one in Rhode Island.[26,55–57]

Step Five: Selecting Channels of Communication

The fifth step in intervention design is selecting communication channels to reach the intervention populations. The two primary communication channels are face-to-face and media communications. Face-to-face communications include both one-on-one and small group discussions. Media communications include *mass* media, such as television, radio, and newspapers, and *small* media, such as newsletters, pamphlets, and limited–use videotapes.

Both face-to-face and media communications can and should be tailored to specific intervention populations. Both types of channels can also be used simultaneously in all of the intervention sites discussed previously. In fact, they should be designed so that they complement each other, because one of the major roles of media communication is to stimulate and influence face-to-face communication.[58]

One of the major differences between face-to-face and media communications is cost per unit time. Delivering 30 minutes of one-on-one discussion between a volunteer and a smoker is far less costly than delivering a nationally televised, 30-second public service announcement against smoking. Cost is a deceptive measure, however, because the 30-second public service announcement may reach millions of viewers during prime time and thus be more cost-effective than the one-on-one approach. Another factor to consider is the far greater control over content and quality intervention designers have with media communications than with face-to-face communications.

Most intervention efforts include both face-to-face and media communications, and each plays to the relative strengths of the other. In general, face-to-face communications are more effective than media communications at changing individuals' knowledge, attitudes, and behaviors. Media communications, on the other hand, are more effective at complementing or stimulating face-to-face communications; promoting interventions, such as "quit smoking" contests; and supporting lifestyle changes by portraying them in a positive light.[59,60]

Learning from political campaigns, public health interventionists are also working more effectively to advocate through and with the media rather than simply using the media to transmit advertising or other messages.[58,59,61] These media advocacy efforts aim to educate media organizations, develop strong relationships with them, and create news. Examples include efforts to educate television news staff about the health care and societal costs of smoking and to hold press conferences that coincide with the release of new public reports on smoking costs.

Step Six: Evaluating and Modifying the Intervention

The last step in intervention is evaluating the activities and making modifications based on the evaluation results. Three principles guide evaluation: begin with baseline data, take ongoing measurements of both inputs and outputs, and keep the evaluation simple.

Baseline Data. The evaluation should begin before the intervention, with the collection of baseline data. Readily available data may be adequate for determining the baseline, but reliance on available data should always be an active decision, not a passive decision driven by the failure to plan for a baseline.

Ongoing Measurements. The evaluation should be ongoing and should include measurement of both the inputs (structure and process) and the outputs (outcomes and impact) of the intervention. Information on inputs provides early feedback, before output data are available and when midcourse corrections may still be relatively easy. Information on inputs is also crucial to understanding information on outputs. For example, a failed smoking intervention among Boy Scouts may result from the fact that only a small proportion of scout troops ever implemented the intervention. Information on outputs is, of course, key to determining whether the intervention is meeting its ultimate objectives.

Evaluation. The evaluation should also be kept as simple as possible, and designers must decide whether they will conduct evaluation research or program evaluation. The choice will depend on what they hope to gain from the evaluation. Evaluation research is designed to be generalizable and to answer questions of general interest, so it is often more complex. Program evaluation, on the other hand, tends to be simpler because it is designed to answer only *specific* questions relating to the program in question. Detailed discussions of these two types of evaluation are published elsewhere.[62,63]

All too often, program evaluation efforts lie at either end of a spectrum that ranges from no evaluation to so much evaluation that the effort is abandoned as insupportable. A frequent mistake in chronic disease interventions is to target biological outcomes that cannot be reached with the time and funds available.[64] For example, it would be inappropriate for the program evaluation of a one–year, workplace–based, smoking intervention to specify coronary heart disease targets, particularly given that the relationship between smoking and coronary heart disease is well established.

Summary of the Six–Step Intervention Approach

Interventions against chronic disease have shown some evidence of success, but much remains to be learned. Most interventions involve efforts to change human behavior. Careful planning, with specification of theoretical approaches, behavioral objectives, intervention populations and sites, and communication channels, is likely to pay off. Evaluation should begin before the intervention, and it should be designed to provide feedback on both the ongoing process of intervention and the achievement of desired outcomes.

PROGRAMS

This section moves from the ideal situation of designing interventions to the reality of chronic disease prevention and control programs, as they have been implemented with effective technologies. Local, state, and national chronic disease prevention and control programs can be conceptualized and organized in many different ways. The programs described here are offered as examples or alternatives only. They are not necessarily the best models.

Because several risk factors contribute to more than one disease or health problem, many control efforts—including school and workplace health education programs and health care setting interventions—are more efficient and effective when delivered as part of an integrated program. For example, developing and delivering different school health curricula on tobacco, drugs, alcohol, and nutrition is not efficient or effective, in terms of either outcomes or cost. Similarly, to make the most of the sometimes difficult task of getting a person to a health care setting, program planners should not limit the encounter to a blood pressure exam or the evaluation of a sore throat. All preventive measures that can and ought to be done at the same visit—such as Pap smears and mammograms—should be encouraged or at least scheduled. Procedures recommended by the United States Preventive Services Task Force are the types of activities that can be grouped by age or risk association and delivered efficiently.[37]

Unfortunately, obtaining funding for integrated public health programs has been difficult. Disease-specific programs are more easily described and understood by policy makers and legislators. In addition, organized activist groups focus on specific diseases, such as cancer, heart disease, and women's health problems, and they are able to generate political and financial support for their interest areas.

At the federal and state levels, chronic disease prevention and control activities are often organized not only by disease (for example, heart disease, cancer, diabetes), but also by risk factor (smoking, unhealthy diet, physical inactivity) and by intervention group (schoolchildren, adolescents, women, older Americans). All chronic diseases place a greater burden on, and in many cases have a higher incidence in, populations of low socioeconomic status.[65,66] Therefore, all public health chronic disease programs should also place particular emphasis on these populations in their intervention efforts.

Disease-Based Efforts

There are many intervention programs that focus on heart disease, cancer, or diabetes. Some of these are described next.

Heart Disease Prevention

Heart disease prevention programs focus on reducing the major risk factors for coronary heart disease: lowering smoking rates; changing diets to include more fruits and vegetables and fewer calories, less total fat, and less saturated fat; increasing physical activity; and controlling elevated blood pressure.

In the United States, chronic disease programs have had some success in promoting cardiovascular health by working closely with groceries and restaurants to promote healthy eating habits (Minnesota), extensively using mass media to promote key messages (California), taking advantage of community interest and organizations (New York), and influencing dietary patterns though cholesterol screening and consumer education.[67] However, more states need to develop comprehensive, well-funded, and well-evaluated cardiovascular disease control programs. Heart disease exacts the greatest health toll of all illnesses, and the risk factors have been identified that must be changed to prevent a considerable proportion of the death, morbidity, and disability associated with the disease.

Few United States programs can match the aggressiveness, completeness, intensity, community support, and perseverance of the North Karelia Project in Finland that was mentioned above. The researchers sought to influence cardiovascular disease risk factors through a variety of approaches and in a variety of sites. They worked with food manufacturers to decrease the fat content of processed foods; conducted mass media campaigns to reach large audiences; targeted schools, clubs, workplaces, and the health care delivery system; and maintained a highly visible community presence.[25,68]

Global efforts to prevent cardiovascular disease are also under way. For example, *The Victoria Declaration on Heart Health* is a blueprint for action on preventing heart disease that was developed by an international group of public health professionals and preventive cardiologists.[69] Participants in the International Heart Health Conference, held in Victoria, Canada, in 1992, are now striving to put the declaration's recommendations into practice in their home countries.

Cancer Control

In the past five years, interest and activity in cancer control have increased markedly, in part due to a growing concern about women's health issues, particularly breast and cervical cancers. CDC's National Breast and Cervical Cancer Early Detection Program, which has established partnerships with 45 states, aims to bring screening services to all women, particularly those who are older, have low incomes, are underinsured or uninsured, or are members of racial/ethnic minority populations. This comprehensive program focuses on increasing women's access to screening and follow-up services, educating women and health care providers, and improving quality assurance measures for mammography and cervical cytology.[70,71]

In addition, at the national and state levels, small-scale activities are being developed to detect prostate and skin cancers. Screening for prostate-specific antigen is being used to permit early detection of prostate cancer, although such an approach has not been demonstrated to be effective at reducing prostate cancer mortality. A more primary preventive approach has been taken to prevent the increasing rates of various types of skin cancers, especially malignant melanoma.[72,73] Australia has instituted a large-scale effort that includes environmental support, such as increased availability of covered areas at sports sites, beaches, and bus stops; and efforts to change behaviors, such as encouraging people to wear hats and use sunscreen when outdoors and to stay out of the sun during the hours of strongest radiation.[74] Some of these approaches are being discussed and applied in southern parts of the United States.

Diabetes Control

Although there is only limited evidence that the onset of diabetes can be prevented, it is known that the rate of complications can be reduced through relatively simple and inexpensive interventions. Diabetes is the leading cause of lower extremity amputations and of blindness, both of which are associated with considerable disability and cost.[75,76] Attention to proper foot care and footwear reduces the rate and severity of infections that lead to amputations,[75] and regular retinal examinations can identify early diabetic retinopathy. The latter can then be managed with laser therapy to prevent or delay visual loss. Moreover, the recently completed Diabetes Control and Complications Trial shows that tighter glycemic control is associated with a lower rate of microvascular complications among persons with type I insulin-dependent diabetes mellitus.[77,78]

All of these diabetes interventions can be promoted through public health programs that focus on both health care providers and patients. Providers need to be kept current in their knowledge of diabetes and in standards of care for the disease. Patients need to be well informed of self-care techniques and helpful services their providers can offer them. Health departments in 40 states now have cooperative agreements with the CDC to reduce the burden of diabetes through health system and community-based interventions.

Risk Factor Control Programs

Risk factor control programs have been implemented for tobacco use, nutrition, and physical activity. Some of these programs are reviewed next.

Tobacco Use Control

There has been a marked increase in state health department activities focused on the prevention and control of tobacco use. This growth has resulted from a variety of factors:

- increased public intolerance of environmental smoke as a health hazard and unpleasant annoyance
- state legislation to restrict indoor smoking
- increased excise taxes on cigarettes, with funds going to support tobacco control programs
- financial support from the National Cancer Institute, the American Cancer Society's American Stop Smoking Intervention Study (Project ASSIST), and the CDC's Office on Smoking and Health activism by consumer groups

In addition, public health activities to prevent and control tobacco use include mass media campaigns, school-based prevention curricula, workplace–based smoking cessation programs, and the provision of technical support for legislative action. California has had much success with its legislation. Proposition 99 raised the excise tax on a pack of cigarettes by 25 cents and originally designated some of the tax revenues for tobacco use control activities. Since the excise tax was raised in 1989, the prevalence of smoking in California declined from an estimated 26.5 percent in 1988 to 20.0 percent in 1993.[79]

Nutrition

Only in recent years have state nutrition programs expanded beyond their traditional maternal, infant, and childhood nutrition activities, which have focused primarily on undernutrition. Increasingly, overnutrition is being recognized as the major contemporary nutritional issue in the United States. Most Americans, including children, need to reduce their intake of calories, fat, salt, and sugar and to increase their intake of grains, fiber-containing foods, fruits, and vegetables.[80] Such a healthful diet would help prevent many chronic diseases, including coronary heart disease, hypertension and stroke, non-insulin-dependent diabetes mellitus, and several types of cancer. Such a diet would also help prevent overweight and obesity.

Results of the National Health and Nutrition Examination Surveys indicate that about 33.4 percent of adults in the United States age 20 years or older were overweight during the period 1988 to 1991. These results reflect a 33 percent increase from the previous decade in obesity among adults in the United States.[81] Public interest in weight loss is great, but few weight loss programs have yielded sustainable results. Experts in the field generally agree that sustainable weight loss depends on a combination of balanced diet and increased physical activity.[82]

Physical Activity

Nearly 60 percent of Americans are sedentary according to the results of Behavioral Risk Factor Surveys conducted in 1991.[83] An increasing body of evidence shows that being sedentary is unhealthy and that even moderate amounts of low-intensity physical activity improve health outcomes.[84] Increased physical activity is associated with better outcomes for such diverse conditions as coronary heart disease, diabetes, hypertension, colorectal cancer, depression, and osteoporosis.[85–92] Despite such findings, limited public health attention and resources have been devoted to promoting physical activity. Public health interventions that have been tried include environmental approaches that encourage increased activity as a part of daily life, such as attractive and accessible stairwells and sidewalks, safe neighborhoods, and affordable neighborhood facilities

for leisure time exercise. Mass media campaigns, health provider incentives, school programs, and activities to increase strength and mobility among older Americans should also be components of public health interventions to promote physical activity.

Programs for Special Populations

Some chronic disease control interventions are geared to reach special populations, such as schoolchildren, older Americans, or persons with low incomes. For example, school-based health activities, including comprehensive school health education programs, are effective public health tools that deal with a wide range of health issues and risk factors, such as drug and alcohol abuse, risky sexual behavior, and activities that result in injuries. Another example are programs that aim to prevent or control chronic diseases among older Americans. These programs focus on health problems such as incontinence, for which preventive opportunities exist, as well as on diseases such as arthritis and Alzheimer's disease that can be managed better to minimize their impact. More detailed descriptions of prevention programs for special populations are published elsewhere.[41,93–95]

Changing Demographic and Economic Factors

In designing and evaluating chronic disease prevention and control programs, other issues must be considered, such as demographic and economic trends. The United States has an aging population, and two segments—all persons over 65 years of age and specifically those over 80 years of age—are growing rapidly.[96] Given the nature and age of onset of chronic diseases, this demographic change will inevitably lead to continued growth in the incidence and prevalence of chronic health conditions, regardless of the success of prevention programs.[97]

CONCLUSION

Chronic diseases constitute a considerable burden of illness by all the usual measures—mortality, morbidity, disability, and cost. In the future, these diseases will continue to incur a large proportion of America's ever increasing health care costs. Primary, secondary, and tertiary prevention programs offer a cost-effective approach to decreasing this burden and improving the quality of life of Americans. However, many of the interventions that have been shown to be cost-effective continue to be underemployed.[22] The effectiveness of chronic disease prevention and control activities must be rigorously evaluated if these programs are to gain broad acceptance and financial support.[98]

Interventions also must be as far-reaching as possible. Some preventive activities can be provided one-on-one in a clinical setting, but such a limited medical approach can never be as efficient or as sweeping as community-based public health efforts. Public health departments have been slow to expand their programs and redirect their efforts to the major killers and cripplers affecting Americans today. A survey of state health departments in 1989 showed that only three percent of public health surveillance expenditures went to chronic disease prevention and control.[99] Support must be strengthened for these activities if public health is to regain a substantive role in improving America's health.

ACKNOWLEDGMENT

We are deeply indebted to Valerie R. Johnson for her editorial assistance and to Delle B. Carey for help with database research.

REFERENCES

1. Centers for Disease Control and Prevention. Chronic disease prevention and control activities—United States, 1989. *MMWR.* 1991;40:697–700.
2. McGinnis JM, Foege WH. Actual causes of death in the United States. *JAMA.* 1993;270:2207–2212.
3. Bartecchi CE, MacKenzie TD, Schrier RW. The human costs of tobacco use. *N Engl J Med.* 1994;330:907–912.
4. Hahn RA, Teutsch SM, Rothenberg RB, Marks JS. Excess deaths from nine chronic diseases in the United States, 1986. *JAMA.* 1990;264:2654–2659.
5. Fries J, Green LW, Levine S. Health promotion and the compression of morbidity. *Lancet.* 1989;1:401–484.

6. National Center for Health Statistics. *Annual Summary of Births, Marriages, Divorces, and Deaths: United States, 1992.* Hyattsville, Md: Public Health Service; 1993. Monthly Vital Statistics Report 41(13):1–9.
7. Hartunian NS, Smart CN, Thompson MC. The incidence and economic costs of cancer, motor vehicle injuries, coronary heart disease, and stroke: a comparative analysis. *Am J Public Health.* 1980;79:184–197.
8. Brown ML. The national economic burden of cancer: an update. *J Natl Cancer Inst.* 1990;82:1811–1814.
9. National Center for Health Statistics. *Health, United States, 1991.* Hyattsville, Md: US Dept of Health and Human Services, Public Health Service; 1992.
10. Boring CC, Squires TS, Tong T. Cancer statistics, 1993. *CA Cancer J Clin.* 1993;43:7–26.
11. Farr W. *Vital Statistics: A Memorial Volume of Selections from the Reports and Writings of William Farr.* Metuchen, NJ: Scarecrow Press; 1975.
12. Farr W. *Vital Statistics.* Reprinted ed. New York, NY: New York Academy of Medicine; 1975.
13. Frost WH, Maxcy KF, eds. *Collected Papers.* New York, NY: Commonwealth Fund; 1941.
14. Snow J. *On the Mode of Transmission of Cholera.* Reprinted ed. New York, NY: Commonwealth Fund; 1936.
15. Centers for Disease Control. Guidelines for evaluating surveillance systems. *MMWR.* 1988;37(suppl 5):1–18.
16. Tyler CW Jr, Last JM. Epidemiology. In: Last JM, Wallace RB, eds. *Maxcy-Rosenau-Last Public Health and Preventive Medicine.* 13th ed. Norwalk, Ct: Appleton and Lange; 1992: 11–39.
17. Remington PL, Goodman, RA. Chronic disease surveillance. In: Brownson RC, Remington PL, Davis JR, eds. *Chronic Disease Epidemiology and Control.* Washington, DC: American Public Health Association; 1993.
18. Last JM, Wallace RB, eds. *Maxcy-Rosenau-Last Public Health and Preventive Medicine.* 13th ed. Norwalk, Ct: Appleton and Lange; 1992.
19. Brownson RC, Remington PL, Davis JR, eds. *Chronic Disease Epidemiology and Control.* Washington, DC: American Public Health Association; 1993.
20. Lunde AS, Lundeborg S, Lettenstrom GS, Thygeses L, Huebner J. The personal number systems of Sweden, Norway, Denmark, and Israel. *Vital Health Stat 2;* 1980. PHS publication no. 80–1358.
21. West R. Saskatchewan health data bases: a developing resource. *Am J Prev Med.* 1988;4(suppl 2):25–27.
22. Tolsma DD, Koplan JP. Health behaviors and health promotion. In: Last JM, Wallace RB, eds. *Maxcy-Rosenau-Last Public Health and Preventive Medicine.* 13th ed. Norwalk, Ct: Appleton and Lange; 1992:701–714.

23. Davis JR, Schwartz R, Wheeler F, Lancaster RB. Intervention methods for chronic disease control. In: Brownson RC, Remington PL, Davis JR, eds. *Chronic Disease Epidemiology and Control*. Washington, DC: American Public Health Association; 1993:51–81.

24. Green LW. Prevention and health education. In: Last JM, Wallace RB, eds. *Maxcy-Rosenau-Last Public Health and Preventive Medicine*. 13th ed. Norwalk, Ct: Appleton and Lange; 1992:787–802.

25. Puska P, Tuomilehto J, Nissinen A, et al. The North Karelia Project: 15 years of community based prevention of coronary heart disease. *Ann Med*. 1989;21:169–173.

26. Farquhar JW, Fortmann SP, Flora JA, et al. Effects of communitywide education on cardiovascular disease risk factors. *JAMA*. 1990;264:359–365.

27. Novotny TE. Tobacco use. In: Brownson RC, Remington PL, Davis JR, eds. *Chronic Disease Epidemiology and Control*. Washington, DC: American Public Health Association; 1993:199–220.

28. Hornik R. Alternative models of behavior change. In: Wasserheit JN, Holmes KK, Aral SD, eds. *Research Issues in Human Behavior and Sexually Transmitted Diseases in the AIDS Era*. Washington, DC: American Society for Microbiology; 1991:201–218.

29. Rogers EM. *Diffusion of Innovations*. New York, NY: Free Press; 1983.

30. Rosenstock IM. The health belief model: explaining health behavior through expectancies. In: Glanz K, Lewis FM, Bimer BK, eds. *Health Behavior and Health Education: Theory, Research, and Practice*. San Francisco, Ca: Jossey-Bass; 1990:39–62.

31. Bandura A. *Social Learning Theory*. Englewood Cliffs, NJ: Prentice-Hall; 1977.

32. Manoff RK. *Social Marketing: New Imperative for Public Health*. New York, NY: Praeger; 1985.

33. Prochaska JO, DiClemente CC. Stages and processes of self-change of smoking: toward an integrative model of change. *J Consult Clin Psychol*. 1983;51:983–990.

34. Fishbein M, Ajzen I. *Belief, Attitude, Intention, and Behavior: An Introduction to Theory and Research*. Reading, Ma: Addison-Wesley; 1975.

35. Liskin L, Church CA, Piotrow PT, Harris JA. AIDS education—a beginning. *Popul Rep (L)*. 1989;8:1–32.

36. *Smoking and Health in the Americas*. Atlanta, Ga: US Dept of Health and Human Services, Public Health Service, Centers for Disease Control, National Center for Chronic Disease Prevention and Health Promotion, Office on Smoking and Health; 1992. DHHS publication CDC 92-8419.

37. US Preventive Services Task Force. *Guide to Clinical Preventive Services: An Assessment of the Effectiveness of 169 Interventions*. Baltimore, Md: Williams & Wilkins; 1989.

38. Kottke TE, Battista RN, DeFriese GH, Brekke ML. Attributes of successful smoking cessation interventions in medical practice: a meta-analysis of 39 controlled trials. *JAMA*. 1988;259:2882–2889.

39. Bartlett EE. Introduction: eight principles from patient education research. *Prev Med*. 1985;14:667–669.

40. Mullen PD, Green LW, Persinger GS. Clinical trials of patient education for chronic conditions: a comparative meta-analysis of intervention types. *Prev Med*. 1985;14:753–781.

41. Kolbe LJ, Iverson DC. Comprehensive school health education programs. In: Matarazzo JD, Weiss SM, Herd JA, Miller NE, Weiss SM, eds. *Behavioral Health: A Handbook of Health Enhancement and Disease Prevention*. New York, NY: John Wiley & Sons; 1984:1094–1116.

42. National Center for Health Education. *A Compendium of Health Education Programs Available for Use by Schools*. Atlanta, Ga: United States Center for Health Promotion and Education; 1982.

43. Glynn TJ. Essential elements of school-based smoking prevention programs. *J School Health*. 1989;59:181–188.

44. Rundall TG, Bruvold WH. A meta-analysis of school-based smoking and alcohol use prevention programs. *Health Educ Q*. 1988;15:317–334.

45. Fielding JE. Health promotion and disease prevention at the worksite. *Ann Rev Public Health*. 1984;5:237–265.

46. O'Donnell MP, Ainsworth T. *Health Promotion in the Workplace*. New York, NY: John Wiley & Sons; 1984.

47. Sloan RP, Gruman JC, Allegrante JP. *Investing in Employee Health: A Guide to Effective Health Promotion in the Workplace*. San Francisco, Ca: Jossey-Bass; 1987.

48. Sorenson G, Glasgow RE, Corbett K. Involving work sites and other organizations. In: Bracht N, ed. *Health Promotion at the Community Level*. London, England: Sage; 1990:158–184.

49. Fielding JE, Piserchia PV. Frequency of work site health promotion activities. *Am J Public Health*. 1989;79:16–20.

50. Hollander RB, Lengermann JJ. Corporate characteristics and work site health promotion programs: survey findings from Fortune 500 companies. *Soc Sci Med*. 1988;26:491–501.

51. Warner KE, Wickizer TM, Wolfe RA, et al. Economic implications of workplace health promotion programs: review of the literature. *J Occup Med*. 1988;30:106–112.

52. Lasater TM, Wells BL, Carleton RA, Elder JP. The role of churches in disease prevention research studies. *Public Health Rep*. 1986;101:125–131.

53. Levin JS. The role of the black church in community medicine. *J Natl Med Assoc*. 1984;76:477–483.

54. Bracht N, Kingsbury L. Community organization principles in health promotion: a five-stage model. In: Bracht N, ed. *Health Promotion at the Community Level*. London, England: Sage; 1990:66–88.

55. Blackburn H, Luepker RV, Kline FG, et al. The Minnesota Heart Health Program: a research and demonstration project in cardiovascular disease prevention. In: Matarazzo JD, Weiss SM, Herd JA, Miller NE, Weiss SM, eds. *Behavioral Health: A Handbook of Health Enhancement and Disease Prevention.* New York, NY: John Wiley & Sons; 1984:1171–1178.

56. Farquhar JW, Maccoby N, Wood PD, et al. Community education for cardiovascular health. *Lancet.* 1977;1:1192–1195.

57. Lasater T, Abrams D, Artz L, et al. Lay volunteer delivery of a community-based cardiovascular risk factor change program: the Pawtucket experience. In: Matarazzo JD, Weiss SM, Herd JA, Miller NE, Weiss SM, eds. *Behavioral Health: A Handbook of Health Enhancement and Disease Prevention.* New York, NY: John Wiley & Sons; 1984:1166–1170.

58. Wallack L. Media advocacy: promoting health through mass communication. In: Glanz K, Lewis FM, Rimer BK, eds. *Health Behavior and Health Education: Theory, Research, and Practice.* San Francisco, Ca: Jossey-Bass; 1990:370–386.

59. Flora JA, Cassady D. Roles of media in community-based health promotion. In: Bracht N, ed. *Health Promotion at the Community Level.* London, England: Sage; 1990: 143–157.

60. Rice RE, Atkin CK, eds. *Publication Communication Campaigns.* Newbury Park, Ca: Sage; 1989.

61. Erickson AC, McKenna JW, Romano RM. Past lessons and new uses of the mass media in reducing tobacco consumption. *Public Health Rep.* 1990;105:239–244.

62. Shortell SM, Richardson WC. *Health Program Evaluation.* St. Louis, Mo: CV Mosby; 1978.

63. Weiss CH. *Evaluation Research.* Englewood Cliffs, NJ: Prentice-Hall; 1972.

64. Mittelmark MB, Hunt MK, Heath GW, Schmid TL. Realistic outcomes: lessons from community–based research and demonstration programs for the prevention of cardiovascular diseases. *J Public Health Policy.* 1993;14:437–462.

65. Adler NE, Boyce T, Chesney MA, et al. Socioeconomic status and health: the challenge of the gradient. *Am Psychol.* 1994;49: 15–24.

66. Adler NE, Boyce WT, Chesney MA, Folkman S, Syme SL. Socioeconomic inequalities in health: no easy solution. *JAMA.* 1993;269:3140–3145.

67. Centers for Disease Control and Prevention. State-specific changes in cholesterol screening—Behavioral Risk Factor Surveillance System, 1988–1991. *MMWR.* 1993;42:663–664.

68. World Health Organization, Cardiovascular Diseases Unit. Review of community intervention studies on cardiovascular risk factors. *Clin Exp Hypertens.* 1992;14:223–237.

69. Advisory Board of the International Heart Health Conference. *The Victoria Declaration on Heart Health.* Victoria, Canada: Health and Welfare Canada; 1992.

70. Centers for Disease Control and Prevention. *Implementation of the Breast and Cervical Cancer Mortality Prevention Act: 1992 Progress Report to Congress.* Atlanta, Ga: US Dept of Health and Human Services, Public Health Service; 1993.

71. Centers for Disease Control. Update: National Breast and Cervical Cancer Early Detection Program, July 1991-July 1992. *MMWR.* 1992;41:739–743.

72. Miller DL, Weinstock MA. Nonmelanoma skin cancer in the United States: incidence. *J Am Acad Dermatol.* 1994;30: 774–778.

73. Setlow RB, Woodhead AD. Temporal changes in the incidence of malignant melanoma: explanation from action spectra. *Mutat Res.* 1994;307:365–374.

74. Brooks J. Threat of skin cancer changing the way Australians live. *Can Med Assoc J.* 1993;148:2027–2029.

75. Bild DE, Selby JV, Sinnock P, Browner WS, Braveman P, Showstack JA. Lower-extremity amputation in people with diabetes: epidemiology and prevention. *Diabetes Care.* 1989; 12:24–31.

76. American Diabetes Association. *Direct and Indirect Costs of Diabetes in the United States in 1992.* Alexandria, Va: American Diabetes Association; 1993.

77. Diabetes Control and Complications Trial Research Group. The effect of intensive treatment of diabetes on the development and progression of long-term complications in insulin-dependent diabetes mellitus. *N Engl J Med.* 1993;329: 977–986.

78. American Diabetes Association. Position statement: implications of the Diabetes Control and Complications Trial. *Diabetes.* 1993;42:1555–1558.

79. Pierce JP, Evans N, Farkas AJ, et al. *Tobacco Use in California: An Evaluation of the Tobacco Control Program—1989–1993.* La Jolla, Ca: University of California-San Diego; 1994.

80. *The Surgeon General's Report on Nutrition and Health.* Washington, DC: US Dept of Health and Human Services, Public Health Service; 1988. DHHS publication 88-50210.

81. Kuczmarski RJ, Flegal KM, Campbell SM, Johnson CL. Increasing prevalence of overweight among US adults. *JAMA.* 1994;272:205–211.

82. Committee on Diet and Health, Food and Nutrition Board, Commission on Life Sciences, National Research Council. *Diet and Health: Implications for Reducing Chronic Disease Risk.* Washington, DC: National Academy Press; 1989.

83. Centers for Disease Control and Prevention. Prevalence of sedentary lifestyle—Behavioral Risk Factor Surveillance System, United States, 1991. *MMWR.* 1993;42:576–579.

84. American College of Sports Medicine. Position stand: physical activity, physical fitness, and hypertension. *Med Sci Sports Exerc.* 1993;25:i–x.

85. Powell KE, Thompson PD, Caspersen CJ, Kendrick JS. Physical activity and the incidence of coronary heart disease. *Annu Rev Public Health*. 1987;8:253–287.

86. Centers for Disease Control. Protective effect of physical activity on coronary heart disease. *MMWR*. 1987;36:426–430.

87. Berlin JA, Colditz GA. A meta-analysis of physical activity in the prevention of coronary heart disease. *Am J Epidemiol*. 1990;132:612–628.

88. Blair SN, Kohl HW III, Paffenbarger RS Jr, Clark DG, Cooper KH, Gibbons LW. Physical fitness and all-cause mortality: a prospective study of healthy men and women. *JAMA*. 1989;262:2395–2401.

89. Thompson WG. Exercise and health: fact or hype? *South Med J*. 1994;87:567–574.

90. Gordon NF, Scott CB, Wilkinson WJ, Duncan JJ, Blair SN. Exercise and mild essential hypertension: recommendations for adults. *Sports Med*. 1990;10:390–404.

91. Byrne A, Byrne DG. The effect of exercise on depression, anxiety, and other mood states: a review. *J Psychosom Res*. 1993;37:565–574.

92. Thompson WG Jr. Exercise, age, and bones. *South Med J*. 1994;87:S23–S25.

93. Kolbe LJ. Developing a plan of action to institutionalize comprehensive school health education programs in the United States. *J School Health*. 1993;63:12–13.

94. Cortese PA. Accomplishments in comprehensive school health education. *J School Health*. 1993;63:21–23.

95. *Healthy People 2000: National Health Promotion and Disease Prevention Objectives*. Washington, DC: US Dept of Health and Human Services; 1991. PHS publication no. 91-50213.

96. Manton KG, Corder LS, Stallard E. Estimates of change in chronic disability and institutional incidence and prevalence rates in the US elderly population from the 1982, 1984, and 1989 National Long Term Care Survey. *J Gerontol*. 1993;48:S153–S166.

97. Helfand AE. Who are the elderly? A profile of older patients. *Clin Podiatr Med Surg*. 1993;10:1–6.

98. Thacker SB, Koplan JP, Taylor WR, Hinman AR, Katz MF, Roper WL. Assessing prevention effectiveness using data to drive program decisions. *Public Health Rep*. 1994;109:187–194.

99. Association of State and Territorial Chronic Disease Program Directors. *Reducing the Burden of Chronic Disease: Needs of the States*. Washington, DC: Public Health Foundation; 1991.

CHAPTER

17

Tobacco Control

John P. Elder, Ph.D., M.P.H.
Christine C. Edwards, M.P.H.
Terry L. Conway, Ph.D.

This chapter discusses both individual and community level tobacco control strategies. It shows how to plan and organize a tobacco control strategy and points out the highlights of California's groundbreaking, statewide tobacco control program.

BACKGROUND

The 1964 surgeon general's report[1] about the dangers of tobacco warned the smoking public that their tobacco use was killing them. The decade following the release of this report witnessed a proliferation of smoking cessation programs for the increasing numbers of people, predominantly upper–class white males, who wanted to quit. At the same time, a small but growing outcry ensued against the marketing of tobacco, resulting in mass media antitobacco campaigns funded by private donations.

As with many other scientific and social developments against the tobacco-using practices of Americans, the tobacco industry successfully countered each antitobacco action with a variety of countercontrol strategies. At the political level, members of the tobacco industry worked with friendly legislators from tobacco states and elsewhere to introduce mildly worded legislation to limit tobacco advertising, with the agreement that antitobacco ads, which research was beginning to show were effective, would also be limited.

This political maneuvering resulted in the Public Health Cigarette Smoking Act of 1969, which banned (effective in 1971) cigarette advertising on television. Although this seemed like a victory for the prohealth advocates, in reality the ban resulted in the loss of valuable, free antitobacco advertising on television. At the same time, the tobacco industry quickly turned their enormous budgets toward print advertising and promotion and sponsorship activities, while the antitobacco forces were left looking for new ways to convince the public not to smoke.

The tobacco industry then introduced a variety of lower tar and nicotine cigarettes, which suggested that, whereas the previous brands might be a little harmful, the new products were not. Since then, this powerful industry has continued to introduce marketing innovations in attempts to bolster diminishing sales. For example, a current controversy involves the sale of single cigarettes, which in many places violates both health and tax laws. Always one step ahead of the game, the tobacco industry is now in the process of developing a prepackaged single cigarette in a tube that would comply with health and tax regulations.

Public health administrators can and should take a leadership role in combatting tobacco use, which is the largest preventable cause of death in the United States. In order to take on this mantle, public health officials must learn to think like the tobacco industry. Its highly funded research and marketing efforts have sapped antitobacco energies. It is safe to assume that the industry would like nothing better than for public health practitioners to continue to spend their time on multisession, small-group quitting classes with modest cessation rates. What undoubtedly concerns the tobacco industry more are policies and prevention programs focusing on occasional smokers, young nonsmokers, and that great majority—passive smokers. To make any further gains in tobacco control, public health practitioners must move out of the traditional domain of health education and make difficult decisions about how best to use tobacco control resources. These difficult decisions may include ignoring the already addicted smoker in favor of more aggressive, community-wide strategies.

ORGANIZING AGAINST TOBACCO

During the 1980s, the domestic and international marketing of tobacco products continued relatively undiminished, with laissez-faire government policies coinciding with the probusiness governments of the United States, United Kingdom, Germany, and elsewhere. The freedom of the tobacco industry to promote its product continued unabated, while public health and tobacco control efforts were spotty at best.

On the other hand, this period also witnessed the development of a somewhat less conservative approach to tobacco control, partly in recognition of the fact that the decline in smoking rates in Western populations was unacceptably gradual, especially for certain groups, such as those of lower socioeconomic status. Priority goals and objectives related to tobacco control were set by the United States surgeon general,[2] as shown in Table 17.1. Community- and organization-wide programs were subsequently developed, as exemplified by the Minnesota and Pawtucket Heart Health Programs.[3,4]

These community-wide programs recognized that very few adults use formal cessation programs to improve their chances of quitting but instead generally "quit on their own"—if they quit at all. Therefore, incentives to quit were used in "Quit and Win" and similar lottery-based efforts. At the same time, prevention programs based on developing refusal skills continued to proliferate and were adopted and implemented by entire school systems.

Also in the 1980s, there was an awakening of societal forces that sought to impose restrictions on the tobacco industry and promote smoke-free societies more aggressively. During this decade, 500 ordinances restricting smoking in restaurants, stores, and workplaces were passed in the United States.[5] In California, 51 percent of cities had enacted local smoking-control ordinances by 1992.[6] In Scandinavian countries, the concept of the smoke-free class of 2000 was promoted in an attempt to rid these nations of the tobacco epidemic by the turn of the century. Other nations as well started to interpret "health for all by the year 2000" as "freedom from tobacco by the year 2000."

In the United States, groups such as Doctors Ought to Care (DOC), the Advocacy Institute, Americans for Non-Smokers' Rights, and Stop Teenage Addiction to Tobacco (STAT) coordinated antitobacco activities nationwide while supporting or even enjoining lawsuits against tobacco companies. The plaintiffs were smokers who were seriously ill or had died from tobacco use. A major milestone in antitobacco efforts was reached in 1987 with the ban on smoking during domestic airline flights.

TABLE 17.1 *Healthy People 2000:* Tobacco Control in the United States

Objectives

1. Reduce cigarette smoking to a prevalence of no more than 15 percent among people age 20 and older (from 29.1 percent in 1987).
2. Reduce the initiation of smoking by youth to no more than 15 percent, as measured by the prevalence of smoking among people ages 20 to 24 (from 29.5 percent in 1987).
3. Increase to at least 50 percent the proportion of current smokers age 20 and older who made a serious attempt to quit smoking during the preceding year, with one-third or more of these attempts resulting in abstinence for at least three months.
4. Increase smoking cessation during pregnancy so at least 60 percent of women who are cigarette smokers at the time they discover they are pregnant will quit smoking and maintain abstinence for the remainder of their pregnancy.
5. Reduce to no more than 25 percent the proportion of children age 6 and younger who are exposed to cigarette smoke at home.
6. Reduce smokeless tobacco use to a prevalence of no more than 4 percent among men ages 18 to 24.
7. Increase to at least 85 percent the proportion of adolescents ages 12 to 17 who perceive social disapproval and great risk or harm to their health from smoking cigarettes.
8. Increase to at least 75 percent the proportion of all primary care providers who routinely advise cessation and provide assistance and follow-up for all of their tobacco-using patients.
9. Include tobacco use prevention in the curriculum of all elementary, middle and secondary schools, preferably as part of comprehensive school health education.
10. Increase to at least 75 percent the proportion of work sites with a formal smoking policy that prohibits or severely restricts smoking in the workplace.
11. Enact in all states comprehensive laws on clean indoor air that prohibit or strictly limit smoking in enclosed public places.
12. Enact and enforce in all states laws prohibiting the sale and distribution of tobacco products to youth younger than age 18.
13. Eliminate exposure to tobacco product advertising and promotion among youth younger than age 18.
14. Ensure that all tobacco product packages and advertisements provide information on all major health effects of tobacco use, including addiction, and will identify product ingredients and the harmful tobacco smoke constituents.
15. Increase to at least 80 percent the proportion of people with time-and/or cost-limited health insurance coverage for services to overcome nicotine addiction.

Advertising

Despite all the cessation, prevention, and society level initiatives, western countries, especially the United States, still comprise "tobacco cultures." In the United States, billboards and magazines are dominated by both the Marlboro Man and Joe the Camel, among other attractive characters. Insidious presentations of ads frequently appear in the background of Hollywood movies and other popular media.

Availability

Adults and youth alike have ready access to cigarettes from vending machines, convenience stores, and nearly every other conceivable retail outlet. A recent study in 18 United States communities showed that an average of 50 percent of youth under the legal age to purchase cigarettes were nonetheless successful at doing so.[7] Although selling individual cigarettes is illegal, many re-

tailers sell them singly for the convenience of those who do not have enough disposable income to purchase an entire pack or for those trying to quit who want "just one more." Also, in spite of the salutary public health effect of increasing taxes, tobacco taxes are seldom increased in the United States or its constituent states, and cigarettes remain affordable to the majority of the population.

Intervention Strategies for Tobacco Control

Intervention strategies for tobacco control include cessation strategies, prevention programs, social marketing strategies, and policy and ordinance activities.

Cessation Strategies

Beginning in the late 1950s, as more medical research began showing a relationship between smoking and disease, many different types of cessation approaches became increasingly available. Therapies have included drug treatments (such as tranquilizers, amphetamines, and, more recently, nicotine gum and patches), hypnosis, acupuncture, professional counseling, aversive conditioning procedures (such as rapid smoking and satiation smoking), and various behavioral self-management strategies (see Schwartz[8] for a review and evaluation of various smoking cessation methods).

The availability and popularity of these treatment approaches have varied over the decades with conditioning-based approaches emphasized in the 1960s, cognitively based self-management procedures emphasized in the 1970s, and relapse prevention and pharmacologic interventions emphasized in the 1980s. Newer strategies are focused largely on relapse prevention with special attention given to weight gain, high-risk situations, and cognitive and behavioral coping strategies.[9]

Different types of smoking cessation strategies (for example, conditioning-based or cognitively based) have experienced more or less popularity throughout the years. Although a few new strategies have been added over the years, many strategies have changed very little over time. There has been a gradual shift away from cessation approaches that require smokers to seek out assistance toward more aggressive strategies that actively seek out smokers to get them to quit.

More importantly, a great deal of sophistication has been gained in the packaging and marketing of these programs, with an increased emphasis on targeting specific groups of smokers (such as pregnant women, Hispanics, and African-Americans). National voluntary agencies (such as the American Cancer Society, the American Lung Association, and the American Heart Association) have played a very important role in educating the public about the hazards of tobacco use. These agencies have sponsored a wide variety of interventions and cessation programs, distributed tremendous amounts of educational materials, and produced and disseminated numerous stop-smoking programs and public service announcements carrying antismoking messages.

Reliance on the Mass Media. In recent years, there has been a much greater reliance on the mass media in broad-based public health cessation strategies for influencing the smoking behavior of large numbers of smokers. An example of one of the most promising public health approaches to cessation, which is facilitated by mass media efforts, is community-wide cessation contests—the most commonly used being the "Quit and Win" approach.[10]

An effective variation of this cessation contest approach was Bloomington, Minnesota's "Quit Date '88." Following a recruitment promotion through print and interpersonal channels, smokers were eligible to enter the contest at any point in an eight-month period, as long as they pledged a quit date. All participants who had quit in the current or previous month during the contest were eligible for a $200 prize at the end of each month. At the end, all participants were eligible for a grand prize trip for two to Mexico. Smokers could quit on their own or obtain help through materials or programs offered by the sponsoring Minnesota Heart Health Program. A total of 918 smokers entered the program (in a city of 85,000), 347 by the first month and 203 in the last month before the grand prize was drawn. An intermediate follow-up showed an abstinence rate of 16.7 percent.[11] Although it may seem low, this rate compares favorably to rates found in more intensive programs, especially given the large numbers of individuals participating in the Minnesota program.

Medical Involvement. During the last decade there has also been an increasing interest in involving physicians and other health care professionals to a greater extent in smoking cessation efforts. Medical organizations have played a more prominent role in smoking and health during the 1980s than they had in the past. The National Cancer Institute has taken an active role in developing and disseminating guidelines for physicians and their office staff that outline procedures that have been shown to be cost effective in helping smoking patients quit.[12–14]

With the popularity of pharmaceutically assisted cessation approaches (for example, gum and patches that release nicotine into the body and presumably reduce withdrawal symptoms), physicians are already involved at some level in patient cessation efforts. The additional application of a few relatively simple techniques by primary providers and their office staff can result in significantly greater numbers of patients quitting.

Prevention Programs

Beginning with the work of Evans and his colleagues at the University of Houston,[15] researchers began to realize the relative futility of trying to get people to give up a drug (tobacco) to which they were seriously addicted. Thus, attention shifted to preventing first or regular use of cigarettes. Previous *educational* programs had emphasized the dangers of smoking, but this new generation of programs emphasized the process of beginning to smoke and sought to counter the social influences that lead to smoking.

Specifically, these were refusal skills training programs, and they stemmed from the belief that most children do not actively seek to try smoking but are pressured to do so by their friends, older siblings, and others. Projects developed by Evans and others focused on developing in-school programs to teach children how to refuse an offer of a cigarette.[16] San Diego's Project SHOUT represents a current version of this type of program.

Project SHOUT. Project SHOUT (Students Helping Others Understand Tobacco) was launched in junior high schools throughout San Diego County, California. It was designed to work with a multischool group of students as they progressed from seventh through ninth grade. SHOUT used a combination of educational, motivational, and community activities, in addition to resistance skills training, to create the optimal environment-behavior relationships to help students resist offers of tobacco use. The intervention was conducted by trained undergraduate students selected to be classroom leaders. Intervention activities included refusal skill training, ad de-bunking, and letter writing, both to city council members and to youth-oriented magazines that advertised cigarettes.

Participation in all of the project SHOUT activities was reinforced with raffle tickets, exchangeable for a variety of prizes donated by local businesses and organizations. Prizes included sports equipment, movie passes, T-shirts, record albums, and others). At the end of the year, a "Fresh Mouth" contest was held as an additional way to win raffle tickets. For this contest, students wrote their names on a sheet of paper if they had not been smoking or chewing tobacco and wanted to enter the drawing. Students whose names were drawn received a carbon monoxide test to see whether they indeed had not been smoking. (All students tested showed themselves to be smoke free.) Fresh Mouth contests were held on a random, unscheduled basis to maximize the effectiveness of this reward contingency.

In its third and final year of tobacco use prevention, SHOUT conducted a home-based intervention consisting of bimonthly newsletters mailed to the subjects' homes, alternating with phone conversations with a new group of undergraduate leaders. Newsletters were designed to provide tobacco information as well as opportunities for the students to express their views about tobacco distribution and use. In addition, twice during the year parents of each SHOUT student received a newsletter similar in content to the student newsletters. Results of this intensive intervention were promising. At the end of the third year of intervention, the prevalence of tobacco use within the previous month was 14.2 percent of the intervention students, compared with 22.5 percent of the control students.[17]

Public Health Impact. Prevention programs represent a substantial improvement over individual-based cessation programs in terms of potential for public health impact. Children are caught before they become addicted to the use of cigarettes. They are typically treated in group (usually classroom) situations that allow the target audience to deal with the potential problem in the same context in which it is likely to occur, that is, in front of their peers. Whereas standard cessation programs have implicitly "blamed" individuals for picking up the smoking habit and thus placed responsibility for giving it up on their shoulders, prevention programs are based on the assumption that children do not exercise freedom of choice when smoking their first cigarette.

The goals of prevention are to manipulate the peer environment, that is, to change any reinforcement for smoking into reinforcement for not smoking, and to develop students' skills to such an extent that experimenting with cigarettes becomes unlikely. These goals are extremely important and challenging, especially considering that the tobacco industry has cleverly modernized their strategies by heavily marketing products in ways that appeal to young children.

Social Marketing Strategies

Social marketing is a term that implies the use of marketing procedures to change social behavior. However, its goal is not necessarily to sell a product or service but to change the attitudes and behaviors of a population.[18] In the area of tobacco control, the bulk of early antitobacco social marketing (and motivational) efforts went into advertising the benefits of smoking cessation and, later, the importance of not starting to smoke. Gradually, the messages became more strident, with posthumous pleas to avoid tobacco from lung cancer victims such as Yul Brynner.

The state of California began an aggressive antitobacco media campaign in 1990 that differed from traditional antitobacco advertising, which simply promoted the benefits of quitting. This media campaign targeted the tobacco industry to expose it as comprised of greedy, profit-motivated liars who would say anything to get children hooked on tobacco. This was a decided shift away from placing the responsibility on the individual smoker.

Media Advocacy. The major tool of social marketing is media advocacy. As discussed in Chapter 13, media advocacy is the strategic use of the mass media for advancing social or public policy initiatives.[19] Media advocates continuously monitor the media to take advantage of any opportunity expected or unexpected, to further health promotion objectives. For example, in southern California, when the 1993 Philip Morris Marlboro Adventure Team trucks began offering merchandise outside convenience stores and gas stations, advocates quickly rallied the news media. The team's activities were broadcast while young people carried antitobacco protest signs around the trucks. The Marlboro Adventure Team soon packed up their trucks and moved on as the negative coverage mounted.

Media advocacy is an important and effective tool for those involved in the field of tobacco control because it provides opportunities for *unpaid* television, radio, and print coverage. It is particularly important to remember, in an era of waning funding, that free public service announcements are not the only social marketing tool available to health educators.

Policy and Ordinance Activities

Restrictions on smoking for fire and safety reasons in the form of ordinances and policy actions have existed for much of this century, but restrictions based on health and annoyance have been implemented largely just over the past two decades.[20] The federal government has not been as successful as state and local governments in enacting smoking control ordinances due to the overwhelming influence of the tobacco industry lobby.

The one notable exception was when Congress successfully acted to restrict smoking on commercial airliners. In 1987, Congress passed legislation banning smoking on all domestic flights of two hours or less. In 1989, they managed to increase that ban to all domestic flights of six hours or less. While this was a major national victory for nonsmokers' rights, the remainder of the successes in policy and ordinance actions have been at the local level.

Smoking Control at the Local and State Level. With few exceptions, smoking control ordinances at the local level are stronger and more comprehensive than state laws. Indeed, they are often enacted because of difficulties in passing strong state laws. Action at the state level is more difficult to achieve for a number of reasons, the primary one being the powerful tobacco industry lobby. Adding to the difficulty is the state legislative process, which makes it much easier to kill a bill than to pass one.

Local officeholders, by contrast, are much less likely to be dependent upon tobacco industry money and therefore much more likely to see passage of a bill all the way through the legislative process.[5] Because most local officeholders do not receive tobacco industry money, the tobacco industry is exposed as an outsider whose sole interests are profits, not the good of the community. Additionally, locally enacted ordinances are generally more palatable to the voter, because community members are more likely to have input and thus a sense of local autonomy.

California has been a leader in the area of locally enacted smoking control ordinances. In 1982, San Diego was the first large California city to enact an ordinance regulating smoking in the workplace.[19] By 1992, over 250 of California's 468 cities had enacted local smoking control ordinances.[5]

Workplace Policies. Voluntary workplace policies have evolved over the years from general *accommodation* policies to complete bans. Early workplace policies may have required no smoking sections in public areas or bans in elevators and hallways, but most private offices were exempt. These policies proved to be inadequate as more nonsmokers began to demand their right to a smoke-free workplace. Recognizing that smoke from designated areas still pollutes other work areas and given the classification by the EPA of secondhand smoke as a class A carcinogen,[21] many work sites have placed a total ban on smoking.

Communities across the nation have begun to use ordinances and policies to prevent the purchase of tobacco by youth. Because more than three million children and youth under the age of 18 still regularly smoke cigarettes, many tobacco control advocates have recognized both the need for ordinances that enforce youth access laws and ban vending machines. In several studies designed to assess the extent of underage youth access to tobacco, children succeeded about 70 percent of the time in purchasing tobacco from stores and 90 to 100 percent of the time in purchasing tobacco from vending machines.[6]

Several approaches can be taken to decrease vending machine sales to minors, such as locking devices or placement only in areas where they can be supervised by an adult. However, the only truly effective measure is a total ban on tobacco vending machines. To date in California, 49 local jurisdictions have passed partial or total vending machine bans. Although a total ban may seem drastic, it seems reasonable when one considers what might happen if alcohol could be sold in vending machines. Individuals of any age could buy it even though one must be 21 years old to buy alcohol legally. One must be 18 years old to purchase tobacco, so it is equally inappropriate to have tobacco readily available for purchase by anyone from a vending machine.

Community Organizational Strategies

Organizational strategies for tobacco control include coordination, social planning and policy, and social action at the community level.

Coordination

In most communities and regions, some coordination of prevention, cessation, and other programs is already occurring. Groups of local people meet formally or informally to discuss existing activities and plan new initiatives. Generally, the groups consist of representatives from voluntary health organizations (such as the American Lung Association, the American Cancer Society, and the American Heart Association); government offices (for example, county and regional health departments); schools; professional associations (for example, medical societies); and other organizations. Such groups are immeasurably important for long-term community ownership and success in tobacco control, but they can often benefit from fresh ideas and new directions.

To improve coordination and enhance effectiveness of existing tobacco control efforts, local smoking control groups should consider the following questions:

1. Is the community truly represented among the group's membership? For example, do blue-collar workers, high-risk teens, women, and minorities have a voice in developing directions and priorities? Do their efforts represent effective and appropriate locality development, such as process-oriented grass roots efforts in the community?
2. Is the group aware of current research developments in tobacco control? Well-meaning groups have been known to adhere to ineffective approaches.
3. Does the group know what role the tobacco industry plays in their community?
4. Are antitobacco activists in communication with the group? Are sufficiently aggressive policy and ac-

tivism strategies being considered, in addition to prevention, cessation, and media efforts?

Social Planning and Policy

Policy initiatives may have two components: *development* of new tobacco control policies and *enforcement* of existing policies. Much of policy-related tobacco control is designed to "protect the innocent." Young people, who are exposed to tobacco advertisements and have access to purchasing the product, either through vending machines or over the counter, may be well on their way to addiction before they are sufficiently mature to consider the consequences. Other nonsmoking individuals may suffer from passive smoking at the work site or other places that legally should be smoke free. Indeed, research in the United States has shown passive smoking to be the third most preventable cause of death.[20] Restricting advertisements, eliminating access and sales to youth, and protecting nonsmokers from passive smoke are priorities for policy development and enforcement.

Finally, overall tobacco control efforts cannot be complete without recognizing the need for further restrictions on the international trade of tobacco. Phillip Morris, R.J. Reynolds, British American, and other tobacco companies make huge profits promoting their products abroad, increasingly in underdeveloped countries. As the populations of these regions often have neither the knowledge nor the power to restrict tobacco imports and marketing, people in tobacco-exporting countries are obligated to lead the way.

Social Action

A minister of a church in Harlem was disgusted with the excessive amount of alcohol and tobacco billboard advertising near his church and the local public schools. He and his parishioners used paint and brushes, and after a long day, many of these ads had disappeared. The "Bugger Up" efforts in Australia promoted a similar concept, resulting in the defacement of tobacco ads throughout the country.

Recently, a group of Latino health promoters and students, armed with cameras and antitobacco fliers, appeared at a Chicano festival in a San Diego park, correctly anticipating that representatives of Camel cigarettes would be there in force. First, they followed "roamers" walking around the park giving out free packs of Camels, placing the antitobacco fliers in the hands of people who had just received a pack and taking pictures of the process. Feeling harassed, the roamers eventually gave up and returned to a central promotional stand. At this location, people were lined up to spin a wheel that yielded "prizes" of Camels and promotional products. The protesters continued to snap pictures of the process, inviting complaints and derisive comments from the Camel representatives operating the stand. Frustrated, one of the representatives pushed a camera into a protester's face—an act widely observed by the public. After a brief staff conference, the Camel team decided to pack up their promotion (and their hundreds of cartons of cigarettes) and leave.[17]

Social action strategies such as this can generate free publicity around a particular controversial topic, invite an industry counterresponse that may backfire and elicit even more public sympathy for the antitobacco cause, and crystallize public opinion for or against the cause. While social action is energizing, it can also be exhausting, and it requires a tremendous amount of dedication and work to be effective. Even with this commitment, care must be taken to prevent specific actions from backfiring and producing greater sympathy for the industry.

Summary

In summary, community organizational strategies include coordination of antitobacco efforts, development and implementation of policy, and antitobacco activism. These efforts hold the greatest potential for meeting the threat to health posed by tobacco (or more appropriately, the tobacco industry). The validity of this assertion is assured by the vigorous counterattacks of the tobacco industry against policy and activism, while it ignores or even expresses support for cessation and prevention efforts.

TABLE 17.2   Advantages and Disadvantages of Various Tobacco Control Strategies

Priority Area	Example	Advantages	Disadvantages
Cessation	Quit and Win Smoking Cessation Contests	1. Noncontroversial	1. Addiction generally firmly in place; high relapse rates 2. Physical damage to smoker may already have been done 3. Intensive intervention may be required 4. Much doubt about public health impact
Prevention	Project SHOUT	1. Noncontroversial 2. Targets children before addiction sets in	1. Some doubt about long-term efficacy
Media	California (Prop 99) Tobacco Control Media Campaign	1. Broad reach (in some applications) 2. Can be used to complement any of the other four activities	1. Can be very expensive 2. Not sufficient by itself
Policy	Banning smoking at the work site	1. Potentially highly effective 2. Protects the innocent (such as passive smokers)	1. Controversial—likely to provoke response from tobacco industry (for example, through Smoker's "Rights" Groups), which will need to be countered 2. Requires support of frequently conservative bureaucracy or elected officials (some of whom may receive financial support from the tobacco industry)
Activism	Doctors Ought to Care	1. Can be highly visible—creates own media through news coverage, etc. 2. Can be effective—establishes cutting edge for others to follow	1. Highly controversial 2. May include activities of questionable legality 3. May offend some elements of the public or be seen by them as the "radical fringe"

Antitobacco activism slingshots will continually be met with the industry's nuclear counterstrikes. Very careful community assessment, research, and the integration of complementary prevention, cessation, marketing, and policy-oriented efforts are a must if tobacco use is to be eliminated in our culture. Table 17.2 summarizes some of the advantages and disadvantages of the various tobacco control strategies that might be considered.

THE CALIFORNIA EXPERIENCE: PROPOSITION 99

In California voters realized that strong, government-sponsored antitobacco efforts were unlikely, given that the tobacco industry is a major contributor to nearly every legislator's and government executive's campaign fund. In 1988, following the leadership of major voluntary health organizations, California voters opted to increase the tax on a pack of cigarettes from the low level of 10 cents to 35 cents. Moreover, this voter-initiated proposition, called Proposition 99, mandated that one-fourth of the tax revenues realized in this increase would be spent on antitobacco education and tobacco-related disease research. This was $150 million per year for a state of 25 million people. The sum was especially important, given the relative decline of federal funding for such research and educational efforts. Despite the fact that the tobacco industry spent well over 10 times as much in anti-Proposition 99 media advertising as the coalition spent promoting the proposition, Proposition 99 was passed by the voters by nearly a two-to-one margin.

The effects of the increased tax were immediate. Tobacco consumption dropped nearly 10 percent from the previous year despite the fact that the actual anti-tobacco campaign had not yet begun.[22] The educational effort then shifted into high gear with extensive mass media, local health department-sponsored efforts, school-based programs, and innovative individual and community initiatives.

A good example of an innovative, locally initiated program funded by Proposition 99 is Project TRUST (Teens and Retailers United to Stop Tobacco). Project TRUST is a county-wide educational effort designed to encourage supermarkets, gasoline stations, convenience stores, liquor stores, and independently owned retailers to decrease tobacco sales to children under 18 years of age, decrease access to tobacco products by children under 18, and decrease tobacco advertising inside and outside stores. Volunteer adults and teens teamed up with Project TRUST staff to develop a community strategy. Teens under 18 (who are too young to purchase tobacco legally) went into stores and attempted to purchase cigarettes. In baseline purchasing attempts, 75 percent of these 12-to-17-year-olds purchased cigarettes with "no questions asked." An intervention is currently in progress whereby stores that refuse to sell tobacco to minors receive free advertising for their high level of social responsibility, whereas clerks and owners of all tobacco-selling stores are given special training in how to check for identification and politely refuse to sell tobacco to teens. Finally, continuing violators will be warned by county officials that they are breaking the law.

Other programs funded by Proposition 99 include highly aggressive antitobacco media campaigns, large-scale smoking cessation and prevention contests, and policy changes promoting increased restrictions on public consumption of tobacco. Special emphasis has been placed on efforts that specifically target the Latino, African-American, and Asian communities, which are also heavily targeted by the tobacco industry. The African-American Tobacco Education Network sponsored a letter-to-the-editor campaign for youth in conjunction with Black Music Month entitled, "Smoking Made Them History." Youth were encouraged to identify an African-American legend such as Nat King Cole, Duke Ellington, or another who died from smoking-related illnesses, and write a letter to the editor of a local paper describing the legend, the cause of death, and their desire that people they care about stop smoking. This event not only heightened awareness of the toll tobacco has taken on African-Americans, but it also encouraged action by youth.

California has been a leader in advancing local level policies and ordinances to restrict or ban tobacco use. The California Smokefree Cities Project, for example, is a statewide program funded to help cities and public health agencies promote healthful community environments. This project provides an extensive bank of information about local tobacco control policy and leadership. It also provides a comprehensive technical assistance network to give immediate service and information to municipal officials. The project is unique in that staff work with nonhealth entities, such as cities and city managers, and bring together the two worlds to facilitate local level change in tobacco use policies.

CONCLUSION

Tobacco use cessation and even prevention programs are of limited public health utility unless subordinated to more aggressive and extensive interventions. These interventions include restricting sales to minors and enforcing these restrictions, protecting nonsmokers through clean indoor air policies, and in other ways implementing policies that make it more difficult for the smoker to casually light up and at the same time encourage him to quit. Interventions also include increasing the costs of tobacco to the consumer, which will at least temporarily suppress purchasing. Finally, aggressive anti-industry advertising makes it more difficult for tobacco interests to defend their credibility and legitimacy. Hopefully, the time is approaching when a concerted nationwide approach, modeled in funding and style after the Proposition 99 experience, will push America's unacceptable tobacco-related mortality to modern-day record low levels.

REFERENCES

1. *Smoking and Health. Report of the Advisory Committee to the Surgeon General of the Public Health Service.* Washington, DC: US

Dept of Health, Education, and Welfare; 1964. PHS publication no. 1103.

2. *Healthy People 2000: National Health Promotion and Disease Prevention Objectives.* Washington, DC: US Dept of Health and Human Services; 1990. PHS publication no. 91-50212.

3. Mittelmark M, Luepker R, Jacobs D, et al. Community-wide prevention of cardiovascular disease: education strategies of the Minnesota Heart Health Program. *Prev Med.* 1986;15:1–17.

4. Elder J, McGraw S, Abrams D, et al. Organizational and community approaches to community–wide prevention of heart disease: the first two years of the Pawtucket Heart Health Program. *Prev Med.* 1986;15:107–117.

5. US Dept of Health and Human Services. *Major Local Tobacco Control Ordinances in the United States.* Bethesda, Md: Public Health Service, National Institutes of Health, National Cancer Institute; May 1993. NIH publication no. 93-3532. Smoking and Tobacco Control Monograph no. 3.

6. Fourkas T, ed. *Tobacco Control in California Cities: A Guide for Action.* Berkeley, Ca: California Healthy Cities Project in partnership with the League of California Cities, Americans for Nonsmokers' Rights, Health Officers Association of California; December 1992.

7. Altman D, Foster V, Rasenick-Douss L, Tye J. Reducing the illegal sale of cigarettes to minors. *JAMA.* 1989;261:80–83.

8. Schwartz, JL. *Review and Evaluation of Smoking Cessation Methods: The United States and Canada, 1978–1985.* Bethesda, Md: US Dept of Health and Human Services; 1987. NIH publication no. 87-2940.

9. *Reducing the Health Consequences of Smoking: 25 Years of Progress. A Report of the Surgeon General.* Washington, DC: US Dept of Health and Human Services; 1989. DHHS publication CDC 89–8411.

10. Elder J, McGraw S, Rodrigues A, et al. Evaluation of two community-wide smoking cessation contests. *Prev Med.* 1987;16:221–234.

11. Lando H, Hellerstedt W, Pirie P, Fruetel J, Huttner P. Results of a long–term community smoking cessation contest. *Am J Health Prom.* 1991;5:420–425.

12. Glynn TJ, Manley MW. *How to Help your Patients Stop Smoking: A National Cancer Institute Manual for Physicians.*

Bethesda, Md: US Dept of Health and Human Services; 1989. NIH publication no. 89-3064.

13. Glynn TJ, Manley MW, Pechacek TF. Physician-initiated smoking cessation program: The National Cancer Institute trials. In: Engstrom PF, Rimer B, Mortenson LE, eds. *Advances in Cancer Control: Screening and Prevention Research.* New York, NY: Wiley-Liss Inc; 1990. Vol. 339:11–25.

14. Manley M, Epps RP, Husten C, Glynn T, Shopland D. Clinical interventions in tobacco control: a National Cancer Institute training program for physicians. *JAMA.* 1991;226:3172–3173.

15. Evans RI. Smoking in children. Developing a social psychological strategy of deterrence. *Prev Med.* 1976;5:122–127.

16. Evans RI, Perry CL, Maccoby N, McAllister AL. Adolescent smoking prevention: a third year follow-up. *World Smoking & Health.* 1980;5:41–45.

17. Elder J, Wildey M, de Moor C, Sallis J, Eckhardt L, Edwards C, et al. The long-term prevention of tobacco use among junior high school students: classroom and telephone interventions. *Am J Public Health.* 1993;9:1239–1244.

18. Elder JP, Geller ES, Howell MF, Mayer JA. *Motivating Health Behavior.* Albany, NY: Delmar Publishers Inc; 1994.

19. Butler J. *How to Counteract the Tobacco Industry's Advertising and Promotion.* Stanford, CA: Stanford Health Promotion and Resource Center; August 1993.

20. US Dept of Health and Human Services. *Strategies to Control Tobacco Use in the United States: A Blueprint for Public Health Action in the 1990's.* Bethesda, Md: Public Health Service, National Institutes of Health, National Cancer Institute; October 1991. NIH publication no. 92-3316. Smoking and Tobacco Control Monograph no. 1.

21. US Environmental Protection Agency. *Respiratory Health Effects of Passive Smoking: Lung Cancer and Other Disorders.* Washington, DC: Office of Health and Environmental Assessment, Office of Research and Development; December 1992. EPA 600-6-90/006F.

22. Flewelling R, Kenney E, Elder J, Pierce J, Johnson M, Bal D. First-year impact of the 1989 California cigarette tax increase on cigarette consumption. *Am J Public Health.* 1992;82:867–869.

CHAPTER

A Public Health Approach to Alcohol and Other Drug Problems: Theory and Practice

James F. Mosher, J.D.

This chapter seeks to lay the groundwork for building a citizen–based public health agenda for addressing alcohol and other drug problems. It addresses both policy and practice issues. In keeping with public health theory, it focuses particularly on prevention as a primary goal of public health policy.

Specifically, a theoretical perspective for addressing alcohol and other drug problems is presented, followed by an examination of the legal–illegal dichotomy that dominates current policies. Next, available data on the prevalence of alcohol and other drug use and their related problems are reviewed. Then public health prevention strategies are outlined. The chapter concludes with implications of the previous sections for public health practice and policy development.

Some caveats should be mentioned first, however. The phrase *alcohol and other drugs* is used in this chapter to emphasize alcohol's status as a psychoactive drug. This is in conformity with preferred practice, as defined by the Substance Abuse and Mental Health Services Administration and the American Public Health Association. Tobacco should be included in the phrase and is omitted here only because a separate chapter in this volume discusses tobacco problems and policies. Due to space limitations, the chapter does not address inappropriate uses of prescription drugs.

BACKGROUND

In 1993, the new Clinton administration issued its *1993 Interim National Drug Control Strategy,*[1] which

243

questioned the strategies and tactics of the war on drugs initiated by President Reagan in 1986. The report concluded that the dominant focus of the previous administration's policies on international drug interdiction had failed to stem the flow of drugs in this country and that federal policy should shift its focus to domestic law enforcement and demand reduction. The findings came as no surprise to public health professionals, researchers, and citizen activists seeking effective strategies for preventing alcohol and other drug problems. Numerous studies have documented the failure of strategies that rely on the drug interdiction and incarceration of drug users, which have been the cornerstones of the drug war.[2,3]

In fact, sufficient evidence existed even prior to the initiation of the most recent drug war in 1986 that the strategies chosen to address the problem would fail. This country has witnessed a whole series of drug wars during the last 100 years with striking resemblances and consequences: excess reliance on criminal law and drug interdiction; definition of the problem as one of morality rather than public health; focus on drug use among disenfranchised groups, usually communities of color; deflection of policy focus from economic, social, and public health issues underlying the drug use; lack of attention to legal drugs; and, ultimately, failure of the drug war to address drug problems effectively.[4–6]

Perhaps most striking from the perspective of this volume is that public health theory and practice have played only a marginal role in defining federal alcohol and other drug policies in this country. This has been particularly true during the drug wars, when public attention has been at its height. During the early 1980s, for example, funding for public health prevention and treatment programs was cut at the same time that funding was increased dramatically for criminal justice and drug interdiction efforts.[5] As a result, treatment was significantly less available in 1987 than in 1976.[7]

Recent developments, particularly at the community level, bring hopes of changing this troubling picture of federal drug policy. Various citizen and professional groups have become increasingly effective at promoting public health strategies for addressing alcohol and other drug problems. These include: a shift of the policy focus away from criminal justice and interdiction strategies to public health strategies; increased attention to the legal drugs, alcohol and tobacco; greater accountability from the legal drug industries; and increased prevention and treatment services, particularly for low income groups and communities of color.[8–10] This activism began to have an impact during the waning years of the Bush-Reagan drug war and provided the public health field an important opportunity, not only to influence drug policy, but also to build a citizen base for action in wider public health arenas.

A PUBLIC HEALTH PARADIGM FOR ALCOHOL AND OTHER DRUG PROBLEMS

Alcohol and other drug problems are best understood by examining the interaction of three key components of any public health problem: environment, agent, and host. In general, the **host** is the individual suffering the public health problem and the **agent** (or vector) is that which is necessary or sufficient to cause harm to the host. The **environment** consists of the social, economic, physical, political, and cultural settings in which the host and agent interact.[5]

Drugs, including alcohol, can play differing roles within this public health paradigm. For drug-related illnesses such as alcoholic cirrhosis, for example, the agent can be viewed as alcohol. In the case of alcohol-related trauma, on the other hand, the agent or vector is energy (the impact of an automobile hitting a tree), and alcohol is a significant environmental factor increasing the likelihood that an injurious energy exchange will occur.

The Role of Environmental Factors

Environmental factors—the forces that bring the agent into injurious contact with the host—are critical in this model. A high-risk environment creates myriad opportunities for public health harm. Focusing solely on the host requires as many separate interventions as there are individuals, whereas a single change in the environment may provide protection to large numbers of people by preventing the agent and host from interacting. A comprehensive public health strategy focuses on all three factors within the paradigm, providing care to those who suffer disease or injury, reducing the harmfulness and availability of particular agents, and addressing dangerous conditions or environments that put people at risk for harm.

The Need for a Systems Approach

At the heart of the host-agent-environment triad is the interaction of various causal factors within and between each point of the triangle. These interactions can best be viewed as a system, because changes at one point inevitably alter the other points and the model as a whole. Because the classic triangle model suggests a static rather than dynamic structure, Wallack and Holder[11] have argued for a systems approach that focuses on the dynamic interactions of all factors affecting alcohol and other drug problems.[12,13]

Using a systems model, an individual can be viewed as surrounded by a series of concentric circles representing various forces that impact the individual's drinking and drug-taking decisions. Family, school, workplace, media, community, and economic conditions, among other factors interact with the individual and with each other in a dynamic system. Shifting individual behavior involves an understanding of the entire system. Similarly, strategies that address risk factors must consider the entire system and not just promote changes in the individual host.

Relationship to Alcohol Policy

Until recently, these public health principles had little impact on society's understanding of alcohol and other drug problems. The field has traditionally focused its attention instead on host and agent factors to the exclusion of an examination of environmental risk factors.

Historical Perspective

During the first part of this century, prior to the repeal of Prohibition in 1933, alcohol policy was dominated by a focus on the individual immorality of drinkers and the need to restrict and eventually prohibit the availability of "demon" alcohol. This perspective continues today in policies addressing many illegal drugs.

Following the repeal, policy shifted to a medical and predominantly host perspective. The predominant focus was on identifying and treating alcoholics. Alcohol problems were considered to rest solely with a limited portion of the population, persons who were predisposed to alcoholism, the disease. With this perspective, policies to address environmental risk factors and controls on alcohol were irrelevant. In fact, they were potentially harmful because they could lead to increased criminal activities and create a "forbidden fruit" status for alcohol.

Recent Trends

In the last 20 years, application of a public health perspective to the alcohol field has brought a dramatic shift in these assumptions.[9,14] In part the shift was occasioned by epidemiologic findings that showed that alcohol problems were not experienced by a small, discrete subpopulation of alcoholics but by many others as well. In fact, alcohol problems were reported by those who clearly did not exhibit drinking patterns associated with alcoholism. It was also discovered that individuals may drastically change their problematic drinking patterns over time without alcoholism treatment intervention.[15]

At the same time, researchers became more sensitive to the wide array of health problems associated with alcohol in addition to alcoholism: trauma, alcohol-related birth defects, sexual assaults and other violence, cirrhosis of the liver and other long term health problems, and workplace and school problems, among others.[14–16] Although alcoholics were more likely to report these problems, the problems were also experienced more broadly across the entire society. The recognition of the diversity of problems associated with alcohol also led to a realization of their complexity. It became apparent that alcohol interacts with and contributes to a wide array of social and health problems; the problems occur in the context of a complex system; and strategies for addressing them must take into account the interaction of a diverse set of factors that put people at risk.

As a result of these shifts in perspective, the field has a new and intense concern with alcohol availability, drinking environments, and environmental risk factors. The focus now is on population-based rather than individual-based strategies. In contrast to Prohibition policies, the aim today is to reduce the harm associated with alcohol use rather than reduce use per se. These topics are explored in more detail later in the chapter.

Relationship to Illegal Drug Policy

Current policies regarding illegal drugs are still dominated by the Prohibition perspective that was applied to alcohol prior to the repeal. The focus has been on individual deviance and immorality and the need to abolish the illegal drug trade. As discussed by Zimring and Hawkins[17] and others,[5] the drug policies of the Bush administration, as developed by the drug czar William Bennett, were based on four key assumptions:

1. Illegal drug use is fundamentally a moral problem.
2. Illegal drug policy should focus on deterring use not on reducing associated health problems.
3. All illegal drugs should be treated as the same and different from legal drugs.
4. Punitive measures to stem use and supply should dominate illegal drug policy.

These assumptions were most apparent in the priorities set for the war-on-drugs budget. Between 1986 and 1992, that budget increased fourfold, from approximately $2.8 billion to $12.3 billion.[18] More than 70 percent of the funds were dedicated to law enforcement costs, primarily prison construction, criminal justice costs, drug interdiction programs, and other Department of Justice programs.

Environmental Approach to Drug Policy

An environmental approach to drug policy challenges each of these assumptions. It can be expressed in four basic principles for guiding the development of illegal drug policies:[5,8]

1. Drug use should be treated primarily as a public health issue rather than an issue of individual morality or deviance. Policy should focus on community and societal environments in which individual problems occur.
2. The primary purpose of drug policy should be to reduce drug-related problems. Reducing drug use may be one strategy to reduce drug harm, but it should not be an aim in itself. (Current policies designed to reduce use may actually increase drug-related problems due to the violence they foster.)
3. Priority should be given to those drugs that create the most risk of harm in society. On this basis primary attention needs to be given to alcohol and tobacco, the legal drugs. Drugs that carry a high risk for addiction and/or violent behavior also should receive a higher priority in drug policy than drugs with lower risks of such harm.
4. Prevention, treatment, and recovery measures should dominate drug policy. Punitive measures targeting drug users should be reserved primarily for drug-related behavior associated with other criminal acts.

As with alcohol policy, an environmental approach to preventing illegal drug problems focuses on two basic risk factors: the availability of illegal drugs and the broader family, community, social, cultural, and political contexts in which illegal drug problems occur. These risk factors are addressed by the specific prevention strategies discussed later in the chapter.

The Illegal/Legal Drug Policy Dichotomy

The legality or illegality of a given drug dominates current and past drug policies. If a drug is legal, it is generally widely available at relatively low prices. Powerful economic interests push for ever increasing markets and lower prices. In response to these economic pressures, legal drug policies generally focus on individual deviance without attention to environmental factors. If a drug is illegal, criminal justice strategies dominate policy, with primary attention given to controlling the distribution network and punishing illegal drug users, who are treated as morally weak. Alcohol policy has shifted three times within this dichotomy: legal, to illegal, and back to legal. Other drugs (such as heroin, cocaine, opium, and marijuana) experienced just one shift, from legal to illegal.

The legal/illegal dichotomy in drug policy clearly creates radically different policy responses, which have little or no relationship to the relative risks to public health that the drugs pose. Although they are different, illegal and legal drug policies nonetheless share basic assumptions: drug problems rest primarily in the individual drug user, either because of moral weakness, disease, or immorality; and environmental risk factors are only marginally significant.

The dominance of the dichotomy has also resulted in little experience with strategies that do not fall within one of these two extremes. A drug is either a scourge that must be eradicated and its users imprisoned, or it is a relatively benign substance (except for those few who need to be treated for addiction) that requires no regulation of its availability and marketing.

Numerous individuals and organizations, including respected public officials, have become increasingly vocal in their call for decriminalization or legalization of illegal drugs, arguing many of the principles cited above. Public health principles do indeed suggest a fundamental shift in focus, from criminal justice to public health strategies. However, calls for decriminalization or legalization may be premature or ill advised. Given the lack of experience in effective control of legal drugs and the historical failure to address underlying environmental factors, deliberate planning and caution will be needed in shifting from a criminal justice focus if the public health consequences of drug use are to be minimized.

THE PREVALENCE OF ALCOHOL AND OTHER DRUG PROBLEMS

Alcohol and other drug use is present throughout society among all social and economic classes, ethnic and racial groups, and geographic regions. Rural areas and the southern region of the country in general have lower use rates. Rates of use vary by type of drug, with alcohol by far the most commonly used drug among all groups. Preferences for illegal drugs vary by type of drug, with some groups favoring one drug over another.

According to the 1991 National Household Survey (NHS), the most recent survey for which data are available, nearly 51 percent of the population over 12 years of age use alcohol at least once a month, compared to 6.3 percent for those who use any illegal drug. These data are shown in Table 18.1 Most illegal drug use can be attributed to marijuana, which is used by 4.8 percent of the population at least once a month. Cocaine, crack, heroin, and other illegal drug use rates are extremely low. Only cocaine is used monthly by more than 1.0 percent of the population.[19]

Significance of Alcohol

These higher levels of alcohol use persist when comparing heavy use of drugs. Thirteen percent of those over 18 years of age report drinking 60 drinks or more per month, and 14 percent report binge drinking (defined as five or more drinks on an occasion at least weekly).[20] Heavy illegal drug use is typically defined as use on at least a weekly basis, and data regarding heavier use are not available. These contrasting definitions of heavy use reflect primarily political rather than public health concerns. Even with its stricter definition, however, heavy alcohol use is far greater than heavy use of illegal drugs: only 1.4 percent of respondents in the

TABLE 18.1 Household Population: Illegal Drug and Alcohol Use (Past Month) 1985, 1988, 1991

	Percent of Population		
	1985	1988	1991
Any illegal drug	11.3	7.3	6.3
Cocaine use	3.0	1.5	0.9
Crack use	a	0.2	0.2
Marijuana use	9.4	5.9	4.8
Alcohol use[b]	59.1	53.4	50.9
Heavy alcohol use[c]	6.5	4.9	5.3

[a]comparable data not available

[b]once a month

[c]five or more drinks on the same occasion, five or more times in the last 30 days.

SOURCES: *National Household Survey on Drug Abuse: 1985–1991.*
Institute of Health Policy. *Substance Abuse: The Number One Health Problem.* Princeton, NJ: Robert Wood Johnson Foundation; October 1993:24.

NHS in 1991 reported once a week or more marijuana use, and just 0.3 percent of respondents reported a weekly or more frequent rate of cocaine use.

Prevalence in Young Adults

Young adults ages 18 to 25 are by far the most likely age group to use alcohol and other drugs, with rates decreasing rapidly with age. For example, 15.4 percent of 18 to 25-year-olds used any illegal drug in the previous month as compared with just 3.5 percent of those over 35 years of age.[19] Men are more likely to report alcohol and other drug use than women, with gender differences being most pronounced among those reporting heavy use.

Illegal drug use rates among young adults have declined steadily, by approximately one-half, since the late 1970s.[21] Alcohol use rates have also declined in this age group, but not nearly so sharply, with alcohol remaining by far the drug of choice. The trends among young adults are a major contributor to the declining use of illegal drugs and (to a much lesser extent) of alcohol in the general population. Interestingly, binge drinking among college students has not declined and remains at an alarmingly high rate (over 40 percent). This contrasts sharply with binge drinking rates of those in the same age group who do not attend college, suggesting that college environments may put young people at a greater risk for heavy drinking.

Ethnic and Racial Group Variations

As shown in Table 18.2, the NHS reports higher rates of use among Latino and African–American populations. These results mirror other reports and fuel a popular belief, reinforced by many media reports, that racial or ethnic specific personal factors are critical determinants of illegal drug use. However, as also shown in Table 18.2, income level is a far better predictor of illegal drug use than is racial or ethnic background. Those with lower incomes are far more likely to use illegal drugs, including cocaine, and less likely to use alcohol than those with higher incomes, regardless of racial or ethnic background. Employment status also serves as an important predictor of illegal drug use. Unemployed respondents are more than twice as likely to report illegal drug use than are those who have full-time employment, regardless of race.[5] Interestingly, the NHS does not report the income data as part of its published materials; they were only obtained through a special request to the Office of Applied Studies at the Substance Abuse and Mental Health Services Administration.

A recent study[22] of crack cocaine use reinforces the importance of looking beyond racial and ethnic factors in assessing drug use data. In the study, crack cocaine users from the 1988 NHS survey were grouped into neighborhood clusters, in effect holding constant shared characteristics such as drug availability and social conditions. Certain neighborhoods had higher rates of crack cocaine use, but the rates of use within the neighborhood clusters did not vary by race or ethnic background. In fact, the only statistically significant racial or ethnic association involved teenage African–Americans, who were less likely to smoke crack cocaine than their white counterparts living in similar neighborhood clusters. The authors concluded that, "Given similar social conditions, crack cocaine smoking does not depend strongly on race per se as a personal characteristic of individuals."[22(p997)] They urged greater attention to the social environments in which drug use takes place.

Excluded Populations

The NHS and high school and young adult surveys are the primary source for data on alcohol and other drug use in the United States, as the above discussion suggests. Unfortunately, these data sources are incomplete, because they do not reflect the entire population. As pointed out by Wish,[23] the NHS does not include the two percent of the population that lives in group quarters (for example, in military installations, dormitories, hotels, hospitals, and jails) or who are transient or homeless. The school–based surveys do not include the 15 to 20 percent of young people who have dropped out of school before graduation.[21]

Various fragmentary studies suggest that alcohol and other drug use within these populations is significantly higher than in the general population.[5] The fact that employment status and income levels are significant

TABLE 18.2 Prevalence of Alcohol and Illegal Drug Use Among Full–Time Employed Persons Ages 18 to 40 by Selected Type of Drug, Personal Income, and Ethnicity: 1992

Personal Income by Race/Ethnicity	Percent of Population		
	Past Month Use of Any Illegal Drug	Past Month Use of Cocaine[a]	Past Month Use of Alcohol
All Respondents			
Euro-American	5.9	0.7	52.7
African-American	9.4	1.8	43.7
Latino	6.3	1.6	47.5
Total[b]			
Less than $12,000			
Euro-American	11.0	2.0	56.9
African-American	11.2	0.9	52.0
Latino	8.0	1.9	56.6
Total[b]	10.6	1.8	55.9
$12,000-19,000			
Euro-American	10.4	1.7	64.3
African-American	7.7	0.8	50.9
Latino	8.2	2.1	60.3
Total[b]	9.7	1.6	61.2
$20,000-29,999			
Euro-American	9.3	1.1	65.6
African-American	6.3	1.6	54.7
Latino	9.4	3.9	61.6
Total[b]	8.8	1.4	63.6
$30,000 or over			
Euro-American	7.1	0.4	74.6
African-American	9.1	1.1	58.5
Latino	5.8	0.8	70.8
Total[b]	6.8	0.4	71.3

[a]Includes crack.
[b]Prevalence data of "Other Ethnicities" not reported separately but included in "Total."
SOURCE: Office of Applied Studies, SAMHSA: Unpublished data from the National Household Survey on Drug Abuse.

predictors of illegal drug use (but not alcohol use) provides additional support for this hypothesis, because the excluded populations are likely to have low incomes and be unemployed. African-American, Latino, and other racial and ethnic groups are also likely to be overrepresented. However, accurate estimates of drug use in these high–risk populations are impossible. Although the Office of Drug Control Policy estimates that there are more than twice as many "hard-core" (at least weekly) cocaine users in the two percent nonhousehold-resident population than in the 98 percent household-resident population, this estimate is highly suspect.[24]

Public Health Consequences of Alcohol and Other Drug Use

Differences in the rates of alcohol and other drug use are reflected in data reporting public health and societal problems, with alcohol problems far more prevalent than illegal drug problems. The nature and definition of the problems also differ, reflecting in part the social responses that emerge from their legal or illegal status. These differences make accurate comparisons between problems associated with alcohol and problems associated with other drugs difficult or impossible. In general, illegal drug use itself is defined as a problem, while alcohol use is usually defined as problematic only when it leads to specific behavioral or physical harm.

Mortality and Traumatic Injury

The federal government estimates that alcohol is a direct or indirect cause of approximately 105,000 deaths per year.[25] Alcohol-related traffic fatalities and digestive diseases (including alcoholic cirrhosis of the liver) comprise the largest groups of deaths, totalling approximately 20,000 deaths each.[25] Alcohol is also implicated in other forms of traumatic deaths, including homicide, suicide, burns, poisoning, drowning, and falls as well as other forms of alcohol-related disease, such as cancers of the liver and stomach.

In addition, alcohol is a major contributor to traumatic injury. Alcohol-related motor vehicle injuries are by far the largest category of these, causing approximately 500,000 serious injuries each year.[26] In general, the higher the blood alcohol content of the person causing the injury, the more serious the injury. Tragically, alcohol-related injuries and deaths are most likely to impact young people. In fact, alcohol-related motor vehicle crashes constitute the leading cause of death for those between the ages of 4 and 34 years.[27] Those dying from alcohol-related causes lost 26 years from their normal life expectancy, far higher than other major causes of death in the United States.[28]

Data regarding illegal drug-related deaths are not nearly as reliable or precise as those available for alcohol. The United States National Center for Health Statistics estimates that there are approximately 10,700 deaths that can be directly attributable to all illegal drug use combined, with an additional 7,700 deaths due to drug-associated AIDS.[27] Illegal drugs contribute indirectly to an unknown additional number of deaths. Ravenholt[29] attributed over 30,000 deaths to all drugs other than alcohol and tobacco, including prescription

drugs. The Drug Abuse Warning Network's (DAWN) medical examiner reports[30] provide data regarding drug-related deaths from 27 major metropolitan areas. In 1991, 5,353 deaths were reported to be related to heroin, morphine, or cocaine. By comparison, marijuana was mentioned in only 199 deaths.

DAWN also provides data regarding illegal drug episodes reported in emergency room (ER) visits.[31] Approximately 433,500 emergency room episodes involving drugs other than alcohol (including prescription and over-the-counter drugs) were reported in 1992. Among illegal drugs, cocaine was mentioned approximately 120,000 times, and heroin and morphine were mentioned 48,000 times. These were by far the leading substances mentioned. By comparison, marijuana was mentioned 24,000 times. There are sharp increases in illegal drug mentions in the DAWN reports between 1990 and 1992 after reductions in the late 1980s. DAWN does not provide a means to compare these data with data on alcohol-related ER episodes. Based on estimates of alcohol-related traumatic events, however, it is probable that alcohol accounts for several times the already alarming numbers reported for illegal drugs.

The relationship of alcohol and other drugs to violent episodes has become an increasing concern, reflecting the high rates of violence in our society. Available studies suggest that illegal drug-related violence is concentrated in African-American and Latino inner-city communities, with young people in these communities having, by far, the highest rates of homicide.[5] Drug-related violence is closely associated with the illegal drug trade. Domestic violence, sexual violence, and child abuse and neglect are all closely associated with alcohol consumption.

Alcohol and Drug Dependence

Based on an analysis of a variety of data, an Institute of Medicine Committee estimated that on a typical day in 1987 to 1988 there were nearly 5.5 million individuals in need of treatment for illegal drug dependence and abuse.[7] The study found that those with low incomes were far more likely to be in the need for treatment. The need for treatment, according to the committee, depends in part on ". . . the kinds of social advantages and supports available to the individual."[7(p91)] By contrast, for the entire year of 1989 only 344,500 persons, or about six percent of those needing treatment, were actually enrolled in a treatment program.[32]

The federal government estimates that approximately six percent of the adult population over 18 years of age are alcohol dependent and that an additional 4 percent are nondependent problem drinkers.[20,27] Using these estimates, more than 18 million adults, or three times the estimates of those needing drug treatment, are either alcohol dependent or have alcohol problems (the data do not address whether those with alcohol problems need to be enrolled in formal treatment programs). Approximately 374,000 persons were actually enrolled in alcoholism treatment units in 1989, about two percent of those the government identifies as having alcohol problems.[32] There has been a long-term shift from publicly funded to privately funded treatment programs, which has led to long waiting lists for low-income individuals who cannot afford the privately funded programs.[5]

Other Public Health Problems

Alcohol and other drug use is associated with a wide array of other public health problems. Alcohol-related birth defects (ARBD) constitute the number one preventable form of birth defects in the United States, and fetal exposures to maternal illegal drug consumption is a serious and growing concern.[33] Although illegal drug use is common in all racial and socioeconomic groups, the impact on infant health appears to be concentrated among women of color and those with lower incomes. This is due to their lack of other basic health and social support systems and the higher likelihood that their illegal drug use will be reported to authorities.[5]

The use of injection to administer illegal drugs has become a significant factor in the spread of AIDS. Alcohol use has been shown to increase the likelihood of unsafe sexual practices, thus contributing to the spread of AIDS.[5,34] Workplace and family disruptions are also closely associated with heavy alcohol consumption.[27,35] While these problems affect all demographic groups,

they are concentrated most heavily among those with low incomes who live in inner-city communities.[5]

Alcohol, Other Drugs, and the Criminal Justice System

Alcohol and other drug use has an enormous impact on the criminal justice system. In 1992, over 2.4 million arrests were made for alcohol-related crimes (including, driving under the influence, liquor law violations, and public drunkenness), and another 1.1 million arrests were made for illegal drug crimes.[18,36] More than two-thirds of illegal drug arrests involve drug possession, with 24 percent involving marijuana possession.[37] The remainder involve the manufacture and sale of drugs. Alcohol and other drug arrests constituted more than 28 percent of all arrests made in 1992.

Alcohol and other drugs also contribute to other crimes. Surveys suggest that one-half or more of those committing most types of crime, but particularly crimes against people, such as violent and public disorder offenses, were under the influence of alcohol at the time of the offense.[28] Between 30 percent to 78 percent of arrestees report being under the influence of illegal drugs at the time of the offense, with higher rates reported for crimes against property.[28,37]

Although alcohol offenses account for a greater number of arrests than illegal drug offenses, there are striking differences in both the trends and the consequences of the two types of offenses. Arrests for alcohol offenses decreased nearly 20 percent between 1983 and 1992, while arrests for illegal drug offenses increased by over 50 percent, even though during that same period illegal drug use declined.[37] Drug offenses actually declined after 1989, when arrests peaked at 1.36 million.

Incarceration rates for drug offenders skyrocketed during this same period. As shown in Figure 18.1, in state prisons incarcerations for drug offenses increased from approximately 38,100 to 149,000 between 1986 and 1991, which is nearly a fourfold increase.[38] Approximately 200,000 people were incarcerated for illegal drug offenses on a given day in 1991. This figure does not include the more than 7,000 juvenile offenders also in custody.[37] Drug offenders now account for 21

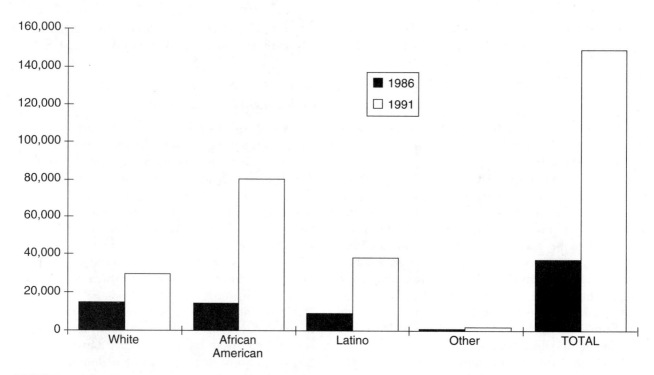

FIGURE 18.1 State Prison Incarcerations for Illegal Drug Offenses 1986, 1991 SOURCE: *Survey of State Prison Inmates*, US Department of Justice, Bureau of Justice Statistics 1991.

percent of all state inmates (up from 9 percent in 1986) and for 57 percent of all federal inmates.[18,37,38] By contrast, public order offenses, which include all alcohol offenses, only total about 5 percent of all incarcerations.

Perhaps most disturbing is the racial and ethnic makeup of those in prison for illegal drug offenses. As shown in Figure 18.1, African-Americans and Latinos are far more likely to be incarcerated for illegal drug offenses, a trend that has accelerated dramatically since 1986. Approximately 86 percent of the increase in state incarcerations for illegal drug crimes between 1986 and 1991 involved African-American, Latino, or other people of color. This trend is even more marked among juvenile offenders. According to one study of state juvenile court records in twelve states, the drug case rates for Euro-American juveniles decreased 15 percent between 1985 and 1988, while those for juveniles of color increased 88 percent during the same time period.[37]

Economic Costs of Alcohol and Other Drug Problems

As the data in this section suggest, alcohol and other drug problems create staggering costs for society in terms of human suffering. The impact is enormous for individuals, families, communities, and institutions within communities, as well as for society as a whole. The suffering associated with these problems also produces economic costs. As shown in Figure 18.2, the federal government estimates that in 1990 alcohol problems caused $98.6 billion and illegal drug abuse caused $66.8 billion in societal costs, including the costs of treatment, medical care, criminal justice, and prevention.[39,40] Nearly three-quarters of drug problem costs are related to crime and criminal justice, with only one-quarter of the costs related to health. By comparison, core health-related costs account for more than

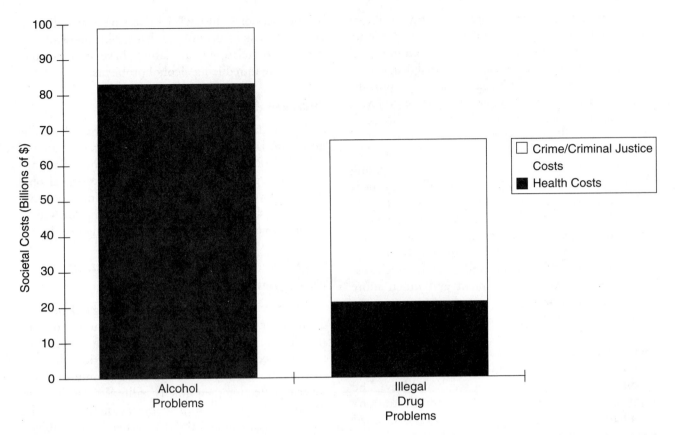

FIGURE 18.2 Economic Costs of Alcohol and Illegal Drug Problems. SOURCES: Rice, D. The economic cost of alcohol abuse and alcohol dependence: 1990. Alcohol, Health & Research World. 1993; 17:10–11. Institute of Health and Aging, UCSF, 1990 (unpublished data).

80 percent of the costs associated with alcohol problems.[39,40] In other words, alcohol problems result in nearly four times more core health costs than illegal drug problems ($58.1 billion compared to $14.6 billion), and the bulk of economic costs ($46.0 billion) associated with illegal drugs are the direct result of the criminal justice response to the problems.

A PUBLIC HEALTH AGENDA FOR ADDRESSING ALCOHOL AND OTHER DRUG PROBLEMS

The preceding sections paint a distressing picture regarding the state of alcohol and other drug problems and related policy in the United States today. Alcohol and other drugs are widely used throughout society, and problems resulting from their use are causing enormous suffering and economic costs, ranking among the most serious societal health problems. Society's response to the problems, however, has not been effective and in some cases has served to exacerbate underlying social, political, and economic injustices.

Although alcohol and other drug use rates are spread throughout all demographic groups in society, problems associated with that use are concentrated disproportionately among those with the least resources. This reflects, in part, underlying environmental factors (for example, racism, poverty, lack of employment, and neighborhood deterioration), which increase the prevalence and severity of alcohol and other drug problems.

Societal responses have focused primarily on illegal drugs despite the fact that alcohol problems are far more serious in terms of human suffering and economic costs than the problems associated with all illegal drugs combined. Individual-based strategies focusing on punishing individuals have predominated in social policy, with environmental risk factors virtually ignored. This societal response to illegal drugs has created its own costs.

The war on drugs has dramatically increased the likelihood of incarceration, particularly for young African-American and Latino men. At the same time it has reduced the availability of treatment programs to those with low income. In general, someone who is Euro-American and middle- or upper-class and suffers an alcohol or other drug problem will probably receive treatment; someone of color and poor is much less likely to have access to treatment and much more likely to be imprisoned.

In short, current policy has largely ignored the public health priorities for both alcohol and other drugs discussed above. Despite the improved rhetoric of the Clinton administration, a fundamental change in policy direction in the near future seems unlikely. The funding priorities delineated in that administration's 1994 national drug control strategy suggest continued heavy reliance on criminal justice and drug interdiction programs and the usual lack of attention to alcohol problems and environmental prevention strategies.[18]

Specific policy reform agendas that need to be incorporated into the nation's agenda regarding alcohol and other drug problems are presented next. The discussion focuses on environmental prevention strategies. They should be viewed as complementing other strategies that address individual risk factors, such as educational campaigns and treatment/recovery programs, which are beyond the scope of this chapter.

Alcohol Availability

As previously mentioned, alcohol and other drug availability is a critical policy variable, with striking contrasts between drugs that are illegal and those that are legal. In general, alcohol is widely and increasingly available, the result of public policy measures supported by the alcohol industry.[9,12] Increasing availability increases the risk of alcohol problems. The following policy measures relating to availability have been shown to be effective in reducing alcohol problems.

Increase Alcohol Taxes

The relative price of alcohol has decreased steadily during the last four decades, primarily because state and federal alcohol taxes have been eroded by inflation.[41] Research suggests that substantially increasing alcohol taxes (to levels reflecting the impact of inflation since 1967) will sharply reduce alcohol consumption and alcohol problems, particularly among young people.[41]

Regulate the Number, Concentration, and Types of Alcohol Outlets

Recent research has established a strong link between the number of alcohol outlets in a community or state and the risk of alcohol problems.[42] Alcohol outlets are concentrated in low-income communities, thus increasing the risk of problems in these communities and adversely affecting their quality of life.[43,44] Alcohol outlets come in various forms—bars, liquor stores, and public arenas, among others. In general, the proliferation of new types of outlets should be avoided, and outlets that closely connect alcohol with food and adult events should be encouraged over those that do not. Control on retail availability involves both state and community action.

Encourage Responsible Practices Among Alcohol Retailers

Unsafe alcohol retail practices, including happy hours and service to minors and intoxicated persons, increase the risk of alcohol problems.[45] For example, approximately 50 percent of drinking while driving events originate from licensed establishments, a figure that can be reduced if serving practices in high-risk establishments are reformed and training is given to managers and servers.[45,46] Industry practices can be reformed through voluntary action or regulation at state and community levels. Civil liability statutes (so-called "dram shop laws") can also provide incentives for the implementation of responsible serving practices.[47]

Increase the Minimum Drinking Age

During the early 1970s, 29 states reduced their minimum–age drinking laws (MADL) from 21 to 18 or 19 years of age. This trend was reversed in the 1980s, and now all states prohibit possession of alcohol by those under 21 years of age. Research shows that the increases in MADLs resulted in a substantial reduction of alcohol-related motor vehicle crash deaths, with study results ranging from 5 to 28 percent reductions.[48]

Regulate the Types of Alcoholic Beverages on the Market

The alcohol industry is continuously developing new types of beverages as well as new packaging for existing products. Some new products have raised serious public health concerns, particularly when young people appear to be targeted. African-American communities, for example, have protested the marketing of malt liquor products because the marketing appears to target young people and saturates their communities.[49] Young people are purchasing these products in 40-ounce bottles and drinking them as single servings, thereby increasing the risk of intoxication.[49] Regulations at the state and/or federal level can control these marketing practices.

Regulate Alcohol Availability in Institutional and Public Settings

Alcohol service is not limited to commercial alcohol establishments. Drinking occurs in a wide variety of public and private settings—community fairs, public parks, sports stadia, private clubs, and churches, among others. Every community institution has a policy regarding alcohol service, although in many cases that policy is unwritten and unspoken. A community-based prevention strategy should include the development of alcohol policies in these settings and institutions. It should address such questions as: Is alcohol service appropriate in the given setting? If so, how should it be

made available? What steps will be taken to reduce the risk of intoxication and service to minors?[50]

Implement Alcohol Production Reforms

Several state and federal policies actively encourage and subsidize alcohol production and marketing. For example, special tax incentives have encouraged the replanting of agricultural lands with wine grapes in California and the production of rum in the Virgin Islands.[12] A variety of production reforms should be instituted to end subsidies to the alcohol industry, encourage nonalcohol–producing crops, and lessen the profitability of alcohol production.

Many or most of these proposed reforms were included in the recommendations of former Surgeon General C. Everett Koop in his workshop on preventing drunk driving.[51] The philosophy underlying the reforms and many of the recommendations themselves are incorporated into other policy documents, including reports by the American Assembly,[52] the National Academy of Sciences,[16] and the American Public Health Association.[8]

Illegal Drug Availability

Only limited options are available for addressing the availability of illegal drugs as long as they remain illegal. Their illegality also hampers the ability to research the drug trade, making an understanding of its structure and of the impact of changes in policy more difficult.[12] Moreover, as policies shift from a predominantly criminal justice focus to a public health focus, drug availability is likely to increase, thereby increasing the risk of drug problems. Despite these difficulties, four policy reforms can be delineated. Implementation should be instituted with caution, with the impact carefully assessed.

Discontinue the Heavy Reliance on Border Interdiction and Incarceration of Drug Users

These strategies have created enormous economic and social costs and have not been effective in reducing the availability and use of drugs. Their use should be greatly limited or discontinued and the resources they use redirected to public health reforms. Treatment should be readily available for those in need without regard to income, and treatment availability should be a high priority for those who are incarcerated. Alternatives to incarceration, such as fines and community service, should be investigated.

Redirect Drug Eradication and Control Efforts

Drug eradication and control efforts should focus on the violence associated with the drug trade, on large producers and retailers, and on those drugs causing the greatest public health harm, such as cocaine and heroin. As discussed above, the reduction of harm should be the primary goal of a public health drug policy.

Promote Drug Control Programs that Limit Availability at the Community Level and Address Community Safety

Illegal drugs create unsafe community environments. Drug sales and drug use may concentrate in public areas (for example, parks, liquor stores, sidewalks), adversely affecting the quality of life of the neighborhood and community and increasing the risk of violence. Drug sales and use at private residences may have a similar impact. Various programs have organized community action to address these problems, thereby building a constituency for broader public health reforms.[53] This in turn supports environmental interventions, which are discussed below.

Promote the Use of Various Civil Sanctions as Possible Alternatives to Criminal Sanctions

Civil sanctions are preferable to criminal sanctions because they are easier to administer and enforce, they are cheaper, and they do not carry the moral overtones inherent in criminal justice proceedings.[12] For example, public nuisance statutes can be used to close down crack houses; forfeiture, civil liability, and tax laws can deter drug production; and local zoning ordinances can deter businesses from allowing loitering and drug dealing in and around their premises.

Addressing Alcohol and Other Drug Environmental Factors

As discussed above, an individual's environment affects her alcohol and other drug use behavior. The environment can be conceptualized as expanding levels of influence over individual behavior, with each level interacting with the others. Prevention efforts will be more effective if they operate across differing environmental levels. The availability of alcohol and other drugs at each level is a critical environmental factor, and it interacts with each of these other major aspects of the environment: family systems; school, peer, and neighborhood environment; workplace environment; community environment; alcohol marketing and mass media; and social, economic, and political environments.

Family Systems

Family experience with and parental attitudes towards alcohol and other drug use and their related problems affect a child's likelihood of developing alcohol and other drug problems.[54] Poor family management, lack of family bonding, poor monitoring of a child's behavior, and physical abuse or neglect have all been identified as risk factors.[55]

School, Peer, and Neighborhood Environment

Schools that maintain and enforce clear, strict policies toward alcohol and other drug use report less use among students.[56] Peer use of alcohol and other drugs has consistently been found to be a strong predictor of use among young people. Neighborhoods with high-density housing, high residential mobility, physical deterioration, and high unemployment rates have high rates of juvenile crime and illegal drug trafficking.[5,57]

Workplace Environment

Workplaces and occupations with high availability of alcohol, unclear rules and expectations regarding drinking on the job, high stress, and limited supervision create high risks for alcohol problems among workers.[58]

Community Environment

The above factors interact and are included in the community environment. Current prevention planning stresses the need to plan and implement programs at the community level. This permits programs to address the multiplicity of factors in a coordinated fashion.[5,53]

Alcohol Marketing and the Mass Media

Industry marketing programs play a major role in shaping the alcohol environment, in turn affecting children's beliefs, attitudes, and intentions to drink.[59] Wallack describes alcohol advertising as the single most important source of alcohol education in our society today.[60] The alcohol industry spends over $1 billion annually in mass media advertising[61] and probably at least that much on promotional and sponsorship campaigns. Its primary purpose is to impact on social norms, practices, beliefs, and expectations.[60] The mass media also play a major role in shaping the alcohol and other drug environment. Portrayals of alcohol and other drug use in entertainment programming and the presentation of alcohol and other drug issues in public affairs programming are all important environmental factors.[60]

Social, Economic, and Political Environments

Social, economic, and political forces interact and share the more immediate environments surrounding individual behavior. Economic and political conditions and social norms have a dramatic effect on all other environmental levels.[5]

Summary

As this brief review and the data above suggest, many of the poorest communities face multiple risk factors for alcohol and other drug problems. Many inner-city communities, for example, have high levels of alcohol and other drug availability; lack basic educational, housing, health care, child care, and employment opportunities; and face institutional racism. These circumstances have put communities, neighborhoods, and families in stress and established the crack cocaine trade as an attractive economic alternative.[5,62] In short, these communities face a set of conditions identified in the literature as creating a high-risk environment for violence and alcohol and other drug problems.

Addressing these environmental concerns requires attention to broad economic, political, and social forces, including the development of a viable social support system, an economic base that is community controlled, and an end to institutional racism. Ironically, funds for some of these purposes were diverted to the war on drugs during the late 1980s, thereby exacerbating the very problems the war on drugs was attempting to address.

IMPLICATIONS FOR PUBLIC HEALTH PRACTICE

The ambitious public health agenda just outlined calls for fundamental changes in current alcohol and other drug policies. This call for reform is based on careful examination of data regarding use and problems and the application of a public health model of prevention. The proposed reforms are not new; indeed, as documented in previous sections, numerous authors and public policy officials are now calling for basic public health reforms. Why, then, has the public health field had so little impact on the public policy debate?

Addressing environmental risk factors, including availability, requires a fundamental shift in orientation in the field of public health, which has traditionally addressed alcohol and other drug problems primarily at the individual level and developed programs to be delivered to those at risk. The recommendations here, however, require changes in public policy. This requires very different skills. For success, the lobbying power of the alcohol industry must be neutralized. The powerful coalition that views the war on drugs as only one aspect of a broader social agenda must also be confronted. These goals require political and policy skills in addition to the program skills traditionally associated with the public health field. Three sets of skills are particularly important in this endeavor: community organizing, coalition building and political advocacy, and media advocacy skills.

Community Organizing

Public health's strength lies in its service to masses of citizens. Building a grassroots network of citizens to advocate for and support new alcohol and other drug policies must be a top agenda for the field. Only democratic action by large numbers of people can be effective in changing the current balance of power.[5,63] Community organizing begins at the neighborhood and community level. This serves to emphasize the need to address problems at these levels.

Coalition Building and Political Advocacy

Bridges across communities and among diverse groups within a community are needed to reform public policies at all levels—local, regional, state, and federal. Coalition building complements community organizing, stimulating community involvement and building on the power of numbers and diversity in a community.[9] Political advocacy and policy analysis skills involve learning to operate effectively within the policy arena. Public health data need to be presented effectively to policy makers, and arguments for reform need to be presented concisely and powerfully. A keen sense of political timing must also be developed.

Media Advocacy Skills

Public health professionals also need to become effective in the mass media, reframing issues and advancing alternative solutions. Wallack, Dorfman, and Woodruff provide an excellent overview of media advocacy in this volume.

CONCLUSION

The public health field provides a unique and powerful set of tools for conceptualizing and addressing alcohol and other drug problems in our society. These problems constitute a crisis for our society, causing untold tragedies in the lives of individuals, families, and communities. Their solution requires confronting some of the basic inequities and injustices afflicting our nation. Public health provides a foundation for action. It is up to those in the field to build on that foundation.

ACKNOWLEDGMENT

Preparation of this manuscript was supported in part by grants from the Beryl Buck Memorial Trust and the California Wellness Foundation.

REFERENCES

1. Office of National Drug Control Policy. *Breaking the Cycle of Drug Abuse: 1993 Interim National Drug Control Strategy*. Washington, DC: White House; September 1993.

2. Reuter P, Crawford G, Cave J. *Sealing the Borders*. Santa Monica, Ca: RAND Co; 1988.

3. Nadelmann E. US drug policy: a bad export. *Foreign Policy.* 1988;70:83–108.

4. Morgan P, Wallack L, Buchanan D. Waging drug wars: prevention strategy or politics as usual. *Drugs & Society.* 1989;3/4:99–124.

5. Mosher J, Yanagisako K. Public health, not social warfare: a public health approach to illegal drug policy. *J Public Health Policy.* 1991;12:278–323.

6. Musto D. *The American Disease: Origins of Narcotic Control.* New York, NY: Oxford University Press; 1973.

7. Gerstein D, Harwood H, eds. *Treating Drug Problems.* Washington, DC: National Academy Press; 1990.

8. A public health response to the war on drugs: reducing alcohol, tobacco and other drug problems among the nation's youth. *Am J Public Health.* 1989;79:360–364. American Public Health Association Position Paper 8817.

9. Mosher J, Jernigan D. New directions in alcohol policy. *Annu Rev Public Health.* 1989;10:245–279.

10. *Media Advocacy in African American and Latino Communities and On-line.* Washington, DC: US Dept of Health & Human Services; 1994. CSAP draft publication.

11. Wallack L, Holder H. The prevention of alcohol-related problems: a systems approach. In: Holder H, ed. *Control Issues in Alcohol Abuse Prevention: Strategies for States and Communities.* Greenwich, Ct: JAI Press; 1987.

12. Mosher J. Drug availability in a public health perspective. In: Resnik H, ed. *Youth and Drugs: Society's Mixed Messages.* Rockville, Md: Office of Substance Abuse Prevention; 1990:129–168. OSAP Prevention Monograph no. 6.

13. Mosher J. Alcohol and poverty: analyzing the link between alcohol-related problems and social policy. In: Samuels S, Smith M, eds. *Improving the Health of the Poor: Strategies for Prevention.* Menlo Park, Ca: Henry J Kaiser Family Foundation; 1992:97–121.

14. Room R. Alcohol control and public health. *Annu Rev Public Health.* 1984;5:293–317.

15. Cahalan D. *Problem Drinkers: A National Survey.* San Francisco, Ca: Jossey-Bass; 1970.

16. Moore M, Gerstein D, eds. *Alcohol and Public Policy: Beyond the Shadow of Prohibition.* Washington, DC: National Academy Press; 1981.

17. Zimring R, Hawkins G. *What Kind of Drug War?* Berkeley, Ca: Earl Warren Legal Institute; 1990. Working Paper no. 16.

18. Office of National Drug Control Policy. *National Drug Control Strategy.* Washington, DC: White House; 1990, 1991, 1992.

19. *National Household Survey on Drug Abuse: Population Estimates 1991.* Washington, DC: US Dept of Health & Human Services, Nat. Inst. Drug Abuse; 1992.

20. Clark W, Hilton M. *Alcohol in America: Drinking Practices and Problems.* Albany, NY: SUNY Press; 1991.

21. Johnston L, O'Malley P, Bachman J. *National Survey Results on Drug Use from the Monitoring the Future Study, 1975–1992,* I and II. Rockville, Md: National Institute on Drug Abuse; 1993.

22. Lillie-Blanton M, Anthony J, Schuster C. Probing the meaning of racial/ethnic group comparisons in crack cocaine smoking. *JAMA.* 1993;269:993–998.

23. Wish E. US drug policy in the 1990's: insights from new data from arrestees. *Int J Addict.* 1990–91;25:377–409.

24. Reuter P. Prevalence estimation and policy formulation. *J Drug Issues.* 1993;23:167–185.

25. Alcohol-related mortality and years of potential life lost—United States. *MMWR.* March 23, 1990;173–187.

26. *Drunk Driving Facts.* Washington, DC: National Highway Traffic Safety Administration, National Center for Statistics and Analysis; 1989.

27. *Seventh Special Report to the US Congress on Alcohol and Health.* Rockville, Md: US Dept of Health & Human Services, National Institute on Alcohol Abuse and Alcoholism; 1990.

28. Brandeis University, Institute for Health Policy. *Substance Abuse: The Nation's Number One Health Problem.* Princeton, NJ: Robert Wood Johnson Foundation; 1993.

29. Ravenholt R. Addiction mortality in the United States, 1980: tobacco, alcohol and other substances. *Population and Development Review.* 1984;10:697–743.

30. *Data from the Drug Abuse Warning Network Annual Medical Examiner Data 1991.* Rockville, Md: US Dept of Health and Human Services; 1991. National Institute on Drug Abuse Series I no. 11-B.

31. *Estimates from the Drug Abuse Warning Network: 1992 Estimates of Drug-Related Emergency Room Episodes.* Rockville, Md: US Dept of Health and Human Services, Office of Applied Studies; 1993.

32. *National Drug and Alcoholism Treatment Unit Survey 1989: Main Findings Report.* Rockville, Md: US Dept of Health and Human Services, National Institute on Drug Abuse; 1990.

33. Trends: survey finds 250,000 pregnant women need treatment. *Alcoholism and Drug Abuse Week.* 1990;2:4–5.

34. Cooper M. Alcohol and increased behavioral risk for AIDS. *Alcohol, Health & Research World.* 1992;16:64–71.

35. Ames G. Research and strategies for the primary prevention of workplace alcohol problems. *Alcohol, Health & Research World.* 1993;17:19–28.

36. *Crime in the United States, 1992: Uniform Crime Reports.* Washington, DC: US Dept of Justice, Federal Bureau of Investigation; 1992.

37. *Drugs, Crime and the Justice System.* Washington, DC: US Dept of Justice, Bureau of Justice Statistics; 1992.

38. *Justice Survey of State Prison Inmates, 1991.* Washington, DC: US Dept of Justice, Bureau of Justice Statistics; 1993.

39. Rice D. The economic cost of alcohol abuse and alcohol dependence: 1990. *Alcohol, Health & Research World.* 1993;17:10–11.

40. Fulco CE, Liverman CT, Earley LE, eds. *Development of Medications for the Treatment of Opiate and Cocaine Addictions: Issues for the Government and Private Sector.* Washington, DC: National Academy Press; 1995.

41. Chaloupka F. Effects of price on alcohol–related problems. *Alcohol, Health & Research World.* 1993;17:46–53.

42. Gruenewald P, Millar A, Treno A. Alcohol availability and the ecology of drinking behavior. *Alcohol, Health & Research World.* 1993;17:39–45.

43. Troutt D. *The Thin Red Line.* San Francisco, Ca: Consumer's Union of the US, West Coast Regional Office; 1993.

44. Calhoun S, Calhoun V. *Alcohol Availability and Alcohol-Related Problems in Santa Clara County.* San Jose, Ca: Santa Clara County Health Dept, Bureau of Alcohol Services; 1989.

45. Saltz R. Server intervention and responsible beverage service programs. *Surgeon General's Workshop on Drunk Driving: Background Papers.* Rockville, Md: Office of the Surgeon General; 1989.

46. O'Donnell M. Research on drinking locations of alcohol–impaired drivers: implication for prevention policies. *J Public Health Policy.* 1985;6:510–525.

47. Mosher J. Legal liabilities of licensed alcoholic beverage establishments: recent developments in the United States. In: Single E, Storm T, eds. *Public Drinking and Public Policy.* Toronto, Canada: Addiction Research Foundation; 1985: 235–256.

48. *Drinking Age Laws: An Evaluation Synthesis of Their Impact on Highway Safety.* Washington, DC: General Accounting Office: 1987. GAO/PEMD-87-10.

49. Marriott M. Cheap high lures youths to malt liquor '40s'. *New York Times.* April 16, 1993;A1,A12.

50. Mosher J. *Responsible Beverage Service: An Implementation Handbook for Communities.* Palo Alto, Ca: Health Promotion Resource Center, Stanford University; 1991.

51. *Surgeon General's Workshop on Drunk Driving: Proceedings.* Washington, DC: US Dept of Health and Human Services, Office of the Surgeon General; 1988.

52. The American Assembly. *Alcoholism and Related Problems: Issues for the American Public.* Englewood Cliffs, NJ: Prentice–Hall Inc; 1984.

53. Gerstein D, Green L. *Preventing Drug Abuse: What Do We Know?* Washington, DC: National Academy Press; 1993.

54. Hawkins D, Lishner D, Catalano R, Howard M. Childhood predictors of adolescent substance abuse: toward an empirically grounded theory. *J Children Contemporary Society.* 1986;18: 1–30.

55. Dembo R, et al. Physical abuse, sexual victimization, and illegal drug use: a structural analysis among high risk adolescents. *J Adolesc.* 1987;10:13–33.

56. Moskowitz J, Jones R. Alcohol and drug problems in the schools: results of a national survey of school administrators. *J Stud Alcohol.* 1988;49:299–305.

57. Bowser B. Bayview-Hunter's Point: San Francisco's black ghetto revisited. *Urban Anthropology.* 1988;17:383–400.

58. Ames G. Research and strategies for the primary prevention of workplace alcohol problems. *Alcohol, Health & Research World.* 1993;17:19–27.

59. Grube J, Wallack L. Television beer advertising and drinking knowledge, beliefs, and intentions among school children. *Am J Public Health.* 1994;84:254–260.

60. Wallack L. Drinking and driving: toward a broader understanding of the role of mass media. *J Public Health Policy.* 1984;5:471–496.

61. Gallo H. Ad spending a mixed bag in 1992. *Impact.* September 1, 1993;23:1–10.

62. Bourgois P. In search of Horatio Alger: culture and ideology in the crack economy. *Contemp Drug Problems.* 1989;16: 619–650.

63. Wechsler R. Community organizing principles and local prevention of alcohol and drug abuse. In: Mecca A, ed. *Prevention 2000—A Public/Private Partnership.* San Rafael, Ca: California Health Research Foundation; 1988:41–52.

CHAPTER

Oral Diseases: The Neglected Epidemic

Myron Allukian, Jr., D.D.S., M.P.H.

You're not healthy without good oral health.

C. Everett Koop, M.D.
former United States Surgeon General

Oral diseases are a neglected epidemic for millions of Americans who suffer unnecessarily from them, even though many oral diseases are preventable. The combination of high prevalence, high morbidity, and relative inattention from the health community make oral diseases a significant public health problem in need of a public health solution.

Public health practitioners have the responsibility and opportunity to include oral health as an integral component of health in the development of policies and programs. Oral health is an essential component of health and well-being. When a needs assessment is done of a community or group of individuals, oral health must be included.

This chapter explains why oral health is a neglected epidemic, why oral health is important, and how public health can help promote good oral health. It also describes the epidemiology of oral disease and discusses

the preventive programs that can improve dental health. It concludes with a discussion of dental personnel in the United States.

BACKGROUND

Unfortunately, beginning in the early 1800s and due to a variety of factors, the mouth was disconnected from the rest of the body in health sciences, education, and practice. After the first dental school in the world, the Baltimore College of Dental Surgery, was founded in 1840, dentistry became a separate health profession from medicine with separate schools, organizations, institutions, and programs. As dentistry evolved, many physicians, nurses, and even public health professionals were left without an understanding or appreciation of the impact oral diseases have on individuals and society.

When public health practitioners properly assess the major health needs of a target population, they usually find that the need for better oral health is a significant public health problem from the perspectives of both prevention and treatment. Major oral diseases and conditions include:

- dental caries (tooth decay)
- periodontal diseases (gum diseases)
- malocclusion (crooked teeth)
- edentulism (complete tooth loss)
- oral cancer
- craniofacial anomalies including cleft lip/cleft palate
- soft tissue lesions
- orofacial injuries
- temporomandibular dysfunction (TMD)

Dental expertise is also of value in promoting and protecting the general health of communities. Examples of health concerns in which dental public health expertise has been invaluable to society are infection control, mercury toxicity, tobacco control, school-based programs, maternal and child health, primary care, AIDS, hepatitis B, tuberculosis, occupational health, needs assessment, policy development, quality assessment, community organization, and prevention on both the individual and community levels.

THE NEGLECTED EPIDEMIC

Although there has been substantial improvement in oral health on a national level in the last 20 years due to water fluoridation, topical fluorides, and an emphasis on prevention, oral diseases are still pandemic in the United States, as the following statistics show:

- Twenty-nine percent of adolescents have severe or very severe malocclusion.[1]
- Sixty percent of adolescents experience gum infections.[2]
- Eighty-four percent of 17-year-old school children have had tooth decay, with an average of eight affected surfaces.[3]
- Ninety-nine percent of adults aged 40 to 44, have had tooth decay, with an average of 30 affected surfaces.[4]
- Forty-one percent of those aged 65 and older have no teeth at all.[4]
- Nearly 30,000 Americans are diagnosed with oral cancer each year and about 8,000 die annually.[5]
- One out of 700 Americans are born with cleft lip/cleft palate.[6]

For vulnerable populations, such as children, minorities, the elderly, and those with low incomes, oral diseases are especially problematic. Selected studies have shown that up to 97 percent of the homeless need dental care.[7] Over half of some Head Start children have had baby bottle tooth decay.[8] Almost half of abused children have orofacial trauma.[9] Thirty percent of the first signs of HIV infection may appear in the oral cavity.[10] Sixteen percent of emergency room visits are for orofacial injuries.[11] Low-income seniors age 65 to 74 are almost four times as likely to be edentulous than high-income seniors.[12] African-American, low-income, and Native American children, respectively, have 65 percent, 91 percent, and 265 percent more untreated tooth decay than their peers.[13] Finally, more than 50 percent of the homebound elderly have not seen a dentist for 10 years.[14]

Fortunately, most oral diseases can be prevented. Unfortunately, once they occur they usually do not resolve themselves without the physical intervention of a dental provider. Two exceptions to this are an incipient carious lesion that is reversible when exposed to fluoride and mild gingivitis.

Untreated dental caries usually progresses to an infection of the nerve and blood supply to the involved tooth, which may result in an abscess, cellulitis (an infection of the soft tissue), and sometimes even death. When dental caries is treated, a dentist must physically remove the bacterial infection, reshape the infected area of the tooth, and then restore the tooth with an artificial substance to retain its function. Restored teeth are weaker than intact healthy teeth and subject to fracture and additional caries attack.

IMPORTANCE OF ORAL HEALTH

Oral health is an integral component of total health. The maintenance of good oral health is important for:

- freedom from pain, infection, and suffering
- ability to eat and chew food, thus for proper digestion and nutrition
- ability to speak properly
- social mobility
- employability
- self-image and self-esteem
- quality of life and well-being

Poor oral health may compromise individuals in school, work, or daily living.[15] People with poor oral health may suffer unnecessarily with pain, have difficulty in interpersonal relationships, and have diminished job opportunities. One study estimated that about 20 percent of Americans experience orofacial pain in a six-month period.[16] For the young, elderly, and medically compromised, good oral health is even more important to function and thrive.

Social Cost of Oral Disease

The social cost of oral diseases to the individual and society are great. For example, in 1989 over 51 million hours of school were lost due to oral health problems, almost 1.2 hours per school child.[17] Also in 1989, over 164 million hours were missed from work, an average of 1.48 hours per employed adult.[17] In 1991, school age children had almost 4.8 million restricted activity days and 2.2 million bed days.[18] In the same year, individuals aged 16 to 64 years had over 8 million restricted activity days and nearly 4 million bed days.[18]

Economic Cost of Oral Disease

The economic cost of oral diseases is also significant. Dental services consumed about $38.7 billion, or 5.3 percent of all health expenditures, in 1992.[19] Dental expenditures are expected to reach $62.3 billion by the year 2000, or about 4 percent of personal expenditures. Most dental expenditures are from private sources, such as private insurance, or out-of-pocket. Only about 95 million Americans have some form of dental insurance, most often through an employer.[12]

Public programs providing dental insurance are few. Medicaid includes dental services, primarily for children as part of the Early Periodic Screening Diagnosis and Treatment (EPSDT) Program. Over $790 million were expended for all dental care to over 5.2 million recipients of Medicaid in 1991.[20] This is less than one percent of the total amount, $77 billion, spent on Medicaid that year. Fewer than 17 percent of Medicaid eligible recipients actually received dental care. In addition, many Medicaid programs do not adequately reimburse for effective preventive procedures such as dental sealants. Dentistry is an optional service for

adults under Medicaid, and many states provide only limited services to adults. Unfortunately, Medicare, which provides health care to individuals over age 65, does not include dental services at all unless they are related to trauma or oral cancer.

AN OVERVIEW OF ORAL HEALTH PROBLEMS

Major oral health problems include dental caries, periodontal diseases, and oropharyngeal cancer. The prevalence and public health significance of these problems are addressed next.

Dental Caries

Dental caries, or tooth decay, is the most prevalent oral disease in the United States. It is a bacterial infection that is influenced by a variety of factors in the host, agent, and environment.

Prevalence

Prevalence of dental caries increases progressively with age throughout life, especially during the first two decades, as shown in Table 19.1. At age six when the 32 permanent teeth usually begin erupting, only about 5.6 percent of school children have had tooth decay in their permanent teeth.[3] Not only does the prevalence of the disease increase with age, but the number of affected tooth surfaces also increases. By age 17, 84 percent of 17-year-olds have had tooth decay, with an average of eight affected tooth surfaces, and by age 40 to 44, almost 99 percent of adults have had tooth decay, with an average of 30 affected tooth surfaces.[3,4] For all children in the United States, 75 percent of the dental caries actually occur in only about 25 percent of children.[3]

Types of Caries

There are three general types of tooth decay: **coronal**, which occurs on the crowns of teeth; **root surface**, which occurs on the roots of teeth; and **recurrent**, which is reoccurring tooth decay. Root surface decay usually occurs in older individuals. A study of New England elders showed that 52 percent of individuals over age 70 years had root caries. For 22 percent of

TABLE 19.1   Prevalence of Tooth Decay and Mean Number of Permanent Tooth Surfaces Affected, United States School Children, 5 to 17 Years of Age, 1986 to 1987

Age	% Prevalence	Mean Number Affected Tooth Surfaces
5	2.7	0.07
6	5.6	0.13
7	15.8	0.40
8	25.0	0.71
9	34.5	1.14
10	44.3	1.69
11	55.0	2.33
12	58.3	2.66
13	66.0	3.76
14	72.3	4.68
15	78.2	5.71
16	80.0	6.68
17	84.4	8.04
all ages (5 to 17)	49.9	3.07

SOURCE: National Institute of Dental Research. *Oral Health of United States Children. The National Survey of Dental Caries in US School Children, 1986–1987.* Bathesda, Md: US Dept of Health and Human Services; 1989. DHHS publication NIH 89–2247.

them, the disease was untreated.[21] The level of untreated dental caries is much higher among minorities and those with low income and less education. People who have lived in fluoridated communities since birth experience much lower rates of dental caries.

Baby Bottle Tooth Decay (BBTD)

The 20 primary teeth begin erupting at about six to nine months of age, and by about two years of age they have all erupted. *Baby bottle tooth decay*—also called nursing or infant caries—is tooth decay that occurs primarily in the upper anterior primary teeth when a baby is given a bottle at bedtime or nap time with sugar added to the contents. Juices or milk alone can cause BBTD if they are given over extended periods of time.

About 8.3 percent of children in the United States age two to five years still use a baby bottle, and of these 48.3 percent were reported as having gone to bed with a bottle containing something other than water.[22] The prevalence of BBTD has averaged as high as 53 percent for Head Start children who were rural Native Americans or Alaskan Natives, and up to 11 percent for children in urban areas. BBTD is higher in preterm, low-birth weight infants and those that are malnourished. This may be due to poor tooth development of the fetus in utero when the mother is malnourished. Other possible causes include bacteria transferred from the caregiver after birth and improper baby feeding practices.

BBTD may be painful and expensive. The treatment may cost about $2,200 to $6,000 per child because general anesthesia and therefore the use of an operating room are often required. It is much more cost effective to prevent it. BBTD can be prevented by educating parents and caretakers about the dangers of giving infants bottles for prolonged periods of time unless they are filled with plain water. Bottle-fed infants should not be given bottles with juices, milk, or sweetened fluids when they are going to bed or otherwise using the bottle as a pacifier. Once a child has been fed by bottle, the teeth should be wiped clean. In general, breast-feeding should be encouraged over bottle-feeding, and parents should be taught to wean from the breast to the cup, rather than the bottle, at around age one year. If BBTD is prevalent in a given population, widespread prevention requires the development of a comprehensive, multidisciplinary, community-oriented edcation program.[8]

Periodontal Diseases

There are essentially two types of infections of the soft tissues (gums) surrounding a tooth: gingivitis and periodontitis. Both are quite common.

Gingivitis

Gingivitis is a localized infection or inflammation of the soft tissues surrounding a tooth that results in swelling and bleeding of the gums. It may or may not be self-limiting. Poor oral hygiene is the major contributing factor to gingivitis; therefore, good self-care is important in its prevention. Some forms of gingivitis, such as acute necrotizing ulcerative gingivitis (ANUG), or trench mouth, can be extremely painful. ANUG is often associated with stress, lack of sleep, poor nutrition, and poor oral hygiene.

Gingivitis occurs in about 60 percent of adolescents and about 40 to 50 percent of adults.[2,4] Among certain high-risk populations, the prevalence is even higher. For Native American and Alaskan Natives, as many as 95 percent may have the disease, and it is found in up to 82 percent of Puerto Ricans and 50 percent of low-income individuals.[23]

Periodontitis

Periodontitis is an infection or inflammation of the soft tissues *and* of the supporting alveolar bone around teeth with loss of periodontal attachment. When left untreated, periodontitis usually results in teeth becoming loose, necessitating extensive treatment and possible removal. For persons with AIDS or HIV infection, periodontitis can progress quite rapidly.

The prevalence of periodontitis increases with age. About 24 percent of people aged 35 to 44 have periodontitis, with the prevalence higher in high-risk populations such as minorities and low-income individuals.[4]

Prevention

Successful prevention of periodontal disease is oriented more to the individual than to the community. Prevention measures are similar for gingivitis and periodontitis, but gingivitis responds better to preventive measures. Patient compliance with proper oral hygiene procedures and regular mechanical removal of dental plaque with a toothbrush and floss helps prevent periodontal disease. It also usually responds well to a thorough professional cleaning, prophylaxis, scaling, and root planing performed by a dentist or dental hygienist.

Educational programs need to be developed as part of comprehensive health education for school children to reinforce the importance of good oral hygiene. Public awareness also needs to be increased so that individual compliance is improved in the use of proper oral hygiene practices and periodic dental visits.

Oropharyngeal Cancer

About 29,600 new cases of oropharyngeal cancer and 7,925 deaths from oropharyngeal cancer were estimated for the United States for 1994.[5] It is the sixth most common cancer for men and the twelfth most common for women. More Americans die from oral cancer than from cervical cancer. Tobacco and alcohol use are associated with over 70 percent of oral cancers, and they occur most often in men over the age of 40.[24] The increase in the use of smokeless tobacco, especially among teenagers, may result in more individuals with oral cancer in the future. The five year oropharyngal cancer survival rate for Euro-Americans is 55 percent compared with 39 percent for African-Americans. Of all cancer it shows the largest discrepancy in survival between these two races.[5]

Early detection and treatment of oral cancer results in higher survival rates. In 1992 only 14.3 percent of respondents in a national survey reported that they had ever been examined for oral cancer.[25] One study showed that for the two years prior to being diagnosed with oral cancer, patients had a median of 7.5 to 10.5 health care visits, yet 77 percent of the eventual diagnoses were for late-stage cancer.[26] Most of these visits were with physicians considered to be their regular source of care.

It is apparent that physicians and other health care providers need to be motivated and trained in early recognition of oral cancer. Health education programs for children and adults should emphasize the dangers of smokeless tobacco, cigarette smoking, and alcohol use. Policies should be implemented to discourage youth from tobacco and alcohol use. For example, in 1994 the National Collegiate Athletic Association (NCAA) banned student athletes and coaches from using smokeless or any other tobacco product during practices and games.[27] Periodic dental visits should also be promoted for early detection and treatment.

THE UTILIZATION OF DENTAL SERVICES

The utilization of dental care varies with age, income, and race,[12] as shown in Table 19.2. It also varies by insurance status.[12] In 1989 approximately 57 percent of the population in the United States over age two years had seen a dentist in the past year, for an average of

TABLE 19.2 Percent of Persons Two Years of Age and Over with Dental Visits in the Past Year and Number of Visits Per Person Per Year, by Age, Race, and Income: United States, 1989

Characteristics	Persons with Visit In Past Year	Visits per Person Per Year
Age	Percent	Number
All ages	57.2	2.1
2-4 years	32.1	0.9
5-17 years	69.0	2.4
18-34 years	57.0	1.8
35-54 years	57.4	2.3
55-64 years	54.0	2.4
65 years and over	43.2	2.0
Race		
African-American	44.5	1.2
Euro-American	59.3	2.2
Family income		
Less than $10,000	40.9	1.3
$10,000-$19,999	43.4	1.5
$20,000-$34,999	58.3	2.0
$35,000 and over	73.0	2.8

SOURCE: Bloom B, Gift HC, Jack SS. Dental services and oral health; United States, 1989. *Vital Health Stat.* 1992; 10:183.

2.1 visits per year. For 5- to 17-year-olds, 69 percent had been to a dentist in the last year, as compared with only 43 percent of persons over age 65. For individuals with a family income of over $35,000 a year, 73 percent had visited a dentist in the last year compared with 40 percent with family incomes of less than $10,000. About 59 percent of Euro-Americans saw a dentist in the past year, with 2.2 visits on average, as compared with 44 percent of African-Americans, with an average of 1.2 visits.[12]

Dental utilization is the lowest for those over age 65 years, but this age group has been increasing its visits to the dentist over the years. For those over age 65 in nursing homes, the unmet needs are even greater, and access to care is limited. The Omnibus Budget Reconciliation Act (OBRA) of 1989 has regulations requiring an oral examination of patients in long-term care facilities within 14 days of admission and annually thereafter. These regulations became effective in April 1992. The extent of the impact this will have for this neglected population remains to be seen.

THE PUBLIC HEALTH APPROACH TO ORAL DISEASES

The oral disease epidemic presents a unique challenge to the public health professional, who has the responsibility to prevent as much disease as possible and to improve access to care for those least able to obtain such services. A population-based approach centered on the three core functions—assessment of dental needs, policy development for dental disease prevention and treatment, and assurance of access to needed services—is most likely to make an impact on oral disease.[28]

Every local, state, and federal health agency and department should have a dental public health program with properly trained staff to address this neglected epidemic. The national oral health objectives for the year 2000 as defined in *Healthy People 2000* can be achieved more easily with dental public health expertise and the appropriate resources.[13] Smaller local health departments should also utilize such dental expertise. Schools of public health and dental, medical, and nursing schools should also include dental public health expertise to help educate health profession students about oral health needs and programs from the public health perspective.

Dental Public Health

Expertise in dental public health is essential to respond to the oral disease epidemic in a meaningful and effective way. Dental public health has been defined by the American Board of Dental Public Health as:

. . . the science and art of preventing and controlling dental diseases and promoting dental health through organized community efforts. It is that form of dental practice which serves the community as a patient rather than the individual. It is concerned with the dental health education of the public, with applied dental research, and with the administration of group dental programs, as well as the prevention and control of dental diseases on a community basis.[29]

Dental public health is the smallest of the eight dental specialties recognized by the American Dental Association. Public health dentists are trained in program and policy development, management and administration, research methods, health promotion, disease prevention, and delivery of care systems. The competency objectives for dental public health have been delineated,[30] and this expertise is unique in dentistry because of its population-based approach.

Public health dentists have improved the oral health of millions of Americans by their initiatives. There are about 1,600 dentists in the United States who work in public health roles, of which about 1,000 have at least one year of advanced education and over 600 have two years.[31] In 1994, 116 dentists were board-certified in dental public health.[32]

The American Board of Dental Public Health is the certifying board for this specialty, which requires a dental degree, a master's degree in public health, a one-year residency, four years experience in dental public health, and then successful completion of a comprehensive three-day examination.

The five major national dental public health associations are

1. American Association of Public Health Dentistry
2. American Board of Dental Public Health
3. American Public Health Association, Oral Health Section
4. Association of Community Dental Programs
5. Association of State and Territorial Dental Directors

The American Association of Public Health Dentistry and the Oral Health Section of the American Public Health Association are the two major dental public health membership organizations. The Association of State and Territorial Dental Directors (ASTDD) is made up of state dental directors, and the Association of Community Dental Programs consists of local dental directors. In addition, both the National Network for Oral Health Access (NNOHA) and the Community and Preventive Dentistry Section of the American Association of Dental Schools (AADS) have strong community orientations. NNOHA membership is primarily made up of community and migrant health cen-

ter dentists; the AADS section consists primarily of educators. Some dental hygienists also have training in public health and are an important resource for improving the oral health of the public.

Individuals trained in dental public health have the knowledge and education to respond to the oral disease epidemic. Public health leaders and programs can utilize these national public health associations as well as the United States Public Health Service for assistance if they do not have access locally to the expertise of public health-trained dentists or hygienists.

Healthy People 2000

Healthy People 2000 includes oral health as one of 22 priority areas. This area contains 16 objectives and numerous subobjectives for special population groups. Four of the 16 objectives are in risk reduction as follows:[13]

1. Increase to at least 50 percent the proportion of children who have received protective sealants on the occlusal (chewing) surfaces of permanent molar teeth. (baseline: 11 percent of children aged eight and 8 percent of adolescents aged 14 in 1986 to 1987)
2. Increase to at least 75 percent the proportion of people served by community water systems providing optimal levels of fluoride. (baseline: 62 percent in 1989)
3. Increase use of professionally or self-administered topical or systemic (dietary) fluorides to at least 85 percent of people not receiving optimally fluoridated public water. (baseline: an estimated 50 percent in 1989)
4. Increase to at least 75 percent the proportion of parents and caregivers who use feeding practices that prevent baby bottle tooth decay. (baseline: data not yet available)

Healthy Communities 2000: Model Standards

These are the guidelines for community attainment of the year 2000 national health objectives.[33] These guidelines assist community leaders in establishing achievable community health objectives according to local needs and priorities. They should be used by every local and state health agency in partnership with the private sector to promote and protect the nation's health. Oral health and the dental public health perspective must be included in these initiatives and represented in these partnerships.

PREVENTION

Many oral disease prevention measures prevent the disease before it occurs, which is called **primary prevention**, as well as control or respond to the disease after it occurs, which is called **secondary** or **tertiary prevention**. Because dental caries is the most common oral disease, and because the prevention methods for caries have such a well-documented scientific basis and are cost effective, the focus here is on dental caries prevention.

Community and Individual Preventive Measures

Dental caries can be prevented on the community or individual level, as shown in Table 19.3. Community prevention programs are more effective than individual prevention programs because they are population based.

The most effective, economical, and practical preventive measure for dental caries is community water fluori-

dation.[34] The most significant contribution a public health professional can make to improve the oral health of a community is to help that community become fluoridated if natural fluoride levels are too low to be effective. Individual prevention measures are not as effective as community prevention measures in general because they rely on the individual to carry them out, decreasing the effectiveness of these measures on a population or group basis. However, individual prevention measures should be continuously recommended and reinforced in all programs to improve individual compliance.

Systemic and Topical Fluorides

Fluoride may be provided systemically or topically as shown in Table 19.3. Preventive measures that provide fluoride to the teeth systemically by ingestion, such as water fluoridation or fluoride tablets, strengthen the teeth *while they are developing* and protect the teeth after they have erupted into the oral cavity throughout life. Continued exposure to fluoridated water and fluorides after tooth eruption also has a benefit.

Children who live in communities that do not have fluoridation should be given a dietary fluoride supplement. In 1989 about 15.1 percent of children under the age of two used a fluoride supplement in the United States.[35] There are major differences in dietary fluoride supplement use by race, income, and education as

TABLE 19.3 Effective Community and Individual Preventive Measures for Dental Caries and Mode of Application

	Measure	Mode of Application
Community		
	community water fluoridation	systemic
	school water fluoridation	systemic
	school fluoride tablet program	systemic
	school fluoride rinse program	topical
	school sealant program (professionally applied)	topical
Individual		
	prescribed fluoride tablets or drops	systemic
	professionally applied fluoride treatment	topical
	over-the-counter fluoride rinse	topical
	fluoride toothpaste	topical
	professionally applied dental sealants	topical

shown in Table 19.4. About 16.6 percent of Euro-American children use fluoride supplements as compared with 6.5 percent of African-American children and 12.9 percent of Hispanic children. Only 6.4 percent of children below the poverty level use fluoride supplements compared with 18.2 percent at or above the poverty level. Some of the geographic variation in fluoride supplement use may be due to water fluoridation status.

Professionally applied fluoride treatments, school and over-the-counter fluoride rinses, and fluoride toothpaste protect the teeth by providing fluoride to the teeth topically after they have erupted into the oral cavity. These fluorides provide an additional benefit to systemic fluoride, especially for high-risk individuals. The direct application of fluoride helps in the remineralization, or repair, of tooth enamel that is in the early stages of tooth decay. Professionally applied fluoride treatments need to be done periodically as long as the individual is at high risk for dental caries. Fluoride toothpaste should be used by people of all ages at least twice a day, after breakfast and before going to sleep at night. About 93.7 percent of school-age children 5 to 17 years of age in the United States use a fluoride-containing toothpaste.[35]

TABLE 19.4 Percent of United States Children Under Two Years of Age by Selected Characteristics Who Use a Dietary Fluoride Supplement, 1989

	%		%
All children	15.1	Parents' Education:	
Race/Ethnicity:		Some college	19.8
		High school or less	10.8
African-American	6.5		
Euro-American	16.6	Region:	
Hispanic	12.9	North	20.6
Non-Hispanic	15.5	Midwest	7.9
		South	10.4
SES Status:		West	20.6
At/above poverty level	18.2		
Below poverty level	6.4		

SOURCE: Wagener DK, Nourjah P, Horowitz A. Trends in Childhood Use of Dental Care Products Containing Fluoride: U.S. 1983–1989. Hyattsville, Md: National Center for Health Statistics; 1992. Advance data from Vital and Health Statistics no. 219.

Due to the widespread use of fluorides in water supplies, dental offices, and over-the-counter dental products, there has been a national decline in tooth decay in the last 20 years.

Dental Sealants. Because fluorides prevent dental caries most effectively on the smooth surfaces of the teeth, now almost two-thirds of tooth decay occurs on the chewing surfaces of teeth.[3] Dental sealants effectively prevent tooth decay on the chewing surfaces of the teeth. **Dental sealants** are thin plastic coatings placed as liquid plastics on the pits and fissures of the chewing surfaces of teeth and then polymerized. Ideally, susceptible tooth surfaces should be sealed soon after the tooth has erupted. This painless and noninvasive procedure does not require anesthesia or the cutting of tooth structure. A good school-based prevention program should use both fluorides and sealants.

Dental Fluorosis. With the increasing use of fluorides there has been an increase in **dental fluorosis**. This is a chronic, fluoride-induced condition, in which enamel development is disrupted and the enamel is hypomineralized.[36] It occurs when the teeth are forming, primarily from birth to six years of age, due to excessive fluoride intake. A confirmed history of fluoride exposure is needed to validate this diagnosis. In the 1980s, a series of studies showed that the prevalence of fluorosis had increased in both fluoridated and nonfluoridated communities.[36] Fluorosis appears clinically as a bilateral chalky white appearance of the teeth. In severe forms the teeth may be discolored or pitted. Most of the increase in fluorosis is of a very mild or mild form that would probably only be noticed by a dentist. Fluorosis is not a health problem, but may be considered an individual cosmetic problem in its more severe forms. It is correctable with dental treatment.

Individuals and populations with varying levels of dental fluorosis have less decay than those without fluorosis. Fluorosis may be due to inappropriate use of dietary fluoride supplements, ingestion of fluoride toothpaste by children under six years of age, infant formula reconstituted with fluoridated water, and communities fluoridated naturally at higher than the recommended level. In 1978, manufacturers of infant formulas, cereals, and juices voluntarily began processing their baby food products with water containing minimal amounts of fluoride. In 1979 a revised lower fluoride supplement schedule was adopted for children under two years of age by the American Academy of Pediatrics following the guidelines of the American Dental Association. In 1994 a new fluoride supplement schedule is expected which will again lower the dosage for children under six years of age.[37] To prevent fluorosis, health professionals and their patients need to be educated about the proper use of fluoride-containing products, particularly for children six years of age and under.

Community Water Fluoridation

Community water fluoridation should be the foundation for improving the oral health of every community. Community water fluoridation is defined as the upward adjustment of the fluoride content of a community water supply for optimal oral health. It is the most cost-effective preventive measure for preventing tooth decay.[34] Fluoridation is safe, economical, and practical.[34,36,38,39] It has been estimated that for each dollar spent on fluoridation, there is up to an $80 savings in dental treatment costs.[40] Today, fluoridation can be expected to prevent tooth decay in both primary and permanent teeth by up to 40 percent. Before the widespread use of fluorides, fluoridation prevented tooth decay by 50 to 60 percent. It is still a public health bargain, however. Because it has demonstrated benefits for adults, everyone reared in a fluoridated community benefits, regardless of age and also regardless of income, education, race, gender, or access to dental care.

All water supplies contain some fluoride naturally but generally not enough to prevent dental caries. The recommended fluoride level is 0.7 to 1.2 parts per million (ppm), depending on the mean maximum daily air temperature over a five year period.[41] Most water supplies in the United States are fluoridated at about 1.0 ppm. At the recommended level in the water supply, fluoride is odorless, colorless, and tasteless. The mean national weighted cost of fluoridation is $0.51 per capita with a range of $0.12 to $5.41, depending on the size of the

community and the complexity of its water distribution system.[34] For communities with more than 10,000 persons, the range is $0.21 to $0.75 per capita, and for communities with less than 10,000 persons, it is $0.60 to $5.41. Once a community is fluoridated, fluoride levels in the water supply must be monitored on a regular basis so that the population served receives the maximum health and economic benefits at little or no risk.[41]

Historical Perspective. Fluoridation's effectiveness was demonstrated in the United States, and the history of its discovery is one of the great public health success stories. For generations, millions of Americans lived in communities that were naturally fluoridated, though not necessarily at the recommended level. Communities then sought to duplicate the benefits that had been demonstrated by nature. In 1945, the first communities implemented *adjusted fluoridation* on a study basis, and in 1950, adjusted fluoridation was endorsed by the United States Public Health Service as a public health measure.

Fluoridation in the United States Today. By 1992, 10,567 community water systems serving 134.6 million Americans in 8,572 communities had adjusted fluoridation.[42] Another 10 million people live in communities that are fluoridated naturally at the recommended level. Indeed, the United States has the largest number of people in the world living in fluoridated communities. Consider the following statistics:

- In 1992, of the 232 million people on public water supplies, about 144.6 million were served by fluoridated water. This is about 62.2 percent of the United States population on public water systems and 55.9 percent of the total United States population.
- Water supplies of 42 of the 50 largest cities in the United States are fluoridated.

Variation in Fluoridation Rates by State and City. Figure 19.1 shows for each state the percent of the public water supply population that uses fluoridated water. It also shows how the state ranked nationally in 1992. Table 19.5 identifies the five highest and lowest states in terms of fluoridation. Three states, Kentucky, Rhode Island, and South Dakota, along with Washington, D.C.,

Percent Of Public Water Supply Population Using Fluoridated Water And State Rank

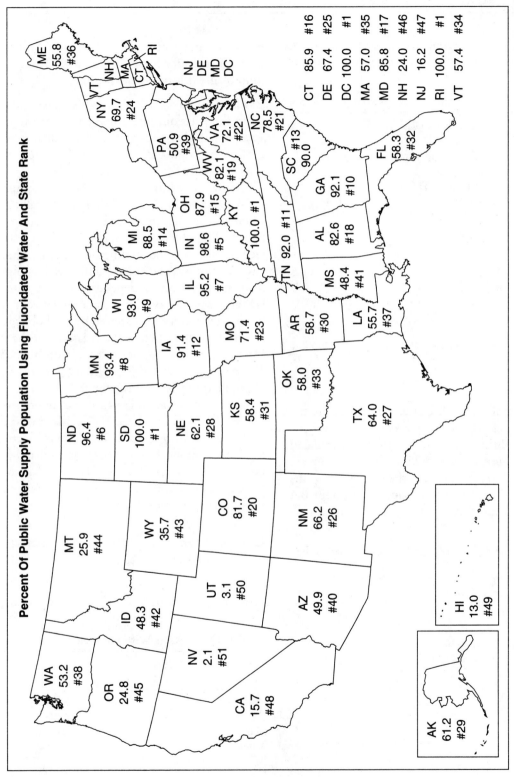

CT	85.9	#16			
DE	67.4	#25			
DC	100.0	#1			
MA	57.0	#35			
MD	85.8	#17			
NH	24.0	#46			
NJ	16.2	#47			
RI	100.0	#1			
VT	57.4	#34			

FIGURE 19.1 SOURCE: *Fluoridation Census, 1992.* Atlanta, Ga: Centers for Disease Control and Prevention, US Public Health Service; 1993.

CDC/NCPS/DOH

TABLE 19.5   Five Highest and Five Lowest Ranking States by Percent of State Population Having Fluoridated Water, 1992*

Rank	State	Percent Fluoridation
	Highest Five States	
1	Kentucky	100.0
1	Rhode Island	100.0
1	South Dakota	100.0
1	Washington, D.C.	100.0
5	Indiana	98.6
	North Dakota	96.4
	Lowest Five States	
47	New Jersey	16.2
48	California	15.7
49	Hawaii	13.0
50	Utah	3.1
51	Nevada	2.1

*include the Washington, D.C.
SOURCE: Centers for Disease Control and Prevention. Public health focus; fluoridation of community water systems. *MMWR.* May 29, 1992; 2(41):372–375, 381.

are 100 percent fluoridated. Nevada and Utah are the least fluoridated at 2.1 and 3.1 percent, respectively.

The 8 cities of the largest 50 that are *not* fluoridated have a total of almost eight million people. They are listed in Table 19.6. Los Angeles, the largest city without fluoridation, is naturally fluoridated at about 0.4 ppm, but this is insufficient to provide maximum ef-

TABLE 19.6   The 8 Cities of the 50 Largest Cities in the United States That Are Not Fluoridated, 1992

City	Rank in Size	Population (1,000s)
Los Angeles, CA	2	3,485
San Diego, CA	6	1,111
San Antonio, TX	10	936
San Jose, CA	11	782
Portland, OR	30	437
Tucson, AZ*	33	405
Sacramento, CA	41	369
Honolulu, HI	44	365
		7,890

*Voted for fluoridation in 1992
SOURCE: *Fluoridation Census, 1992.* Atlanta, Ga: Centers for Disease Control and Prevention, US Public Health Service; 1993.

fectiveness in preventing tooth decay. The Tucson City Council voted for fluoridation in 1992 and is expected to implement it in the near future.

Fluoridation Laws. Eight states have laws that require fluoridation, and these laws vary from state to state. The eight states and their national rank for percent of the population with a public water supply that is fluoridated are given in Table 19.7.

Illinois and Minnesota have the most comprehensive legislation requiring fluoridation. In the fall of 1995 the California legislature passed a law requiring fluoridation of all public water systems with at least 10,000 service connections, depending on funding. Fluoridation laws usually help facilitate public health policy to implement fluoridation, depending on the nature of the law and whether or not it is enforced. On the other hand, a referendum is required by the public in the following five states before fluoridation can be initiated: Delaware, Maine, Nevada, New Hampshire, and Utah. These states rank from 25 to 52 in terms of the percent of population with fluoridated public water.

Mandatory referenda shift the responsibility for public health policy from the legislature or board of health to the voting public. This is an ineffective way to determine public health policy as shown by the low ranks of these states. It is essential that legislators, community leaders, and health policy makers are educated about the benefits of fluoridation.[43]

Comparison of Effective Community Prevention Programs

Community prevention programs are difficult to compare due to wide variation in the studies done.

TABLE 19.7   States With Fluoridation Laws

State	National Rank	State	National Rank
Connecticut	16	Nebraska	28
Georgia	10	Ohio	15
Illinois	7	S. Dakota	1
Minnesota	8	Michigan	14

SOURCE: *Fluoridation Census, 1992.* Atlanta, Ga: Centers for Disease Control and Prevention, US Public Health Service; 1993.

Table 19.8 compares five different community programs that have been shown to be effective. Most of the information (except the data on practicality) comes from the Michigan Conference on Cost Effectiveness on Caries Prevention in Dental Public Health.[34]

Due to the widespread use of fluoridation and fluorides and the halo, or diffusion, effect through processed foods and beverages, all of which result in overlapping benefits and a national decline in dental caries in children, it is difficult to determine the absolute effectiveness of specific fluoride programs. For any given community, a thorough analysis of the literature, consultation with a dental public health expert, and review of the community's needs and resources should be done to determine which type of program is best for that community. As shown in Table 19.8, community fluoridation generally is the most effective and economical of the five effective community prevention programs for dental caries.[34] It is also the most practical.

For communities without a public water supply, school water supply fluoridation program or a school dietary fluoride supplement program would probably be the fluoride preventive measure of choice, depending on the dental health of school children and the community's resources. School–based dental disease prevention programs and clinics are effective because they work with population groups who have not yet had the disease, are readily accessible, and can be reached on a group basis with proven prevention programs. School prevention programs also reinforce the importance of good, regular oral hygiene.

School Fluoridation. **School fluoridation** is the adjustment of the fluoride content of a school's water supply to prevent dental caries. The school water supply is fluoridated at 4.5 times the level recommended for community fluoridation because children are in school only for a limited amount of time during the year. Studies have shown that school fluoridation prevents tooth decay by 20 to 30 percent over 12 years for children aged 5 to 17.[34] This figure may now be too high, as there have been no recent studies since the national decline in dental caries due to the impact of more widely available fluorides. In 1992 there were 117,430 children in 330 schools and 12 states in the United States receiving the benefits of school fluoridation.[42]

TABLE 19.8 Comparison of Five Effective Community Prevention Programs for Dental Caries*

Program	Effectiveness (percent)	Adult Benefits	Cost per Year	Practicality
Community Fluoridation	20-40	demonstrated	$0.51 per capita[a]	excellent; most practical; no individual effort necessary
School Fluoridation	20-30[b]	expected but not demonstrated	$0.85-$9.88 per child	good, if there is no central community water supply; no individual effort necessary
School Dietary Fluoride Daily Supplement Program	30	expected but not demonstrated	$0.81-$5.40 per child	fair; continued school regimen required for 8-10 years
School Fluoride Mouth Rinse Program	25-28[b]	not expected	$0.52-$1.78[c]	fair; continued daily or weekly school regimen required
School Sealant Program	51-67[d]	expected but not demonstrated	$13.07-$28.37 per child	good; primarily done for children age 6-8 and 12-14 years

*This table is a simplified comparison of these prevention programs. A thorough analysis of the literature should be done to understand the relative merits of these programs.
[a] see text for range
[b] this range may now be high; no recent studies
[c] includes using volunteer personnel
[d] first molar chewing surfaces only over a five-year period
SOURCE: Burt B. Proceedings of the workshop: cost effectiveness of caries prevention in dental public health. *J Public Health Dent.* 1989; 49:5. Special Issue.

School Dietary Fluoride Supplements. School dietary fluoride supplement programs, such as fluoride tablet programs, are done on a daily basis during the school year only for children who live in nonfluoridated communities. School dietary fluoride supplements are effective because children are assured of receiving fluoride on a regular basis. These programs should begin at the earliest age possible and continue until the age of 12 to 14 years. The programs are easy to implement and require little classroom time, although achieving compliance in the middle school years can be a challenge.

School Fluoride Mouth Rinses. Topical fluoride programs such as school rinse programs can be done in nonfluoridated communities, those recently fluoridated, or those with children at high risk for dental caries. The effectiveness of school fluoride rinse programs is no longer clear in communities where the amount of new tooth decay is already low due to the widespread use of fluorides in general.

School rinse programs are usually carried out weekly for ease of administration. Nondental personnel may supervise both fluoride tablet and rinse programs. They are easy to carry out and require little classroom time, about three to five minutes per procedure. About one in ten school children, 5 to 17 years of age, participate in a school-based fluoride mouth rinse program.[35]

School Sealant Programs. School sealant programs are recommended in both fluoridated communities and nonfluoridated communities for children age 6 to 8 and 12 to 14 years. School sealant programs are important because they target the 6-and 12-year molars, which are highly susceptible to decay. The 6-year molars are the most important teeth for maintaining the dental arch.

These programs are more cost-effective when sealants are placed by dental hygienists or dental assistants rather than dentists. In 1991, 48 states allowed dental hygienists to place sealants, and 15 states allowed dental assistants to place sealants, under various degrees of supervision by a dentist. About 43 percent of state dental practice acts did not require a dentist to be physically present at all when sealants were placed by auxiliaries in public programs, and 29 states reported having a community-based sealant program. In addi-

tion, Medicaid reimbursement for sealants is provided in 42 states.[44]

Sealants are generally applied to a tooth surface only once, but sometimes they need to be replaced, so they should be checked periodically. Five-year studies show a 51 to 67 percent reduction in tooth decay of the chewing surfaces of first molars to which sealants have been applied.[34] School sealant programs should be done in conjunction with fluoride prevention programs to obtain the maximum protection for children.

Oral Health Education. Oral health education should be incorporated into the school curriculum beginning in kindergarten to reinforce in children the importance of individual and community dental preventive measures and the need for periodic dental visits. Parents, teachers, health professionals, community leaders, and the public in general also need to be informed about dental disease prevention and the significance of oral health.

Physicians, nurses, and other health providers, in addition to dental health providers, play an important role in educating the public about oral health. The United States Clinical Preventive Services Task Force included counseling to prevent dental disease and screening for oral cancer in its recommendations to physicians.[45] It recommended that all patients be encouraged to visit a dental care provider on a regular basis. In addition, primary care clinicians should counsel patients regarding daily tooth brushing and dental flossing, the appropriate use of fluoride for caries prevention, the importance of avoiding sugary foods, and risk factors for developing baby bottle tooth decay. For children living in communities with inadequate water fluoridation, dietary fluoride supplements should be prescribed. While examining the mouth, clinicians should be alert for obvious signs of oral disease.

Screening for Oral Cancer. Although routine screening of asymptomatic persons for oral cancer by primary care clinicians is not recommended, it may be prudent for clinicians to perform careful examinations for cancerous lesions of the oral cavity in patients who use tobacco or excessive amounts of alcohol, as well as those with suspicious symptoms or lesions detected through self-examination. All patients should also be counseled to receive regular dental examinations, discontinue the use of all forms of tobacco, and limit consumption of alcohol. In addition, persons with increased exposure to sunlight should be advised to take protective measures to protect their lips and skin from the harmful effects of ultraviolet rays.[45]

Other Prevention Programs. It is beyond the scope of this chapter to discuss the full range of prevention programs related to oral health. Other examples of successful programs range from mouth guard programs for high school athletes in contact sports[46] to programs to educate dentists about children suffering from abuse or neglect[47] or how dental care providers may help the users of cigarettes and smokeless tobacco quit.[48] Clearly, there are a range of oral health programs to improve oral health that can be utilized in any community depending on their needs and resources.[49–53]

ORAL HEALTH—AN ESSENTIAL COMPONENT OF HEALTH AND PRIMARY CARE

Oral health is an essential component of total health and primary care.[54] Dental and oral diseases may well be the most prevalent and preventable conditions affecting Americans.[55] When any type of health or primary care program is being considered or developed there should be an oral health component. As oral diseases affect most of the population, community–based prevention should always be a very high priority. Unfortunately, the United States does not have national disease prevention or treatment programs, or national health insurance. Regardless of whether an evolving health care system emphasizes oral health services, public health professionals have the responsibility and opportunity to make meaningful contributions to the public's health by including oral health in health programs.

Vulnerable populations, such as those of low income, minorities, migrants, persons with HIV, and the institutionalized, homeless, homebound, elderly, and medically compromised, have the greatest dental needs as well as the least access to dental services. Health programs targeted to vulnerable and high–risk populations must have an oral health component. Although there are some dental programs provided by local, state, and federal agencies for vulnerable populations, they are inadequate.

Low–income groups and minorities suffer a disproportionate share of untreated oral diseases. Community–based prevention, health care reform, and primary care dentistry can help address inequities and access issues for vulnerable populations.[56] The following three specific recommendations have been made by Bolden, Henry, and Allukian:[56]

1. Oral health services must be part of the minimum benefit package for both children and adults in any health care program.
2. Prevention at the individual level and community-based prevention, such as fluoridation, should both be essential components of any health program.
3. Special initiatives need to be developed to improve oral health status and access for low income, minority, and other vulnerable populations.

Examples of such initiatives have also been suggested. They include:[56]

- focusing on recruiting, retaining, and graduating minority dental providers
- providing school-based and outreach programs to underserved communities
- establishing and strengthening incentives for dentists to work in underserved areas
- substantially increasing the number and scope of dental programs in community health centers
- promoting and supporting the use of dental auxiliaries to help provide oral health services efficiently and effectively
- providing funding for minorities and low income individuals to attend schools of dentistry, dental hygiene, and dental assisting
- providing funding to local and state health departments and dental schools so they may develop innovative programs to improve oral health status and access for vulnerable populations

DENTAL PERSONNEL

The total number of dental personnel is adequate to meet the current demand for oral health services but not the need. There is also a maldistribution of dental personnel in certain parts of the United States, with many inner-city and rural areas left underserved. According to a 1994 personal written communication with J. Rossetti of the Health Resources and Service Administration, in FY 1993 there were 1,069 designated dental health professional shortage areas (HPSAs) in the United States, requiring 2,087 dentists to fill the identified gaps.

If there were health care reform in our country that included reimbursement for oral health needs, the demand for service would increase and stress the capacity of the existing dental care delivery system. The best response to the growing need would be to increase the use of dental auxiliaries and incorporate oral health services into existing programs for vulnerable populations. The public health professional, as a leader and policy maker, can play a key role in helping to meet oral health needs by drawing upon four categories of dental personnel for assistance: dentists, dental hygienists, dental assistants, and dental laboratory technicians.

Dentists

Dentists have a minimum of two years of college before going to dental school, and most have a college degree. In 1993, there were fifty-four dental schools in the United States, all but two of which had four-year curricula. Of the remaining two, one had a three-year and the other a five-year curriculum.[57] Dentists receive a doctor of dental surgery (D.D.S.) or the equivalent doctor of dental medicine (D.M.D.) degree.

There were 148,800 dentists in the United States in 1990, for an active dentist-to-population ratio of 59.5 per 100,000.[58] Due to the closure of six dental schools since 1985, a decrease in the applicant pool, and the increasing cost of a dental education, the number of dental school graduates dropped from 5,550 in 1980 to 3,918 in 1991.[58] By the year 2000, the ratio of active dentists to population is expected to decrease to 57.6 per 100,000 and then to 47.0 per 100,000 by 2020.[58]

Most dentists in the United States are general practitioners who work in private practice. Only 18 percent of dentists are active specialists.[57] The eight dental specialties are dental public health, endodontics, oral and maxillofacial surgery, oral pathology, orthodontics, pediatric dentistry, periodontics, and prosthodontics.

Dental Hygienists

Dental hygienists primarily provide preventive services to patients, usually including screening, prophylaxis (cleaning), scaling, root planing, health education, and topical fluoride and dental sealant application. Most hygienists have two years of education and training after high school. Once hygienists are licensed by the state, they are known as registered dental hygienists (RDHs). Some hygienists have four or more years of education. Hygienists who work in public health policy or administration usually have a master's or doctoral degree in public health or health sciences.

In 1990, there were about 98,000 hygienists with active licenses in the United States of which about 81,000 were in active practice.[58] Dental hygienists are an excellent resource for public health initiatives for promoting and implementing prevention programs, health education, screening and referral, school-based programs, community outreach, and improved access to the underserved. Some state dental practice acts unnecessarily restrict what hygienists may do, resulting in access problems, lower efficiency, and higher costs for providing oral health services.

Dental Assistants

A formally trained dental assistant usually has one year of training after high school. Many dentists have trained their assistants on the job, but this is not recommended given the technological advances and challenges in dentistry, including the need for following the Centers for Disease Control and Prevention's guidelines for infection control. Dental assistants usually assist the dentist or hygienist when treatment is provided to the patient. Their duties include but are not limited to history taking, selecting and sterilizing instruments, mixing dental materials, and taking and developing radiographs.

Studies have shown that the productivity of dentists can be improved dramatically by the proper use of dental assistants. When dental assistants are allowed to perform expanded duties, the productivity of dentists increases even more.[59,60] Many state practice acts unnecessarily restrict what dental assistants are allowed to do, thus constraining dental productivity. In 1990, there were about 201,400 active dental assistants in the United States, for a ratio of 1.35 active assistants per active dentist.[58]

Dental Laboratory Technicians

Upon receiving a prescription from a dentist, dental laboratory technicians construct prostheses for the dentist to provide to the patient. These include but are not limited to dentures, crowns, bridges, and space maintainers. Lab technicians usually do not have direct contact with patients. In a few states, such as Oregon, dental laboratory technicians, known as denturists, are allowed to make dentures directly for the public. Lab technicians may have a one- to two-year training period after high school, but many are trained on-the-job. In 1990, there were about 70,000 laboratory technicians in the United States.[58]

CONCLUSION

Oral diseases are a neglected epidemic in our country. The public health professional has the responsibility and opportunity to respond to this epidemic. Oral health is an essential component of total health for both the individual and the community. The challenges to the public health professional for the future have been clearly delineated.[13,27,61] Oral health has 16 objectives in the year 2000 national health objectives and must be included in the three public health core functions of assessment, policy development, and assurance.

Most oral diseases can be readily assessed and prevented. Cost-effective individual and community preventive measures are available. Every local, state, and federal health department and agency should have dental public health expertise to respond effectively to this epidemic. Every health initiative or program should in-

clude an oral health component, from targeted programs for infants, pregnant women, persons with HIV, or the homeless, to health centers, managed care, and local, state, and national programs, including health care reform. The oral health needs of the American people must be addressed by the public health professional for healthier communities and a healthier nation.

ACKNOWLEDGMENT

The author would like to thank Dr. Stephen B. Corbin of the Centers for Disease Control and Prevention and Dr. Alice M. Horowitz of the National Institute of Dental Research for their assistance.

REFERENCES

1. National Center for Health Statistics. *An Assessment of the Occlusion of the Teeth of Youths, 12–17 Years, United States. Vital and Health Statistics.* Washington, DC: US Govt Printing Office; 1977. DHEW publication HRA 77-1644. Series 11 no. 162.

2. Bhat M. Periodontal health of 14-17 year old U.S. school children. *J Public Health Dent.* Winter 1991;51(1):5–11.

3. National Institute of Dental Research. *Oral Health of United States Children. The National Survey of Dental Caries in U.S. School Children, 1986–1987.* Bethesda, Md: US Dept of Health and Human Services; 1989. DHHS publication NIH 89-2247.

4. National Institute of Dental Research. *The National Survey of Oral Health in U.S. Employed Adults and Seniors: 1985–1986.* Bethesda, Md: US Dept of Health and Human Services; 1987. DHHS publication NIH 87-2868.

5. Boring CC, Squires TS, Tong T, Montgomery S. Cancer statistics, 1994. *CA Cancer J Clin.* January/February 1994;44:1.

6. Edmonds LD, James LM. Temporal trends in the prevalence of congenital malformations at birth based on the Birth Defects Monitoring Program, United States, 1979–1987. *MMWR.* 1993;39:19–23.

7. Allukian M, Kazmi I, Foulds SH, Horgan W. The unmet dental needs of the homeless in Boston. Presented at the 112th Annual Meeting of the American Public Health Association; November 13, 1984; Anaheim, Ca.

8. Kelly M, Bruerd B. The prevalence of nursing bottle decay among two Native American populations. *J Public Health Dent.* 1987;47:94–97.

9. Becker DB, Needleman HL, Kotelchuck M. Child abuse and dentistry: orofacial trauma and its recognition by dentists. *J Am Dent Assoc.* July 1978;97(1):24–28.

10. Melnick SL, Engel D, Truelove E, et al. Oral mucosal lesions: association with the presence of antibodies to the human immunodeficiency virus. *Oral Surg Oral Med Oral Pathol.* 1989;68:37–43.

11. Flanders R. Orofacial injuries: prevalence and prevention in Illinois. *Ill Dent J.* May/June 1992:211–216.

12. Bloom B, Gift HC, Jack SS. Dental services and oral health; United States, 1989. *Vital Health Stat.* 1992;10:183.

13. *Healthy People 2000: National Health Promotion and Disease Prevention Objectives.* Washington, DC: US Public Health Service; 1990. PHS publication no. 91-50212.

14. Kaste LW, Marcus P, Monopoli M, Allukian M, Douglass CW. Oral health status of homebound elders in Boston. Paper presented at the 18th Annual Meeting of the American Association for Dental Research; March 15–18, 1989; San Francisco, Ca.

15. Hollister MC, Weintraub JA. The association of oral status and systemic health, quality of life, and economic productivity. *J Dent Educ.* December 1993;57(12):901–912.

16. Lipton JS, Ship JA, Larach-Robinson D. Estimated prevalence and distribution of reported orofacial pain in the United States. *J Am Dent Assoc.* 1993;124(10):115–121.

17. Gift HC, Reisine ST, Larach DC. The social impact of dental problems and visits. *Am J Public Health.* 1992;82(12):1663–1668.

18. Adams PF, Benson V. Current estimates from the National Health Interview Survey, 1991. *Vital Health Stat.* 1992; 10(184):46–47,54.

19. Bruner ST, Waldo DR, Mckusick DR. National health expenditures projections through 2030. *Health Care Finance Review.* Fall 1992;14:1–29.

20. *A Statistical Report on Medicaid.* Baltimore, Md: Health Care Financing Administration, Office of the Actuary; December 1992.

21. Joshi A, Douglass CW, Jette A, Feldman H. The distribution of root caries in community–dwelling elders in New England. *J Public Health Dent.* Winter 1994:15–23.

22. Kaste LM, Gift HC. Baby bottle feeding behavior in children ages 2–5. *J Dent Res.* February 1994;33(2):580.

23. Ismail AI, Breis A, Burt A, Brunelle JA. Prevalence of total tooth loss, dental caries, and periodontal disease in Mexican-American adults: results from the Southwestern Hispanic Health and Nutrition Examination Survey. *J Dent Res.* 1987;66:1188.

24. *Cancers of the Oral Cavity and Pharynx: A Statistics Review Monograph, 1973–1987.* Atlanta, Ga: Centers for Disease Control and the National Institutes of Health; 1991.

25. Centers for Disease Control and Prevention. Examinations for oral cancer—United States, 1992. *MMWR.* March 25, 1994;43(11):198–200.

26. Prout MN, Heeren TC, Barber CE, et al. Use of health services before the diagnosis of head and neck cancer among Boston residents. *Am J Prev Med.* 1990;6:77–83.

27. Palmer C. NCAA forbids tobacco usage. *ADA News.* February 21, 1994;25:4.

28. Institute of Medicine, Committee for the Study of the Future of Public Health. *The Future of Public Health.* Washington, DC: National Academy Press; 1988.

29. Executive summary: application for continued recognition of dental public health as a dental specialty. *J Public Health Dent.* Winter 1986;46(1):35–37.

30. Rozier RG. Competency objectives for dental public health. *J Public Health Dent.* Fall 1990;50(5):338–344.

31. *Application for Continued Recognition of Dental Public Health as a Specialty.* Richmond, Va: American Association of Public Health Dentistry; December 1985.

32. *Annual Report.* Gainesville, Fl: American Board of Dental Public Health; 1994.

33. *Healthy Communities 2000: Model Standards: Guidelines for Community Attainment of the Year 2000 National Health Objectives.* 3rd ed. Washington, DC: American Public Health Association; 1991.

34. Burt B. Proceedings of the workshop: Cost effectiveness of caries prevention in dental public health. *J Public Health Dent.* 1989; 49:5. Special Issue.

35. Wagener DK, Nourjah P, Horowitz A. *Trends in Childhood Use of Dental Care Products Containing Fluoride: U.S. 1983–1989.* Hyattsville, Md: National Center for Health Statistics; 1992. Advance data from Vital and Health Statistics no. 219.

36. *Review of Fluoride: Benefits and Risks.* Washington, DC: US Public Health Service; February 1991.

37. Jakush J. CDT to consider fluoride dosage. *ADA News.* February 21, 1994;25:4.

38. Kaminsky LS, Mahoney MC, Leach JF, Melius JM, Miller MJ. Fluoride: benefits and risk of exposure. *Crit Rev Oral Biol Med.* 1990;1(4):261.

39. National Research Council. *Health Effects of Ingested Fluoride.* Washington, DC: National Academy Press; 1993.

40. Centers for Disease Control and Prevention. Public health focus: fluoridation of community water systems. *MMWR.* May 29, 1992;2(41):372–375,381.

41. Centers for Disease Control. *Water Fluoridation: A Manual for Engineers and Technicians.* Atlanta, Ga: US Public Health Service; 1986:19.

42. *Fluoridation Census, 1992.* Atlanta, Ga: Centers for Disease Control and Prevention, US Public Health Service; 1993.

43. Allukian M, Ackerman J, Steinhurst J. Factors that influence the attitudes of first-term Massachusetts legislators toward fluoridation. *J Am Dent Assoc.* April 1981;104(4):494.

44. Cohen LA, Horowitz AM. Community-based sealant programs in the United States: results of a survey. *J Public Health Dent.* Fall 1993;53:4.

45. US Preventive Services Task Force Report. *Guide to Clinical Preventive Services.* Baltimore, Md: Williams and Wilkins; 1989.

46. Flanders R. Mouthguards and sports injuries. *Ill Dent J.* Jan/Feb 1993:13–16.

47. Missouri Dental Association. Child abuse update 1994. Reprinted from the *Missouri Dent J.* 1994; pp. 1–101.

48. National Cancer Institute. *How to Help Your Patients Stop Using Tobacco: Manual for the Oral Health Team.* Washington, DC: National Institutes of Health; 1991. PHS publication no. 91–3191.

49. Allukian M. Effective community prevention program. In: Depoala DP, Cheney JG, eds. *Handbook of Preventive Dentistry.* Littleton, Ma: Publishing Services Group Inc; 1979.

50. Horowitz AM. Community–oriented preventive dentistry programs that work. *Health Values.* Jan/Feb 1984;8(1):121–129.

51. Allukian M. Community oral health programs. In: Clark JW, ed. *Clinical Dentistry, II.* Philadelphia, Pa: Harper & Row; 1987.

52. Association of State and Territorial Dental Directors. *Guidelines for State Dental Public Health Programs.* 1985.

53. Association of State and Territorial Dental Directors. *Public Health Core Functions: Strategies for Addressing the Oral Health of the Nation.* March 1994. Discussion paper.

54. Isman RE. Integrating primary oral health care into primary care. *J Dent Ed.* December 1993;47(12):846–852.

55. Oral Health Coordinating Committee, Public Health Service. Toward improving the oral health of Americans: an overview of oral health status, resources, and care delivery. *Public Health Rep.* Nov/Dec 1993;108(6):657–672.

56. Bolden AJ, Henry JL, Allukian M. Implications of access, utilization and need for oral health care by low income groups and minorities on the dental delivery system. *J Dent Ed.* 1993; 57(12):888–900.

57. American Association of Dental Schools. *Dean's Briefing Book, Academic Year, 1992–1993.* Washington, DC: AADS; 1993.

58. US Dept of Health and Human Services. *Health Personnel in the United States, Eighth Report to Congress. Allied Health, 1991.* Washington, DC: HRSA/Bureau of Health Professions; September 1992.

59. *Comptroller General: Increased Use of Expanded Function Dental Auxiliaries Would Benefit Consumers, Dentists and Taxpayers. Report to the Congress.* Washington, DC: General Accounting Office; March 7, 1980. Publication HRD-80–51.

60. Liang JN, Ogur JD. *Restrictions on Dental Auxiliaries; An Economic Policy Analysis.* Washington, DC: Federal Trade Commission; May 1987.

61. Corbin SB, Mecklenburg RE. The future of dental public health report: preparing dental public health to meet the challenges and opportunities of the 21st century. *J Public Health Dent.* Spring, 1994;54(2):80–91.

CHAPTER

20

Infectious Disease Control

Alan R. Hinman, M.D.

Historically, infectious diseases have been the major killers of humans. It is only within the last century that they have been replaced as primary threats in the United States by injuries and chronic diseases. The major advances in infectious disease control to date have been through protection of food and water and through immunization.

This chapter begins with general considerations of infectious disease transmission, surveillance, and investigation, and then considers specific topics of immunization, sexually transmitted diseases (STDs, including human immunodeficiency virus [HIV] infection), tuberculosis (TB), and foodborne and waterborne diseases.

GENERAL CONSIDERATIONS

This section introduces the reader to general principles of infectious disease transmission. It also discusses how surveillance and outbreak investigation help control the spread of infectious diseases.

Transmission

Most of the infectious diseases that have a significant impact on the public's health are communicable and may be transmitted in one of four ways: common vehicle, contact, airborne, or vector borne transmission.[1] **Common vehicle** transmission results from contamination of a vehicle (for example, food, water, or intravenous fluids) to which several susceptible individuals are exposed. **Contact** transmission can occur as a result of direct physical contact (for example, in sexual intercourse) or indirect contact (for example, in the fecal-oral spread of enteric organisms, inhalation of large droplets of infected respiratory secretions, or sharing of needles for injection of drugs).

Airborne spread occurs when infectious droplets form droplet nuclei, which may remain suspended in the air for minutes to hours and be dispersed widely. For example, patients in a hospital several rooms away from a patient with varicella have become infected,[2] and measles has been transmitted to a patient visiting a physician's office approximately one hour after the source case had left the office.[3] **Vectors** are typically arthropods that acquire the infectious agent from feeding on an infected individual and subsequently inoculate it into a susceptible host. They may act either as passive carriers of the organism (as, for example, in plague or Lyme disease) or as an integral part of the life cycle of the agent (as, for example, in malaria).

Surveillance

Surveillance is key to understanding the epidemiology of infectious diseases. A simple definition of surveillance is "information for action,"[4] and it generally entails ongoing collection of data about cases of disease, reporting of these data to a central location (typically a health department), analyzing them, and using the resulting analysis to develop interventions and monitor their success. Ongoing surveillance also provides the information needed to determine whether interventions should be modified (for example, changing the age of vaccination or providing additional doses of vaccine to individuals). In addition, surveillance may identify clusters of cases or outbreaks, which warrant further investigation.

Outbreak Investigation

Epidemic investigation involves seven major steps, many of which may be carried out simultaneously. The first step is to confirm that there is, in fact, an outbreak. The classical definition of an epidemic is "the occurrence in a community or region of cases of an illness (or an outbreak) clearly in excess of expectancy."[5] Obviously, it is necessary to know not only how many cases there are, but how many are expected. A single case of paralysis due to wild poliovirus occurring in the United States, for example, would be considered a potential epidemic because there have been no such cases reported since 1979.[6] The second step is to identify the illness involved, often by establishing a clinical case definition if a definitive diagnosis has not been established.

The third step is to enumerate all cases and to categorize them according to time, place, and person. Characterization as to time typically involves construction of an epidemic curve showing the number of cases by time of onset (for example, by hour, day, or week, as appropriate). A common source outbreak with a point contamination of the vehicle typically has an epidemic curve with a single sharp peak centered on the median incubation period following exposure (typically a few hours to a few days). Person-to-person transmission is generally accompanied by an epidemic curve in which there is a gradual build-up of cases, often with a typical incubation period between "generations" of cases, and a gradual decline as susceptibles are exhausted, in the absence of measures to interrupt transmission. Characterization by place often involves constructing a map showing residence (or work site) of individual cases in order to identify any geographic localization. Characterization by person involves the obvious—age and sex—but may also entail race/ethnicity, occupation, and other variables.

The fourth step in epidemic investigation is to confirm the diagnosis in the laboratory or by other means. The fifth step is to formulate a hypothesis about the cause of the epidemic and the means of transmission and to test that hypothesis through further investigation or interview of cases, culture of suspected water or food, or other means. The sixth step is to take control measures to end the epidemic. The final step, and the one most often ignored, is to prepare and disseminate a report about the epidemic, either through formal publication in the literature or through an administratively circulated form. This last step is essential in order to learn from the current situation and prevent recurrences.

IMMUNIZATION

Immunization is one of the most important interventions for the control of infectious diseases. This section addresses vaccines, including their safety and effectiveness, as well as immunization schedules and immunization laws.

Vaccines

Vaccines are suspensions of attenuated live or killed microorganisms (bacteria, viruses, or rickettsiae), or fractions thereof, which are administered to induce immunity and thereby prevent infectious disease. Live, attenuated vaccines are believed to induce an immunologic response more similar to that resulting from natural infection. Inactivated or killed vaccines can consist of:

- inactivated whole organisms (for example, cholera or pertussis)
- soluble capsular material alone (for example, pneumococcal polysaccharide)
- soluble capsular material covalently linked to carrier proteins (for example, *Haemophilus influenzae* type b conjugate vaccines)
- purified extracts of some component or components of the organism (for example, hepatitis B, subunit influenza, or acellular pertussis).

Toxoids are modified bacterial toxins (for example, diphtheria or tetanus) that have been rendered nontoxic but retain the ability to stimulate the formation of antitoxin. They are often included in the general category of vaccines.[7]

Vaccines are among the safest and most effective means available to prevent infectious diseases. Widespread immunization of infants and young children has had a dramatic impact on the occurrence of several infectious diseases. Global eradication of smallpox is certainly the most dramatic public health achievement of any kind to date.

Table 20.1 depicts the maximum annual number of cases ever reported in the United States and the number of cases reported in 1992 for diseases against which most infants and young children are immunized. Reductions of more than 90 percent have been seen for all conditions except hepatitis B, for which universal immunization of newborns has not yet been fully implemented. No cases of paralysis due to wild poliovirus acquired in the United States have occurred since 1979, and a goal has been set for global eradication by the year 2000.[8] The last case of paralysis due to wild poliovirus

TABLE 20.1 Comparison of Maximum and Current Morbidity due to Vaccine–Preventable Diseases

	Maximum Cases	Year	1992	Percentage Change
Diphtheria	206,939	1921	4	−99.99
Measles	894,134	1941	2,237	−99.75
Mumps[a]	152,209	1968	2,572	−98.31
Pertussis	265,269	1934	4,083	−98.46
Polio (paralytic)	21,269	1952	4[b]	−99.98
Rubella[c]	57,686	1969	160	−99.72
CRS[d]	20,000	1964–1965	11	−99.95
Tetanus[e]	1,560	1923	45	−97.12
Haemophilus Influenzae type b	20,000[f]	1984	1,412	−92.94
Hepatitis B	26,611	1985	16,126	−39.40

[a]first reportable in 1968
[b]subject to change due to retrospective evaluation or late reporting; all are vaccine associated
[c]first reportable in 1966
[d]congenital rubella syndrome estimated for the 1964 to 1965 pandemic
[e]cases first reportable in 1947; maximum based on number of deaths
[f]first reportable in 1991; based on five United States population–based studies, 1976 to 1984
SOURCE: Centers for Disease Control and Prevention, unpublished data.

in the Americas had onset in Peru in August 1991.[9] Of particular note in the table is the reduction in invasive disease due to *Haemophilus influenzae* type b (Hib), for which a vaccine was first put into widespread use in 1987. In just six years, there has been more than a 90 percent reduction in the reported incidence of this major cause of bacterial meningitis.[10]

Immunization Schedules

Recommendations for immunization of children in the United States are developed principally by the Public Health Service's Immunization Practices Advisory Committee (ACIP)[7] and the American Academy of Pediatrics Committee on Infectious Diseases ("Red Book Committee").[11] Along with the American Academy of Family Physicians, these two committees have recently agreed on a common immunization schedule, which is shown in Table 20.2. Immunization of all infants in the

TABLE 20.2   Recommended Childhood Immunization Schedule, United States, January–June 1996

Vaccines are listed under the routinely recommended ages. Bars indicate range of acceptable ages for vaccination. Shaded bars indicate *catch-up vaccination:* at 11–12 years of age, hepatitis B vaccine should be administered to children not previously vaccinated, and varicella zoster virus vaccine should be administered to children not previously vaccinated who lack a reliable history of chicken pox.

Age ▶ / Vaccine ▼	Birth	1 mo	2 mos	4 mos	6 mos	12 mos	15 mos	18 mos	4–6 yrs	11–12 yrs	14–16 yrs
Hepatitis B[a,b]	Hep B-1									Hep B[b]	
		Hep B-2			Hep B-3						
Diphtheria, Tetanus, Pertussis[c]			DTP	DTP	DTP	DTP[c] (DTaP at 15+ m)			DTP or DTaP	Td	
H. influenzae type b[d]			Hib	Hib	Hib[d]	Hib[d]					
Polio[a]			OPV[e]	OPV	OPV				OPV		
Measles, Mumps, Rubella[f]						MMR			MMR[f] or	MMR[f]	
Varicella Zoster Virus Vaccine[g]						Var				Var[a]	

[a]*Infants born to HBsAg–negative mothers* should receive 2.5 μg of Merck vaccine (Recombivax HB) or 10 μg of SmithKline Beecham (SB) vaccine (Engerix-B). The 2nd dose should be administered ≥ 1 mo after the 1st dose.
Infants born to HBsAg-positive mothers should receive 0.5 mL Hepatitis B Immune Globulin (HBIG) within 12 hr of birth, and either 5 μg of Merck vaccine (Recombivax HB) or 10 μg of SB vaccine (Engerix-B) at a separate site. The 2nd dose is recommended at 1–2 mos of age and the 3rd dose at 6 mos of age.
Infants born to mothers whose HBsAg status is unknown should receive either 5 μg of Merck vaccine (Recombivax HB) or 10 μg of SB vaccine (Engerix-B) within 12 hr of birth. The 2nd dose of vaccine is recommended at 1 mo of age and the 3rd dose at 6 mos of age.
[b]Adolescents who have not previously received 3 doses of hepatitis B vaccine should initiate or complete the series at the 11–12-year-old visit. The 2nd dose should be administered at least 1 mo after the 1st dose, and the 3rd dose should be administered at least 4 mos after the 1st dose and at least 2 mos after the 2nd dose.
[c]DTP4 may be administered at 12 mos of age, if at least 6 mos have elapsed since DTP3. DTaP (diphtheria and tetanus toxoids and acellular pertussis vaccine) is licensed for the 4th and/or 5th vaccine dose(s) for children aged ≥ 15 mos and may be preferred for these doses in this age group. Td (tetanus and diphtheria toxoids, adsorbed, for adult use) is recommended at 11–12 years of age if at least 5 years have elapsed since the last dose of DTP, DTaP, or DT.
[d]Three *H. influenzae* type b (Hib) conjugate vaccines are licensed for infant use. If PRP-OMP (PedvaxHIB [Merck]) is administered at 2 and 4 mos of age, a dose at 6 mos is not required. After completing the primary series, any Hib conjugate vaccine may be used as a booster.
[e]Oral poliovirus vaccine (OPV) is recommended for routine infant vaccination. Inactivated poliovirus vaccine (IPV) is recommended for persons with a congenital or acquired immune deficiency disease or an altered immune status as a result of disease or immunosuppressive therapy, as well as their household contacts, and is an acceptable alternative for other persons. The primary 3-dose series for IPV should be given with a minimum interval of 4 wks between the 1st and 2nd doses and 6 mos between the 2nd and 3rd doses.
[f]The 2nd dose of MMR is routinely recommended at 4–6 yrs of age or at 11–12 yrs of age, but may be administered at any visit, provided at least 1 mo has elapsed since receipt of the 1st dose.
[g]Varicella zoster virus vaccine (Var) can be administered to susceptible children any time after 12 months of age. Unvaccinated children who lack a reliable history of chicken pox should be vaccinated at the 11–12-year-old visit.

TABLE 20.3 Recommended Immunizations for Adults

Vaccine	Routine Age Group[a]				Special Circumstances						
	18–24	25–49	50–64	≥65	Military Recruits	Travelers	Health Care Workers	Occupation	Immuno-compromised[b]	Pregnancy	Chronic Illness
Adenovirus 4 and 7					X						
Anthrax								S			
BCG							S±				
Cholera						S					
Diphtheria	X	X	X	X	X	X	X	X	X	X	X
Haemophilus influenzae type b									S±		
Hepatitis B						S	X	S			
Influenza				X	X	S	X		X		X
Japanese Encephalitis						S					
Measles	X	X[c]			X	X	X		O	O	

Vaccine								
Meningococcal	O					X		X
Mumps				X	S			X[c]
Plague			S		S			
Pneumococcal	X	X					X	
Polio-inactivated				S	S			
Polio-oral		O		S	S	X		
Rabies			S		S		O	
Rubella	O	O		X	X	X	O	X
Smallpox (vaccinia)	O	O		O	O		O	O
Tetanus	X	X	S	X	X	X	X	X
Typhoid					S			
Yellow Fever		O			S			

Symbol Reference:
X: recommended
±: divided opinion
O: contraindicated
S: selected risk situation
aunless contraindications exist
bMeasles, mumps, and rubella vaccines should be considered for persons with symptomatic HIV infection. They are routinely indicated for persons with asymptomatic HIV infection.
cif susceptible; persons born prior to 1957 generally considered immune

United States is currently recommended against ten diseases: diptheria (D), hepatitis B, Hib, measles, mumps, pertussis (P), poliomyelitis, rubella, tetanus (T), and varicella.

Table 20.3 shows immunization recommendations for adults, who may have special needs for vaccines such as pneumococcal polysaccharide and influenza. Recommendations for use in adults of the recently licensed varicella and hepatitis A vaccines have not yet been finalized.

Immunization Laws

Immunization efforts in the United States have been significantly aided by the enactment and enforcement of laws in each state that require immunization before first entry into school. As a result, at least 96 percent of children entering school are fully immunized. Unfortunately, there has been less success in immunizing infants and young children on schedule. Although precise nationwide figures are not available, it was estimated in 1992 that only 50 to 60 percent of two-year-old children had completed the primary series of immunization, and in some cities the figure was even lower.

Several factors are responsible for this situation, including lack of access to immunization services, high cost of vaccines, and uninformed or poorly motivated parents. One of the most striking factors is that many opportunities to immunize children are missed. This results from provider failure to assess immunization status, failure to administer all needed vaccines at a single visit, and invoking of inappropriate "contraindications" to vaccination, among other problems. An analysis of the problems[12] led to the development of standards for pediatric immunization practice,[13] shown in Table 20.4, and a major initiative in 1993 to improve immunization levels in preschool children.[14]

Vaccine Safety and Effectiveness

Although modern vaccines are safe and effective, they are neither perfectly safe nor perfectly effective. Some individuals who receive vaccine will not be protected against disease and some will suffer adverse con-

TABLE 20.4 Standards for Pediatric Immunization Practices

1. Immunization services are readily available.
2. There are no barriers or unnecessary prerequisites to the receipt of vaccines.
3. Immunization services are available free or for a minimal fee.
4. Providers utilize all clinical encounters to screen and, when indicated, vaccinate children.
5. Providers educate parents and guardians about immunization in general terms.
6. Providers question parents or guardians about contraindications and, before vaccinating a child, inform them in specific terms about the risks and benefits of the vaccinations their child is to receive.
7. Providers follow only true contraindications.
8. Providers administer simultaneously all vaccine doses for which a child is eligible at the time of each visit.
9. Providers use accurate and complete recording procedures.
10. Providers coschedule immunization appointments in conjunction with appointments for other child health services.
11. Providers report adverse events following vaccination promptly, accurately, and completely.
12. Providers operate a tracking system.
13. Providers adhere to appropriate procedures for vaccine management.
14. Providers conduct semiannual audits to assess immunization coverage levels and to review immunization records in the patient populations they serve.
15. Providers maintain up-to-date, easily retrievable medical protocols at all locations where vaccines are administered.
16. Providers practice patient-oriented and community-based approaches.
17. Vaccines are administered by properly trained persons.
18. Providers receive ongoing education and training regarding current immunization recommendations.

sequences. Adverse events may range from minor inconvenience such as local discomfort or fever to serious conditions such as paralysis associated with oral poliovirus vaccine (OPV). The goal is to achieve maximum safety and maximum efficacy.

Assessing the Risks

In developing recommendations for vaccine use, it is essential to consider the risks as well as the benefits of the vaccine. The balance between vaccine benefit and risk, on the one hand, and the risk and severity of the disease, on the other, must continually be reassessed as this relationship may change over time. For example, in the United States, the risk of rare complications of smallpox vaccine outweighed the risk of complications or death associated with possible importation of smallpox even before global eradication was achieved. As a consequence, routine smallpox vaccination was discontinued years before global eradication was certified.[15]

It is often difficult to ascertain whether an adverse event that occurs after immunization was caused by the vaccine or was merely temporally related and caused by some totally independent (and often unknown or unidentified) factor. This is particularly a problem during infancy, when a number of conditions may occur spontaneously. In a given instance it may be impossible to determine whether vaccine was responsible. Adverse events caused by vaccines may be common and minor (for example, fever and transient rash occur seven to ten days following vaccination in 5 to 15 percent of measles vaccine recipients) or rare and severe (for example, paralysis in a recipient of OPV, or in a close contact of a recipient, occurs once for every 2.7 million doses of vaccine distributed). Particularly when dealing with rare events, it may be necessary to carry out large-scale case-control studies or review comprehensive records of large numbers of infants (potentially hundreds of thousands) to ascertain whether those who received vaccine had a higher incidence of the event than those who did not.[16]

The Institute of Medicine (IOM) of the National Academy of Sciences recently completed reviews of adverse events associated with the "traditional" childhood

TABLE 20.5 Summary of Institute of Medicine Findings on the Relationship of Adverse Events to Individual Vaccines

Vaccine	Establishes Causation	Favoring Causation	Favoring Rejection of Causation
DT/Td/T	anaphylaxis	Guillain–Barre syndrome; brachial neuritis	encephalopathy; infantile spasms; death from SIDS
Pertussis* (DTP)	anaphylaxis; protracted, inconsolable crying	acute encephalopathy; shock and unusual shocklike state (hypotonic-hyporesponsive episodes)	infantile spasms; hypsarrythmia; Reye's syndrome; sudden infant death syndrome
Measles (see MMR)		anaphylaxis; death from measles vaccine strain in primarily immunocompromised	
MMR (measles, mumps, and rubella)	anaphylaxis; thrombo-cytopenia		
Mumps (see MMR)			
OPV	poliomyelitis; death from polio vaccine strain—mainly in immuno-compromised individuals	Guillain–Barre syndrome	
IPV			
Hepatitis B	anaphylaxis		
Hib (conjugate)			Early onset *Haemophilus Influenzae* b disease
Rubella* (see MMR)	acute arthritis	chronic arthritis	

*DTP was reviewed by an earlier committee. Initial report categories corresponding to table headings were: evidence indicates a causal relationship; evidence is consistent with a causal relationship; evidence does not indicate a causal relationship.

vaccines (DTP, polio, MMR) and concluded that evidence was insufficient to establish a causal relationship for many conditions about which parents had been concerned (particularly permanent brain damage following receipt of pertussis vaccine). Table 20.5 summarizes the IOM conclusions.[17,18]

Informing the Public

It is important that vaccine recipients (or their parents or guardians) be aware of the potential adverse events associated with vaccination as well as of the benefits. The Centers for Disease Control and Prevention has developed standardized *Vaccine Information Pamphlets* as required by the National Childhood Vaccine Injury Act of 1986 (Section XXI of the Public Health Service Act).[19] Whether in the public or private sector, all providers of the specified vaccines (diphtheria and tetanus toxoids; measles, mumps, pertussis, poliomyelitis, and rubella vaccines) are required to use these materials to notify patients and parents formally of the risks and benefits of these vaccines. Providers are also required to report certain conditions which follow immunization with these vaccines, as listed in Table 20.6. The act also establishes a no-fault compensation mechanism for those who are injured by these vaccines. Information about this pro-

TABLE 20.6   Reportable Events Following Immunization

Vaccine	Event	Interval from Vaccination
DTP;P;DTP/polio combined	anaphylaxis or anaphylactic shock	24 hours
	encephalopathy (or encephalitis)[a]	7 days
	shock collapse or hypotonic–hyporesponsive collapse[a]	7 days
	residual seizure disorders[a]	
	any acute complication or sequela (including death) of above events	No limit
	Events in vaccinees described in manufacturer's package insert as contraindications to additional doses of vaccine[b] (such as convulsions)	(see package insert)
Measles, mumps, and rubella; DT,Td, tetanus toxoid	anaphylaxis or anaphylactic shock	24 hours
	encephalopathy (or encephalitis)[a]	15 days for measles, mumps, and rubella vaccines; 7 days for DT, Td, and T toxoids
	residual seizure disorder[a]	
	any acute complication or sequela (including death)	No limit
	events in vaccinees described in manufacturer's package insert as contraindications to additional doses of vaccine[b]	(see package insert)
Oral polio vaccine	paralytic poliomyelitis	
	in a nonimmunodeficient recipient	30 days
	in an immunodeficient recipient	6 months
	in a vaccine–associated community–acquired infection	no limit
	Any acute complication or sequela (including death) of above events	no limit
	events in vaccinees described in manufacturer's package insert as contraindications to additional doses of vaccine[b]	(see package insert)

TABLE 20.6   (continued)

Inactivated polio vaccine	anaphylaxis or anaphylactic shock	24 hours
	Any acute complication or sequela (including death) of above event	no limit
	events in vaccinees described in manufacturer's package insert as contraindications to additional doses of vaccine[b]	(see package insert)

[a]Aids to interpretation:

Shock collapse or hypotonic-hyporesponsive collapse may be evidenced by signs or symptoms such as decrease in or loss of muscle tone, paralysis (partial or complete), hemiplegia, hemiparesis, loss of color or turning pale white or blue, unresponsiveness to environmental stimuli, depression of or loss of consciousness, prolonged sleeping with difficulty arousing, or cardiovascular or respiratory arrest.

Residual seizure disorder may be considered to have occurred if no other seizure or convulsion, unaccompanied by a fever or accompanied by a fever of less than 102°F (38.9°C), occurred before the first seizure or convulsion after the administration of the vaccine involved. In the case of vaccines containing measles, mumps, or rubella, the first seizures or convulsions must occur within 15 days after vaccination. In the case of any other vaccine, the first seizures or convulsion must occur within 3 days of vaccination or within 1 year after vaccination if two or more seizures or convulsions, unaccompanied by fever or accompanied by fever of less than 102°F, occurred.

The terms seizure and convulsion include grand mal, petit mal, absence, myoclonic, tonic-clonic, and focal motor seizures and signs. Encephalopathy means any significant acquired abnormality of, injury to, or impairment of function of the brain. Among the frequent manifestations of encephalopathy are focal and diffuse neurologic signs, increased intracranial pressure, or changes lasting at least six hours in level of consciousness, with or without convulsions. The neurologic signs and symptoms of encephalopathy may be temporary with complete recovery, or they may result in various degrees of permanent impairment. Signs and symptoms such as high–pitched and unusual screaming, persistent inconsolable crying, and bulging fontanelle are compatible with an encephalopathy but in and of themselves are not conclusive evidence of encephalopathy. Encephalopathy usually can be documented by slow-wave activity on an electroencephalogram.

[b]The health care provider who administered the vaccine must refer to the contraindication section of the manufacturer's package insert for each vaccine.

gram can be obtained from the National Childhood Vaccine Injury Compensation Program (Parklawn Building, 5600 Fishers Lane, Rockville MD 20857, telephone 301-443-6593 or 1-800-338-2382). CDC has also developed *Important Information Statements* for use with other vaccines purchased with federal funds.

Children's Vaccine Initiative

Continuous efforts are underway to improve safety and efficacy of existing vaccines, simplify the vaccination schedule, and develop new immunizing agents. A children's vaccine initiative is underway (with overall coordination by the World Health Organization) to develop a combination vaccine that would include all antigens and be effective when administered in a single oral dose at birth.[20] Although this ideal is a long way off, there are several combined products which should become available in the near future (for example, DTP-hepatitis B-Hib, DTP-IPV) and allow infants to receive fewer injections of different products. In addition, new technology may permit timed release of antigen with

the result that only a single injection might be required of a product that now requires three or four injections administered over a period of months.

Vaccine Efficacy

The fact that vaccines are not perfectly effective means that some vaccinated individuals will develop disease on exposure. A common situation in the United States in recent years has been that approximately half the people with a disease (for example, measles) give a history of vaccination. This leads many persons to question the efficacy of the vaccine.

A simple formula exists to determine *vaccine efficacy (VE)*:

$$VE = (ARU - ARV)/ARU \times 100.$$

In this equation, ARU is the attack rate of disease in unvaccinated individuals and ARV is the attack rate in vaccinated individuals.[21] A nomogram has been constructed, as shown in Figure 20.1, to demonstrate the relationship between the proportion of cases with a

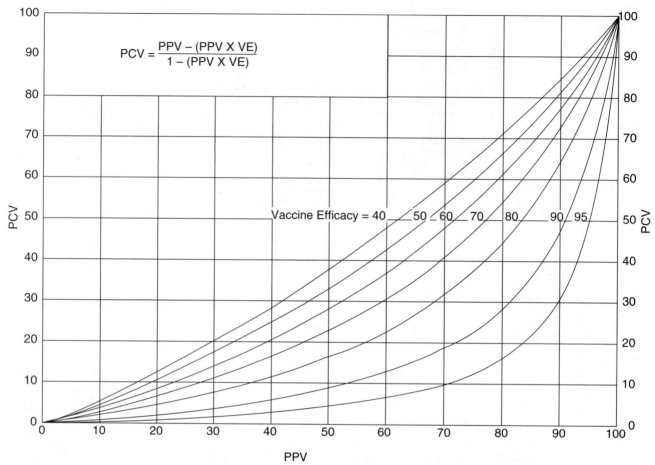

$$PCV = \frac{PPV - (PPV \times VE)}{1 - (PPV \times VE)}$$

FIGURE 20.1 Percentage of cases vaccinated (PCV) by percentage of population vaccinated (PPV), for 7 values of vaccine efficacy (VE). SOURCE: Orenstein WA, Bernier RH, Dondero TJ, et al. Field evaluation of vaccine efficacy. *Bull WHO.* 1985; 63:1055–1068.

history of vaccination (PCV) and the proportion of the population vaccinated (PPV) at varying levels of vaccine efficacy (VE). Simply put, if 90 percent of the population has been vaccinated with a 90 percent effective vaccine, one would expect approximately half the cases to give a history of vaccination, thus supporting a continued high efficacy for the vaccine.

SEXUALLY TRANSMITTED DISEASES (STDs)

All STDs, including human immunodeficiency virus (HIV) infection, are historically, biologically, be-

haviorally, economically, and programmatically related.[22] Intimate sexual contact is the common (but not exclusive) mode of transmission of the causative organisms. Several dozen bacterial, viral, parasitic, and fungal infections are now recognized as being commonly (or predominantly) transmitted through sexual contact. In general, they share the characteristic that women suffer disproportionately from their effects. This is a result of a variety of factors, including the fact that women are generally less able to prevent exposure to STDs than men because of the lack of safe, effective female-controlled preventive measures. Women also are frequently unable to negotiate the conditions under which sexual intercourse occurs. In addition, complications of STDs in women are likely to be more severe: pelvic inflammatory disease (PID), infertility, ectopic pregnancy (the leading cause of maternal mortality in the United States), and cancer.[23]

Efforts to control STDs have been guided by both the magnitude of the problem and the availability of diagnostic and therapeutic measures. The United States began this century focusing on one dominant STD, syphilis, which could be diagnosed with newly developed serologic techniques and treated with a suppressive therapy. Subsequent improvements in the ability to detect and treat syphilis led to a striking decline in its incidence.

Growing awareness of the serious individual and social implications of gonorrhea, accompanied by improvements in diagnostic techniques, led the United States to embark on a major program to control gonorrhea in the 1970s. In the early 1980s, the spectrum of STDs expanded. Concern arose about syndromes associated with *Chlamydia trachomatis*, *Trichomonas vaginalis*, herpes simplex virus, and human papillomavirus. By the mid-1980s, HIV emerged to dominate the field of STDs.

Model of STD Transmission

Anderson and May have developed a simple and very useful model of transmission of STDs based on earlier work by themselves and by Yorke and Hethcote.[24] It is based on the assumption that a disease can only sustain itself when the reproduction rate is greater than one, that is, when each infected person on average transmits the disease to at least one other person. If the reproduction rate is less than one, transmission of the disease cannot be sustained and it will die out. The formula for the reproduction rate is

$$R = B \times c \times D$$

where R is the reproduction rate (the number of new infections produced by an infected individual); B is a measure of transmissibility (the average probability that an infected individual will infect a susceptible partner given exposure); c represents the average number of different partners the infected individual has per unit

time; and D represents the duration of infectiousness of the disease. These three determinants of the reproductive rate are influenced by the interplay of biological and behavioral variables for each STD.

The values for each parameter may vary depending on the STD and the type of sexual contact; estimates have been made for several of them. For example, for gonorrhea the overall estimate for B is 50 percent (50 to 90 percent for male-to-female transmission and 20 to 50 percent for female-to-male transmission). For syphilis, B is estimated at 20 to 30 percent and for HIV at 1 to 10 percent.[25] Additionally, HIV transmissibility is apparently higher for penile-anal intercourse than for penile-vaginal intercourse.

Because not all members of a given population have the same number of sex partners, a refinement can be made in the formula for variable c, using the median number of sex partners and the variance in the number of sex partners instead of a simple average. It appears that a core population of highly sexually active persons (with many different partners) plays a major role in the continued transmission of STDs.

The duration of the infectious period, D, is also quite different for the different STDs, ranging from a few days for gonorrhea (in men), to a lifetime for HIV infection. There are other biological and behavioral factors affecting D, such as health care-seeking behavior, and compliance with treatment, among others.

Elements of Control Programs

Control strategies may aim to modify any of the factors in the equation of transmissibility. In general, control programs include public information and education, professional education and training, screening, prompt diagnosis and therapy, counseling, partner notification, and surveillance. No approach by itself is likely to prevent the spread of STDs, but each contributes to the overall effort.

The aim of public information and education, counseling, and partner notification is to reduce factors B, c, and D by encouraging changes in sexual and health care-related behaviors. Holmes and Aral describe at least three types of behavioral interventions, differing in their objectives:[26]

1. interventions reducing the risk of exposure to and acquisition of STDs through changes in sexual behavior, such as abstinence or postponing sexual activity, monogamy or reducing the number of sex partners, using condoms, and avoiding receptive anal intercourse, among others (affects factors B and c).

2. interventions reducing the risk of transmission and complication of STDs through changes in health care-seeking and compliance behavior by educating people about the manifestations of STDs, increasing the level of suspicion when symptoms occur, increasing awareness of the availability of services, and teaching about the need for consistent condom use and completion of therapy, among others (affects B and D).

3. interventions increasing accessibility and effectiveness of STD services through professional education and training, primarily aimed at reducing the duration of infection (D) but, if counseling is successful, also lowering the risk of transmission (B) and the number of sex partners (c). A major component of most current control programs is the provision of prompt and adequate diagnosis and therapy, which certainly reduces the duration of infection (D) but requires availability of services.

Given the differential importance to overall STD transmission of those who have few and those who have many sex partners, it appears that targeted behavioral change among core group members would have much greater impact on transmission than would behavioral changes in noncore group members.

Through partner notification, the sex (and needle-sharing) partners of persons with STDs are contacted, notified of their risk of exposure (without disclosing the identity of the original patient), educated about risky practices and prevention methods, and encouraged to come in for examination and possible treatment. This activity can affect all three factors in the equation: persons can reduce transmissibility (B) (for example by eliminating receptive anal intercourse or insisting on the use of condoms in all sexual activity); they can reduce the number of their sexual partners (c); or they can

be diagnosed and treated early in the progression of their own infection (D).

Surveillance is essential to assess the magnitude of the problem, identify groups at particular risk, monitor trends, and evaluate the impact of control programs. It is (or should be) a major determinant of program direction.

Control of HIV

With particular regard to HIV, it must be recognized that the HIV epidemic is not a monolithic event. Rather, it is a number of epidemics with varying primary means of transmission and different rates of spread in different areas and in different segments of society.[27] These may call for different approaches. Freedom from discrimination and guaranteed confidentiality are essential to prevention programs. Current HIV prevention efforts focus on: preventing initiation of the behaviors and conditions that put individuals at risk of acquiring or spreading the virus and modifying behaviors to reduce the likelihood of transmission if exposure occurs.

Education

Education, the chief approach for preventing the initiation of risky behaviors, takes place at several levels—societal, group, and individual. Societal approaches may involve mass media efforts to inform the public and prevent discrimination against those infected with HIV. School-based educational programs are another societal approach to primary prevention. These programs may be effective in encouraging students not to use drugs, to delay sexual activity, and to adopt safe sex practices when they do become sexually active. The emphasis should be on skill development as well as on knowledge. It is important to be aware that the impact of these efforts may not be immediate.

Outreach

Perceived social norms within peer groups are also important determinants of behavior. Because some health agencies may not have established ties or credibility with many of the persons who engage in risky behavior, community-based nongovernmental organizations and direct outreach programs have been crucial in reaching these persons with approaches that are culturally sensitive and linguistically appropriate. For example, recovering addicts may be used to contact injecting drug users who are not yet in drug treatment programs. The outreach workers stress the need for behavior change, the need to eliminate or reduce risk of infection or transmission, the benefits of knowing one's HIV infection status, and the need to support others as they attempt to sustain no-risk or low-risk behaviors.

Counseling

Individual educational approaches are another key component. Counseling before and after HIV testing is a critical opportunity to discuss the risk of infection and the ways in which risk can be reduced or eliminated. Counseling and testing are among the largest components of the current HIV prevention program in the United States. The primary public health purposes of counseling and testing are (1) to allow persons at risk of HIV infection to learn their HIV status, (2) to help uninfected persons initiate and sustain behavioral changes that reduce their risk of becoming infected, and (3) to assist those already infected to avoid infecting others. In addition, counseling and testing are a gateway to other services, and they provide the starting point for partner notification, in which sex and needle-sharing partners of infected persons are contacted and offered HIV counseling and testing. Partner notification provides a vital one-to-one education interaction with persons who may be unaware of their risk of infection.

Risk Reduction

The only sure way to prevent transmission of HIV is to avoid sex with an HIV-infected person and to avoid injecting drugs. However, sexual abstinence is rarely achievable, and only a fraction of injecting drug users become permanently drug free. Consequently, it is important to provide information on means of reducing

risk, for example by using condoms, avoiding anal intercourse, not sharing needles, and cleaning "works" with bleach.

Clinical Services

In addition to the education approaches, several clinical services are important in preventing HIV transmission. Of utmost importance is protection of the blood supply through testing of all donor blood. Other clinical services include treatment of other STDs, which may increase the risk of HIV transmission, treatment of drug addiction, treatment of tuberculosis infection, and provision of contraceptive services. These services can be incentives for persons at high risk to participate in prevention programs. Antiviral treatment, when demonstrated to reduce infectivity in persons who are infected, is also an important component of prevention programs. Another important component is the education of health care workers in the use of universal precautions that reduce the risk of nosocomial transmission.

Voltaire's phrase, "the best is the enemy of the good,"[28] applies to HIV prevention and to other preventive measures. In some situations, the insistence on only the "best" solution to a given health problem may interfere with the incremental, partially effective steps that are collectively necessary in mounting effective (but not perfect) prevention programs. In fact, if the imperfect approach is more acceptable to the target population than the perfect one, it may ultimately have a greater effect on the occurrence of disease.

Summary

The HIV epidemic and other major health problems are not monolithic events that happen in the same way or at the same rate in all groups. Nor are they uniformly susceptible to any single intervention. Controlling the HIV epidemic and solving other problems will require different, mutually reinforcing techniques to reach the myriad of groups in this pluralistic society. Until more effective (or even "perfect") approaches are available, partially effective approaches should be more fully implemented. The world is not a perfect place, and the quest for solutions must reflect that fact.[29]

TUBERCULOSIS

At the turn of the twentieth century, tuberculosis (TB) was the leading cause of death in the United States. TB is caused by *Mycobacterium tuberculosis*, a bacterium primarily transmitted through inhalation of airborne bacilli or droplet nuclei. Initial infection is usually not noticed but is accompanied by an immune response manifested by development of a positive reaction to purified protein derivative (PPD) applied intradermally.

Only five to ten percent of immunocompetent infected persons ultimately go on to develop tuberculosis disease at any time in their lives. However, for those with impaired immune systems the risk of developing active TB is much higher (on the order of seven to ten percent per year for those with HIV infection).[30] Clinical manifestations of TB commonly involve fever, weight loss, and cough, reflecting pulmonary infection. Persons with pulmonary TB may develop cavitary lesions visible on chest X ray and may excrete large numbers of organisms when they cough or sneeze.

For those excreting large numbers of bacilli (who are presumably most infectious), it may be possible to visualize characteristic acid-fast bacilli (AFB) on direct smear of the sputum. For others, however, diagnosis of TB is made difficult by the fact that the causative organisms are slow growing and it may take three to six weeks for a culture to become positive and then another three to four weeks to determine antibiotic susceptibility. During this time the patient may remain infectious if not started on appropriate therapy.

Prevention and Control

The approach to TB prevention and control in the United States has two major components. One is the identification and treatment of persons with TB disease. This both cures their infection and prevents transmission to others. The other is the identification and treatment of those with TB infection to prevent their subsequent development of the disease.

Management of TB disease (or latent infection) is made difficult by the fact that treatment (either for infection or disease) involves six months or more of medication. Consequently, patient adherence to therapy is a major problem, and inconsistent adherence to therapy may result in the emergence of organisms resistant to the drugs being administered. Fortunately, directly observed therapy (DOT), in which a health worker personally gives medication to the patient and observes that it is taken, has been shown to be a highly effective way of assuring completion of therapy.[31]

History

Reported mortality from TB has declined steadily since the beginning of the twentieth century as a result of the isolation of infected individuals in sanatoriums and improvements in nutrition and housing. TB first became reportable on a nationwide basis in 1952, and from that time until 1985, there was a steady decline in reported incidence, averaging four to five percent per year. These trends are shown in Figure 20.2. The breaks in the curve in 1963 and 1975 resulted from changes in definitions of reportable cases.

During the late 1960s and early 1970s, virtually all TB sanatoriums were closed. Unfortunately, the savings realized by this action were not matched by a redirection of funds to establish an adequate outpatient management system. Nonetheless, TB rates continued to decline. Because of the favorable trends in TB incidence, it was believed that TB might be eliminated from the United States. An Advisory Committee on the Elimination of Tuberculosis was formed, and in 1989 it released a *Strategic Plan for Elimination of Tuberculosis in the United States*.[32] The plan defined the target as an incidence of TB less than one case per million population by the year 2010. An interim target for the year 2000 was an incidence of 35 cases per million. The plan described three components: (1) more effective use of existing prevention and control methods; (2) development and evaluation of new prevention, diagnostic, and treatment technologies; and (3) technology assessment and transfer.

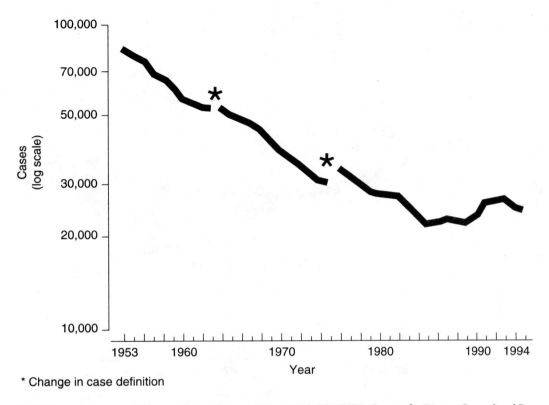

FIGURE 20.2 Reported TB cases United States, 1953 to 1994. SOURCE: Centers for Disease Control and Prevention, unpublished data.

The plan was widely endorsed and increased resources were made available to TB control programs, although not in the amounts felt necessary to fully implement the elimination program. In the late 1980s the incidence of TB plateaued and then began to rise; there was a 20 percent increase in reported numbers of cases between 1985 and 1992. Assuming that the reported incidence should have continued to decline at the rate it did from 1980 to 1985, it is estimated that more than 63,000 *excess* cases of TB occurred during the period 1986 to 1993. These trends are shown in Figure 20.3.

TB in the United States Today

The recent increase in the incidence of TB is ascribed to at least four factors: (1) deterioration of the public health infrastructure; (2) immigration of persons from countries with high prevalence of TB; (3) the HIV epidemic; and (4) outbreaks of TB (particularly multidrug-resistant TB [MDR-TB]) in congregative settings such as hospitals, correctional facilities, and shelters for the homeless, among others.

The deterioration of the public health infrastructure is not easy to document, although it is widely accepted as a fact. One indicator of deterioration is the declining proportion of patients who complete six continuous months of therapy. According to unpublished CDC data, this fell from 86 percent in 1987 to 81 percent in 1991. Between 1986 and 1992, the absolute number of cases of TB occurring in persons born in another country increased by more than 50 percent, and the proportion of all cases they represented increased from 21 percent to 27 percent.[33] Approximately half of these persons had been in the United States for less

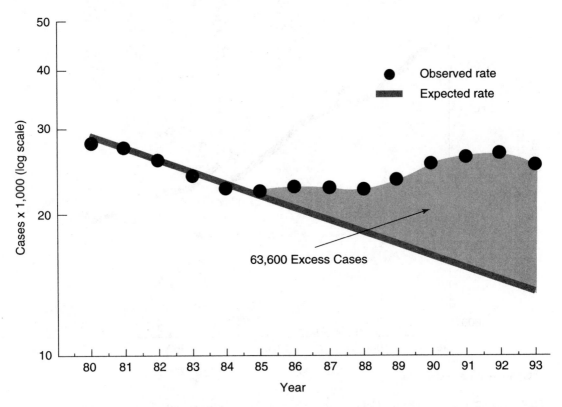

FIGURE 20.3 Expected and observed TB cases United States, 1980 to 1993. SOURCE: Centers for Disease Control and Prevention, unpublished data.

than five years and probably arrived in this country infected with TB.

It is not currently possible to estimate exactly what proportion of TB is related to HIV infection nationwide. However, blinded HIV serosurveys have been carried out in 30 or more TB clinics nationwide. These demonstrate a range of HIV infection in TB patients of from 0 to over 60 percent; the pooled seroprevalence increased from 13.1 percent in 1989 to 21.4 percent in 1991. These figures are based on unpublished data from the CDC. In some areas it is clear that coinfection with HIV plays a major role in recent increases in incidence of TB.

Multidrug–Resistant Tuberculosis

Recent outbreaks of MDR-TB in congregative settings have usually been associated with failures in ap-

propriate infection control procedures, including early diagnosis and treatment, appropriate isolation, use of environmental controls such as negative–pressure isolation rooms and ultraviolet germicidal irradiation (UVGI), and use of appropriate personal respiratory protective devices.[34] The outbreaks have typically involved HIV-infected patients and health care personnel and have been characterized by death–case ratios of 80 percent or greater.

To respond to this challenge, a national task force was formed and developed the *National Action Plan to Combat Multidrug-Resistant Tuberculosis,* first released in April, 1992.[35] The action plan elaborates on the earlier *Strategic Plan to Eliminate Tuberculosis* and has guided governmental activities since its release. It identifies 38 specific problems in nine major areas, defines objectives to address each of the problems, describes implementation steps to achieve the objectives, identifies the responsible organization(s) for carrying out the implementation steps, and gives starting dates for each of the steps. The nine primary areas of activity described in the Action Plan are surveillance and epidemiology, laboratory diagnosis, patient management, screening and preventive therapy, infection control, outbreak control, program evaluation, information dissemination/training and education, and research. Substantially increased federal resources have been made available to implement the plan, although they have not yet reached the amount estimated for full implementation.

Although the emergence of MDR-TB has posed a significant problem in some areas of the country, it should be remembered that approximately 40 percent of all counties in the United States are free of reported TB and that in 25 states and the District of Columbia, the reported incidence in 1992 was lower than that in 1991. In these areas, continuation of currently successful approaches is warranted. In areas that are particularly affected by immigration, HIV-TB, and/or MDR-TB, intensified activities will be needed. Even though the reported incidence of TB rose in this country as a result of identifiable problems, it appears that the elimination target is still realistic if effective implementation of aggressive prevention and control strategies is maintained, although achievement of the target may be slightly delayed.[36] As a result of increased efforts, the reported incidence of TB declined in 1993 and 1994.

FOODBORNE AND WATERBORNE DISEASE

A variety of parasitic, bacterial, and viral diseases can be transmitted through food and water. Disease occurs either from infection or from intoxication. Some diseases, such as giardiasis and typhoid fever, result from ingestion of small numbers of microorganisms which subsequently multiply and cause disease, either local or invasive. Others, such as cholera and diarrhea caused by enterotoxigenic *E. coli*, result from ingestion of living bacteria that multiply and elaborate toxins, which act on intestinal mucosa to cause diarrhea. Some conditions such as botulism or *Clostridium perfringens* food poisoning result from ingestion of toxin formed by organisms multiplying in the food before it is eaten. Finally, some fish and shellfish may contain toxins that cause neuromuscular symptoms. Food and water can also carry natural or synthetic toxins (for example, metals, plant toxins, and insecticides).

These illnesses may vary greatly in symptoms. Some are characterized by mild nausea, vomiting, and diarrhea (most *Salmonella* infections). Others may be associated with life-threatening profuse diarrhea (cholera), hemorrhagic diarrhea with hemolytic-uremic syndrome (*E. coli* 0157:H7), sepsis (typhoid), infectious hepatitis (hepatitis A), miscarriage (*Listeria monocytogenes*), or cranial nerve and respiratory paralysis (botulism).

Waterborne Diseases

Waterborne illness is now relatively uncommon in the United States as a result of the protection of water supplies, prevention of cross–connections between water and sewage systems, and the use of chlorination. If water supplies become contaminated large numbers of persons may become ill. During a 1965 outbreak of waterborne salmonellosis in Riverside, California, an estimated 16,000 persons became ill.[37] More than 400,000 persons became ill with waterborne cryptosporidiosis in Milwaukee in 1992, according to unpublished CDC data.

Foodborne Diseases

Foodborne illness remains common and causes an estimated 6.5 million cases of human illness and 9,000 deaths annually in this country.[38] *Salmonella* is the most commonly reported bacterial cause of foodborne outbreaks, accounting for 28 percent of outbreaks of known etiology and 45 percent of outbreak-associated cases during 1973 to 1987.[39] Foodborne disease outbreaks may range from one or two cases to hundreds or thousands. Outbreaks are often caused by foods of animal origin that become contaminated during slaughter or processing and are subsequently subjected to inadequate cooking or other food handling practices. For example, *E. coli* 0157:H7 lives in the intestines of healthy cattle and can contaminate meat during slaughter. If the meat is not subsequently thoroughly cooked it can cause illness. Recent outbreaks were associated with undercooked hamburger patties.[40]

Prevention of foodborne illness involves preventing initial contamination; cooking foods properly to destroy organisms that are present; preventing cross-contamination or recontamination (as can occur when cooked foods are sliced with a knife or on a cutting board contaminated by raw food or are placed back in containers from which they came before cooking); preventing incubation of microorganisms (keeping cold foods cold and hot foods hot); and ensuring other appropriate food–handling practices.

CONCLUSION

Infectious diseases remain significant causes of human morbidity and mortality. The current low rates in the United States reflect active control measures that range from simple sanitation to vector control to complex schedules of immunization. However, it must be remembered that infectious diseases are merely being kept at bay; relaxation of control efforts can and will lead to a resurgence unless the disease has been eradicated. We also have recent experience with emergence of new or modified diseases (for example, AIDS, and *E. coli* O157:H7), which pose new threats to health and necessitate maintenance of surveillance and response capability.[41]

REFERENCES

1. Hinman AR. Control of communicable diseases. In: Wallace HM, Patrick K, Parcel GS, Igoe JB, eds. *Principles and Practices of Student Health*. Oakland, Ca: Third Party Publishing Co; 1992:53–62.

2. Gustafson TL, Lavely GB, Brawner ER Jr, et al. An outbreak of airborne nosocomial varicella. *Pediatr.* 1982;70:550–556.

3. Bloch AB, Orenstein WA, Ewing WM, et al. Measles outbreak in a pediatric practice: airborne transmission in an office setting. *Pediatr.* 1985;75:676–683.

4. Orenstein WA, Bernier RH. Surveillance: information for action. *Pediatr Clin North Am.* 1990;37:709–734.

5. Benenson AS, ed. *Control of Communicable Diseases in Man,* 15th ed. Washington, DC: American Public Health Association; 1990.

6. Strebel PM, Sutter RW, Cochi SL, et al. Epidemiology of poliomyelitis in the United States one decade after the last reported case of indigenous wild virus-associated disease. *Clin Infect Dis.* 1992;14:568–579.

7. Centers for Disease Control, Immunization Practices Advisory Committee (ACIP). General recommendations on immunization. *MMWR.* 1989;38:205-214,219–227.

8. Wright PF, Kim-Farley RJ, de Quadros CA, et al. Strategies for the global eradication of poliomyelitis by the year 2000. *NEJM.* 1991;325:1774–1779.

9. de Quadros CA, Olive JM, Carrasco P, et al. Update: eradication of paralytic poliomyelitis in the Americas. *MMWR.* 1992;41:681–683.

10. Adams WG, Deaver KA, Cochi SL, et al. Decline of childhood *Haemophilus influenzae* type b (Hib) disease in the Hib vaccine era. *JAMA.* 1993;269:221–226.

11. American Academy of Pediatrics. *Report of the Committee on Infectious Diseases.* 22nd ed. Elk Grove Village, Il: American Academy of Pediatrics; 1991.

12. The National Vaccine Advisory Committee. The measles epidemic: the problems, barriers, and recommendations. *JAMA.* 1991;266:1547–1552.

13. Ad Hoc Working Group for the Development of Standards for Pediatric Immunization Practices. Standards for pediatric immunization practices. *JAMA.* 1993;269:1817–1822.

14. Centers for Disease Control and Prevention. Recommended childhood immunization schedule—United States, 1995. *MMWR.* 1995;44(No. RR-5):1–9.

15. Centers for Disease Control. Vaccination against smallpox in the United States: a reevaluation of the risks and benefits. *MMWR.* 1971;20:339–345.

16. Orenstein WA, Hinman AR, Bart KJ, Hadler SC. Immunization. In: Mandell GL, Douglas RG Jr, Bennett JE, eds. *Principles and Practice of Infectious Diseases.* Fourth edition. New York: Churchill Livingstone; 1995.

17. Howson CP, Howe CJ, Fineberg HV, eds. *Adverse Effects of Pertussis and Rubella Vaccines.* Washington, DC: Institute of Medicine, National Academy Press; 1991.

18. Stratton KR, Howe CJ, Johnson RB Jr, eds. *Adverse Events Associated with Childhood Vaccines: Evidence Bearing on Causality.* Washington, DC: Institute of Medicine, National Academy Press; 1993.

19. Hinman AR. The National Vaccine Program and the National Vaccine Injury Compensation Program. *Food Drug Cosmetic Law J.* 1989;44:633–637.

20. Mitchell VS, Philipose NM, Sanford JP, eds. *The Children's Vaccine Initiative: Achieving the Vision.* Washington, DC: Institute of Medicine, National Academy Press; 1993.

21. Orenstein WA, Bernier RH, Dondero TJ, et al. Field evaluation of vaccine efficacy. *Bull WHO.* 1985;63:1055–1068.

22. Cates W Jr, Hinman AR. Sexually transmitted diseases in the 1990s. *NEJM.* 1991;325:1368–1370.

23. Hinman AR, Wasserheit JN, Kamb ML. Potential impact of STD prevention programmes. In: Rashad H, Gray R, Boerna T, eds. *Evaluation of the Impact of Health Interventions.* Liege: International Union for the Scientific Study of Population; 1995.

24. Anderson RM. The transmission dynamics of sexually transmitted diseases: the behavioral component. In: Wasserheit JN, Aral SO, Holmes KK, Hitchcock PJ, eds. *Research Issues in Human Behavior and Sexually Transmitted Diseases in the AIDS Era.* Washington, DC: American Society of Microbiology; 1992: 38–60.

25. Brunham RC, Ronald AR. Epidemiology of sexually transmitted diseases in developing countries. In: Wasserheit JN, Aral SO, Holmes KK, Hitchcock PJ, eds. *Research Issues in Human Behavior and Sexually Transmitted Diseases in the AIDS Era.* Washington, DC: American Society for Microbiology; 1991: 61–80.

26. Holmes KK, Aral SO. Behavioral interventions in developing countries. In: Wasserheit JN, Aral SO, Holmes KK, Hitchcock PJ, eds. *Research Issues in Human Behavior and Sexually Transmitted Diseases in the AIDS Era.* Washington, DC: American Society for Microbiology; 1992:318–344.

27. Hinman AR. Strategies to prevent HIV infection in the United States. *Am J Pub Health.* 1991;81:1557–1559.

28. Kaplan J, ed. *Bartlett's Familiar Quotations.* 16th ed. Boston: Little, Brown & Co.; 1992:306.

29. Cates W Jr, Hinman AR. AIDS and absolutism: the demand for perfection in prevention. *NEJM.* 1992;327:492–494.

30. Selwyn PA, Hartel D, Lewis VA, et al. A prospective study of the risk of tuberculosis among intravenous drug users with human immunodeficiency virus infection. *NEJM.* 1989;320: 545–550.

31. American Thoracic Society. Intermittent chemotherapy for adults with tuberculosis. *Am Rev Respir Dis.* 1974;110: 374–375.

32. Centers for Disease Control. A strategic plan for the elimination of tuberculosis in the United States. *MMWR.* 1989;38 (No. S-3):1–25.

33. Centers for Disease Control and Prevention. Tuberculosis Morbidity—United States, 1992. *MMWR.* 1993;42:696–697, 703–704.

34. Hinman AR, Hughes JM, Snider DE Jr, Cohen ML. Meeting the challenge of multidrug-resistant tuberculosis: summary of a conference. *MMWR.* 1992;41(No. RR-11):49–57.

35. Centers for Disease Control. National action plan to combat multidrug-resistant tuberculosis. *MMWR.* 1992;41(No. RR-11):1–48.

36. Hinman AR, Hughes JM. The strategic plan to eliminate tuberculosis in the United States and the national action plan to combat multidrug–resistant tuberculosis. In: Rossman MD, MacGregor RR, eds. *Tuberculosis: Clinical Management and New Challenges.* New York: McGraw Hill; 1995.

37. Collaborative Report: A waterborne epidemic of Salmonellosis in Riverside, California, 1965. *Am J Epidemiol.* 1971; 93:33.

38. Bennett JV, Holmberg SD, Rogers MF, Solomon SL. Infectious and parasitic diseases. In: Amler RW, Dull HB, eds. Closing the gap: the burden of unnecessary illness. *Am J Prev Med.* 1987;3(suppl):102–114.

39. Bean NH, Griffin PM. Foodborne disease outbreaks in the United States, 1973-1987: pathogens, vehicles and trends. *J Food Protect.* 1990;53:804–817.

40. Centers for Disease Control. Multistate outbreak of *E. coli* 0157:H7 infections. *MMWR.* 1993;42:258–263.

41. Lederberg J, Shope RE, Oaks SC Jr, eds. *Emerging Infections: Microbial Threats to Health in the United States.* Washington, DC: National Academy Press; 1992.

CHAPTER

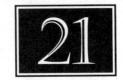

Environmental Health and Protection

Larry J. Gordon, M.S., M.P.H.

Public and scientific concern regarding the quality of the environment and related health and ecological considerations has never been more intense. Civic and political leaders, whether liberal, moderate, or conservative, express the need for effective environmental health and protection measures.[1] There is a challenge to provide effective environmental health and protection services that balance public demands with sound scientific principles.

This chapter provides an overview of the field of environmental health and protection, including its history, scope, and mission. The areas of risk assessment and communication are elaborated upon in particular. Environmental health and protection organizations at all levels are described, and program design and support are discussed. Prevention, personnel, access to services, and continuing education are also addressed. The chapter concludes with a look at future prospects in this field.

OVERVIEW

Environmental health and protection services are integral components of the continuum of health services,

as shown in Figure 21.1. They are essential precursors to the efficacy of the other components of the health services continuum. Other health services include personal public health services (population-based disease prevention and health promotion) and health care (diagnosis, treatment, and rehabilitation of a patient under care on a one-on-one basis).[2]

Environmental health and protection problems range from the transmission of disease agents to a susceptible population through food, water, wastes, and air, to unhealthful exposure to toxic chemicals and radiation. Such problems associated with the modern environment continue to become increasingly complex and, in some cases, may have become intractable.

Environmental problems impact human health as well as ecological relationships, and they are closely interrelated. The basic causes of these problems are population growth and distribution, which in turn create problems associated with resource development and consumption, technology, energy production and utilization, transportation, wastes, and urbanization. The ecological maxim that "everything is connected to

Health Services Continuum: Examples of Issues

Environmental Health and Protection	Health Promotion	Disease Prevention	Health Care
clean air	substance abuse	infectious diseases	diagnosis
clean water	family planning	clinical prevention	primary care
toxic chemicals	nutrition	PKU screening	case management
safe food	health education	glaucoma	outpatient services
radiation	violence	diabetes	clinics
solid wastes	obesity	osteoporosis	treatment
occupational health	tobacco	cancer	surgery
hazardous wastes	mental health	suicides	long-term care
risk assessment	physical activity and fitness	oral health	acute case
risk communication		heart disease and stroke	rehabilitation
risk management	access		cost containment
global degradation		maternal and child health	health insurance
land use		access	mental health and treatment
noise			
disease vectors			developmental disabilities
housing			
ecological dysfunction			alcohol and drug treatment
unintentional injuries			
access			access

FIGURE 21.1 SOURCE: McFarlane D, Gordon L. Teaching health policy and politics in US schools of public health. *J Public Health Policy.* 13(4):428–434.

everything else" has become increasingly apparent. Solutions to society's environmental health and protection problems are as complex as their nature and causes, involving both the public and private sectors.

Such solutions not only impact the health of the public and the quality of the environment, but they impact the economy as well. Solutions require qualified personnel, an informed and supportive citizenry, environmental health and protection leadership, impeccable scientific research, adequate data to measure and understand problems and trends, a healthy economy, rational public and private sector policies, workable legislation, and financing prioritized to deal with the more important problems as determined by sound epidemiology, toxicology, and risk assessment.[3(pp28–32)]

Historical Perspective

Environmental health and personal public health measures have always been the two major components of the field of public health practice. Early public health efforts were developed largely to address serious environmental health problems such as contaminated drinking water, disease-transmitting milk, insects and rodents, garbage, and unsafe food. Sanitary engineers and sanitarians were early-day leaders in designing and implementing effective measures to prevent disease and protect the health of the public.

Selected excerpts from the 1850 *Report of the Sanitary Commission of Massachusetts*[4] indicate a visionary understanding of the importance of environmental health and protection issues. Consider the following:

> We recommend that provision be made for obtaining observations of the atmospheric phenomena, on a systematic and uniform plan, at different stations within the Commonwealth . . . We recommend that measures be taken to prevent, as far as possible, the smoke nuisance.

The report also notes that " . . . the tendency of our people seems to be toward social concentration . . ." The report continues:

> We recommend that, in laying out new towns and villages, and in extending those already laid out, ample provision be made for a supply, in purity and abundance, of light, air, and water; for drainage and sewerage, for paving, and for cleanliness.

The report contains additional recommendations relating to housing, schools, occupational health, and adulterated food and drugs. The report also recommends that persons be specially educated in sanitary science. All of these recommendations are still sound today.

Scope

The scope of environmental health and protection has expanded and become more complex. It is essential to discuss environmental health by using the terminology environmental health *and* environmental protection, rather than environmental health *or* environmental protection. To an undesirable extent, the two have become separated and utilized to denote programs based on organizational settings rather than on logical or definable differences in programs, missions, or goals. This distinction is artificial and has led to inappropriate organizational separation of activities that share the common goals of protecting the public's health and enhancing environmental quality. In some cases, the separate terminology has created organizational barriers rather than essential bridges among the organizations involved in the struggle for environmental quality.

The programmatic scope of environmental health and protection includes, but is not limited to:

- ambient air quality
- water pollution control
- safe drinking water
- indoor air quality
- noise pollution control
- radiation protection
- food protection
- occupational health and safety
- meat inspection
- disaster response
- cross-connection elimination
- shellfish sanitation and certification
- institutional sanitation
- pure food control
- housing conditions

- recreational area sanitation
- poultry inspection
- solid waste management
- hazardous waste management
- vector control
- pesticide control
- land use
- milk sanitation
- toxic chemical control
- unintentional injuries
- prevention of ecological dysfunction.

In addition, there are global environmental health and protection issues, such as habitat destruction, species extinction, possible global warming and stratospheric ozone depletion, planetary toxification, desertification, deforestation, and overpopulation. Indeed, excessive population growth contributes to all of the foregoing problems as well as to famine, war, disease, social disruption, illegal immigration, economic failures, and resource and energy shortages.

Definition

Environmental health and protection can be defined as the art and science of protecting against environmental factors that may adversely impact human health or adversely impact the ecological balances essential to long-term human health and environmental quality. Such factors include, but are not limited to, air, food, and water contaminants; radiation; toxic chemicals; wastes; disease vectors; safety hazards; and habitat alterations.[4] This definition is illustrated by Figure 21.2.

Public health personnel have traditionally justified, designed, and managed environmental programs based on public health components. However, as environmental problems, priorities, public perception and involvement, goals, and public policy have evolved, ecological considerations have become increasingly important. Whatever long-term human health threats exist, both the public and public policy leaders know that pollution is also killing fish, limiting visibility, creating stenches, ruining lakes and rivers, degrading recreational areas, and endangering plant and animal life.

The 1990 report of the United States Environmental Protection Agency's Science Advisory Board, *Reducing Risk: Setting Priorities and Strategies for Environmental Protection,* states:

> . . . there is no doubt that over time the quality of human life declines as the quality of natural ecosystems declines . . . over the past 20 years and especially over the past decade, EPA has paid too little attention to natural ecosystems. The Agency has considered the protection of public health to be its primary mission, and it has been less concerned about risks posed to ecosystems . . . EPA's response to human health risks as compared to ecological risks is inappropriate, because, in the real world, there is little distinction between the two. Over the long term, ecological degradation either directly or indirectly degrades human health and the economy . . . human health and welfare ultimately rely upon the life support systems and natural resources provided by healthy ecosystems.[5]

Mission

Environmental health and protection agencies should have the mission of delivering services in such a manner as to protect the health of the public and the quality of the environment. Additionally, environmental health and protection agencies should have the mission of stimulating interest in related areas where they may not have primary responsibility and technical expertise. For example, it may be desirable to support and promote such environmental health and protection-related activities as long-range community planning, zoning ordinances, plumbing codes, building codes, solid waste systems, economic development, energy conservation, and transportation systems.

Other agencies, such as agriculture departments, have an obvious and appropriate mission to promote and protect a given industry or segment of public interest. Conflicts of interest occur when missions are mixed, thereby resulting in the familiar "fox in the henhouse" syndrome. Such conflicts of interest result in the public being defrauded rather than receiving the protection they deserve. If environmental health and protection agencies do not fully develop and understand the necessity of a mission of protecting the health of the public and the quality of the

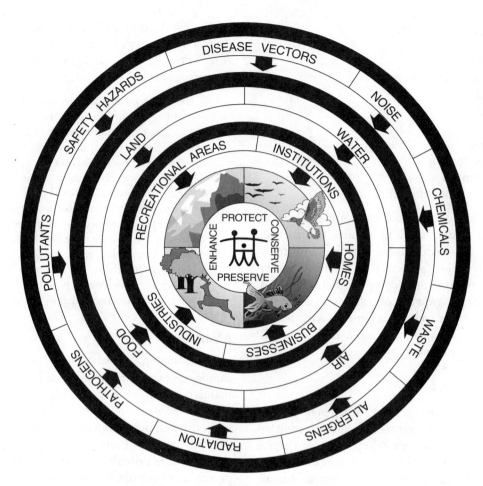

FIGURE 21.2 SOURCE: Gordon LJ. *New Mexico Environmental Improvement Agency Guide.* Santa Fe, NM: New Mexico Environmental Protection Agency; 1972.

environment, they may end up actually protecting or promoting the interests of those they are charged with regulating.

Goal

The goal of environmental health and protection is to ensure an environment that will provide optimal health, safety, ecological well-being, and quality of life for this and future generations. When goals are set, it is important to realize that we do not live in a risk-free society or environment. Therefore, the appropriate goal for many environmental health and protection

programs may not always be *zero risk*. The pursuit of zero risk as a goal is frequently unnecessary, economically impractical, often unattainable, and likely to create unfounded public concern when zero risk is not attained. Additionally, the pursuit of zero risk as a goal for one issue may preclude resource availability for other priorities.

Priorities

Globally, priority environmental health and protection issues include species extinction; wastes; desertification; deforestation; possible global warming and stratospheric ozone depletion (legitimate scientific debate continues over these two issues); planetary toxification; and, most importantly, overpopulation.[3(pp28–32)] Priorities for environmental health and protection programs vary nationally as well as regionally.

In addition, the public and political perceptions of risks and priorities frequently differ from those of environmental health and protection scientists. For example, a December 1991 survey (conducted by the Institute for Regulatory Policy) of nearly 1,300 health professionals in the fields of epidemiology, toxicology, medicine, and other health sciences indicated that over 81 percent of the professionals surveyed believe that public health dollars for reduction of environmental health risks in the United States are improperly targeted.[6]

A 1990 Roper poll determined that at least 20 percent of the United States public considered hazardous waste sites to be the most significant environmental issue. Contrary to this public perception, however, the 1990 report of EPA's Science Advisory Board[5] listed ambient air pollution, worker exposure to chemicals, indoor pollution, and drinking water pollutants as the major risks to human health. Although not EPA programs, food protection and unintentional injuries should be added to this list. Legitimate scientific debate continues over the proper standard and measures for childhood lead poisoning, but many researchers believe that childhood lead poisoning should also be a high-priority issue.

The same EPA report included as risks to the natural ecology and human welfare habitat alteration and destruction; species extinction and overall loss of biological diversity; stratospheric ozone depletion; global climate change; herbicides and pesticides; toxics, nutrients, biochemical oxygen demand, and turbidity in surface waters; acid deposition; and airborne toxics. Among relatively low risks to the natural ecology and human welfare, the report listed oil spills, groundwater pollution, radionuclides, acid runoff to surface waters, and thermal pollution.

Healthy People 2000[7] also suggests environmental health objectives from the viewpoint of the United States Public Health Service.

ASSESSING AND COMMUNICATING RISKS

Considering the serious differences in recommended priorities advocated by scientists as compared with those advocated by the public and by political leaders, risk assessment must be considered a high-priority issue to be understood and practiced by all those involved in protecting the health of the public and the quality of the environment. These individuals must effectively communicate risks to the public and to policy makers.

Risk Assessment

Utilizing sound scientific principles to assess risk is vital to recommending priorities, designing environmental health and protection programs, requesting funds, and evaluating control efforts. In addition to assessing human health risk, risk assessment procedures may also be utilized to determine ecological, economic, and quality of human life impacts. Models used to determine risk commonly consider hazard identification, exposure assessment, amount or dose-response, and risk characterization.

The EPA requests and budgets funds based on relative risk to human health. But it is placing increased emphasis on ecological risk. The effort to base funding on relative risk has not been entirely successful, however, for a number of reasons, including: the impact of public sentiment; the efforts of various environmental activist groups that frequently have their own priorities and agendas; and the nature of the congressional committee system whereby committees jealously protect their own environmental turf.

Risk Assessment Models

Like other statistical processes, the findings of risk assessment models may vary considerably depending on the assumptions, data, and models utilized. Serious debate continues over the validity of risk assessment models and methods. Understandably, such differences are confusing to public policy makers and sometimes create a credibility gap concerning risk assessment as a useful process.

Risk assessment has always been utilized informally and even intuitively by public policy makers and environmental health and protection personnel. Utilizing risk assessment mathematical models is a comparatively recent development. Whenever a decision or recommendation has been made to develop a policy or manage an environmental problem based on available information, a risk assessment has been performed. At times, environmental personnel must make major emergency decisions based on incomplete but compelling information without having the luxury of waiting until incontrovertible evidence is available.

For the most part, human health risk assessment models have been formulated to determine carcinogenic possibilities and are based on single agent exposures. It is necessary that models be developed to assess the effects of multiple exposures, agents, and synergism. Models should also reflect carcinogenicity, mutations, teratogenicity, altered reproductive function, mental health impacts, neurobehavioral toxicity, and other specific organ impacts.

Formal risk assessment procedures require the multidisciplinary involvement of personnel having a wide variety of knowledge and skills from such fields as epidemiology, toxicology, medicine, chemistry, biology, physics, meteorology, geology, mathematics, hydrology, and engineering. Despite such expertise, however, risk assessment remains as much an art as a science, and risk assessment models need significant improvement. Human health and the environment would be better served by having risk assessment recommendations developed by institutions separate from those having risk management responsibilities so as not to unduly skew or politicize the process.[9]

Every environmental health and protection practitioner need not be a technical expert in risk assessment modeling procedures but should understand their usefulness and limitations. Practitioners should understand that the public is barraged with "catastrophe-of-the-week" environmental information regarding risk, coupled with a paucity of critical scientific inquiry. Practitioners should also recognize that there would be many times the actual morbidity and mortality if all these predicted catastrophes were factual. Finally, practitioners should be scientifically critical, routinely questioning existing policies, standards, regulations, and proposals to assure that all measures reflect scientifically valid priorities and needs.

The Role of Other Factors in Risk Assessment

Risk assessment is only one of the factors to be used to determine priorities. Other considerations include social factors, economic factors, political factors, and technical feasibility. Community input and involvement are also essential. Otherwise, risk assessment may be seen by the community as a measure used to avoid community concerns in the absence of continuing risk communication.

Risk Communication

Experience indicates that many environmental health and protection practitioners have not demonstrated adequate knowledge and skills as risk communicators. This is one of the reasons environmental health and protection priorities and policies frequently differ from those recommended by scientists. In the absence of continuing effective risk communication, sound risk assessment is merely an academic exercise. Many practitioners continue to confuse public information and the distribution of public information materials with the art of risk communication.

Risk communication is an art requiring complete openness throughout any planning and decision process. It requires embracing, including, and involving appropriate interest groups. Failures to communicate risk and develop scientifically valid priorities and policies are frequently linked to the failure to involve and educate the public and appropriate interest groups throughout the process and the failure to openly discuss the needs, assumptions, alternatives, and data on which risk has been assessed.

Like risk assessment, risk communication is both interdisciplinary and multidisciplinary. Essential knowledge and skills are derived from such fields as sociology, political science, education, and marketing.

How well the environment is protected and disease and disability prevented in the future will depend less on technical skills alone and more on the ability to listen to, understand, value, and incorporate other community perspectives. It will also depend on how well we are able to communicate our knowledge, not as *the* solution but as *part* of the solution. Those environmental health and protection professionals who are successful at combining technical skills with community skills, including risk communication, will be most successful at developing environmental policies and programs that are supported by the public and therefore effective in the long run. (Personal communication from S. B. Kotchian, December 29, 1993)

ORGANIZATIONS

This section discusses environmental health and protection organizations at all levels—local, state, and federal. The history and diversification of these organizations is also outlined.

History

Until the late 1960s and early 1970s, organizational models for the delivery of environmental health services at the federal, state, and local levels were reasonably standard. At the federal level, most environmental health responsibilities, as they then existed, were lodged within the Consumer Protection and Environmental Health Service of the United States Public Health Service (USPHS). Notable exceptions included water pollution control, which had previously been transferred from the USPHS to the Department of the Interior, as well as the pesticide regulation program of the Department of Agriculture.

In the various states, nearly all environmental health programs were organized within state health departments. At the local level, most environmental health activities were within the purview of local health departments. Significant exceptions included programs, such as air pollution control, that were assigned to special districts or regional authorities. In the western United States, a few jurisdictions created local environmental health departments or agencies in an attempt to assure greater emphasis on environmental

health and protection. Some of these are single purpose agencies, such as the Los Angeles Air Quality Management District; others are comprehensive in environmental health and protection services, including those in Albuquerque, New Mexico; San Bernardino County, California; Ventura County, California; Sacramento, California; and Mecklenburg County, North Carolina.

The Federal Level

During the late 1960s and early 1970s, the public became concerned and aroused over the deteriorating state of the environment. President Richard Nixon's Council on Executive Reorganization (known as the Ash Council), appointed in 1969, conducted extensive hearings and studies regarding establishment of a federal environmental organization and made recommendations to the president. Representatives of the Section on Environment of the American Public Health Association presented testimony to the Ash Committee, recommending that the scope of programs included in the new environmental agency be broader than the scope that was ultimately developed. The APHA section also recommended that the proposed environmental agency *not* be a component of the Department of the Interior, due to the obvious conflict of interest with the resource development responsibilities of the department. The environmental subcommittee of the Senate Committee on Public Works, chaired by Senator Edmund Muskie, also conducted lengthy hearings. Congress was convinced that a new agency should be developed to be the lead environmental agency and to aggressively administer a wide range of environmental programs.

President Nixon created the United States Environmental Protection Agency (EPA) by executive order on September 9, 1970. The order incorporated water pollution control and certain pesticide research functions from the Department of the Interior; water supply protection, solid waste management, air pollution control, radiation protection, and pesticide research from the Department of Health, Education and Welfare; pesticide regulation from the Department of Agriculture; and radiation standards from the Atomic Energy Commission and the Interagency Federal Radiation Council.[10]

In addition to the EPA, other significant environmental health and protection agencies of the federal government include:

- the Occupational Safety and Health Administration of the Department of Labor
- the Public Health Service (including the National Institute of Environmental Health Sciences, the Centers for Disease Control and Prevention, the Indian Health Service, the Food and Drug Administration, the Agency for Toxic Substances and Disease Registry, and the National Institute for Environmental Health and Safety)
- the Coast Guard
- the Geological Survey
- the National Oceanographic and Atmospheric Administration
- the Nuclear Regulatory Commission
- the Corps of Engineers
- the Department of Transportation
- the Department of Agriculture
- the Department of Housing and Urban Development.

Major departments administering proprietary environmental management programs include Defense, Energy, and Interior.

Environmental health and protection risk management largely ceased being a responsibility of state health departments and the United States Public Health Service following the creation of EPA. Citizen environmental activists and elected officials have tended to view EPA as a model for the states to emulate. The increasing emphasis on health care delivery in health departments has altered their role, frequently resulting in reduced visibility of and emphasis on environmental health and protection.

State Agencies

A 1993 study, conducted by the Johns Hopkins School of Public Health under contract with the USPHS Bureau of Health Professions, revealed that approximately 85 percent of state level environmental health and protection activities were being administered by environmental health and protection agencies other than traditional state health departments.[11] Environment-focused agencies developed programs that emphasized enforcement, inspection, monitoring, record keeping, remediation, standard setting, and litigation; by contrast, health department programs tended to emphasize epidemiology, health surveillance, risk assement, toxicology, education, communication, and consultation.

In the same study, every state indicated that multiple agencies were involved in environmental health and protection activities, and many states reported that as many as four agencies had environmental health and protection responsibilities. Data from the study also suggested that states spend approximately the same amounts on environmental health and protection as they do on all other public health activities combined.

Environmental health and protection agencies, regardless of their titles, are still components of the broad field of public health because their programs fall within any common definition of environmental health and protection and are based on achieving public health goals. Such agencies have various titles, such as departments of environment, environmental protection, ecology, labor, agriculture, environmental quality, natural resources, or pollution control.

In general, state environmental health and protection agencies are apt to have responsibilities for water pollution control, air pollution control, solid waste management, public water supplies, occupational health and safety, pesticide regulation, and radiation protection.[12] A number of states have transferred milk and food protection responsibilities to agriculture departments, despite the inherent and dangerous conflict of interest in having consumer protection activities administered by a department devoted to protecting and promoting the agriculture industry and agricultural productivity.

Local Agencies

The majority of local environmental health and protection activities remain the responsibility of local health departments. Local activities tend to be different in nature from those assigned to state agencies, focusing on such traditional programs as milk sanitation, food protection, recreational area sanitation, institutional sanitation, noise pollution control, on-site liquid waste disposal, safe drinking water, insect and rodent control, nuisance abatement, animal control, and, in some jurisdictions, housing conservation and rehabilitation. A few local jurisdictions administer comprehensive indoor and ambient air pollution control programs, and some are active in water pollution control, solid waste management, radiation control, and hazardous waste management.[13]

Many local governments have assigned certain environmental health and protection activities to other agencies, such as public works, housing, planning, councils of government, solid waste management, special purpose districts, and regional authorities.[14]

Federal, State, or Local?

Whenever possible, environmental health and protection services should be delivered by the agency that is closest to the people being served. A local community agency can do a better job of protecting the local environment than can a distant bureaucracy.[14] There are, however, certain issues that must be dealt with at higher levels of government.

Federal Level

Environmental issues best dealt with at the federal level include problems of an *interstate* nature, such as protection of food and food products, solid and hazardous wastes transportation, water pollution control, pesticide regulation, and air pollution resolution. All of these problems are handled by appropriate federal agencies. The federal government also has retained partial or sole authority for many activities that are federally mandated or funded, including but not limited to certain aspects of radioactive waste management, water pollution control and facilities construction, air pollution control, occupational safety and health, and safe drinking water. State and local governments have frequently accepted primacy for some of these activities, but they still must adhere to federal requirements. In addition, the federal government develops criteria, standards, and model legislation.

State Level

State agencies or special districts may find it easier to deal with certain issues on a problem basis rather than on a limited local jurisdiction basis. Examples include water pollution control, air pollution control, solid waste management, and milk sanitation. Also, in sparsely populated states and in rural areas of some other states, the state agency may exercise direct authority in all program areas. In addition, many state agencies provide technical and consultative support to local environmental health and protection agencies. Like federal agencies, state agencies may develop criteria, standards, and model legislation for state and/or local adoption. State agencies may also administer state and federal grant-in-aid funds for local agencies.

Problems at the Local Level

There may be a conflict of interest situation when local environmental health and protection agencies attempt to regulate local government proprietary functions, such as public water supply, solid waste disposal, and sewage treatment. In addition, smaller local agencies may not have expertise in such specialized areas as radiation protection, epidemiology, toxicology, and risk assessment. Thus, the federal government has encouraged states to accept primacy for certain functions, such as occupational safety and health, hazardous waste management, and safe drinking water, although some states have developed memoranda of understanding or joint powers agreements with local governments so that local agencies can play a role.

Diversification

The trend to organizationally diversify environmental health and protection programs and move them to organizations other than the health department will continue in response to several factors: the priority of environmental health and protection; the demands of environmental advocates; and the perception that many health departments have become significantly involved in health care to the detriment of environmental health and protection. That is, the increasing responsibilities of federal, state, and local health departments as providers of health care may translate into inadequate leadership and priority for environmental health and protection within health departments.[3(pp28–32)] Health departments have also found it difficult to deal with the ecological aspects of environmental health and protection.

The diversification of environmental health and protection services may be seen as a part of the nation's evolving governmental system. Such organizational diversification does not mean that environmental health and protection programs are no longer a basic component of the field of public health. While each community or state has only one health department, every community and state has many other public health agencies, including numerous environmental health and protection agencies.

The American Public Health Association's Program Development Board has noted that many public health services are administered by a wide array of agencies, including but not limited to health departments. In response, it has developed the following definitions to clarify relationships:

> A "health department" is an agency of government that includes the words "health department" in its title and is charged with delivering identifiable services designed to prevent or solve health problems.

> A "health agency" is an agency of government charged with delivering identifiable health services designed to prevent or solve health problems. (Written communication from George C. Pickett, Chair, APHA Program Development Board)

Summary

Environmental health and protection, like other components of public health, is not a profession, discipline, or department but a cause and a field engaged in by a wide array of personnel practicing within a broad and complex spectrum of departments and agencies.

Those interested in environmental health and protection should recognize that the public and the environment are also served by agencies other than health departments. Academic institutions preparing students for environmental health and protection careers should orient students to leadership roles in the multitude of agencies involved. Public health leaders should help assure that the programs administered by such agencies are comprehensive in scope and that they are based on sound epidemiology, toxicology, and risk assessment data. They must also help assure that the programs have adequate legal, fiscal, laboratory, epidemiological, and other support they need to be effective.

ENVIRONMENTAL HEALTH AND PROTECTION PROGRAMS

An environmental health and protection program is a rational grouping of activities designed to solve one or more problems. An environmental health and protection problem is a reasonably discrete environmental issue having an impact on human health, safety, or the quality of the environment. Examples of environmental health and protection problems and properly designed environmental health and protection programs are shown in Figure 21.3.

Program Design

A veritable arsenal of program activities are utilized in varying degrees to constitute programs. These include, but are not limited to, inspection, surveillance, sampling, analyses, public information, environmental health and protection planning, pollution prevention, regulation, epidemiology, risk assessment, education of target groups, demonstrations, consultation, training, research, design and plan review, economic and social incentives, warnings, risk communication, hearings, permits, grading, compliance schedules, variances, injunctions, administrative and judicial penalties, embargoes, and environmental impact statements.

In designing programs, activities must be organized in such a manner as to address most effectively the problem(s) being considered. Some selection and mix of such activities are utilized to develop programs for all

		Environmental Health Problem Examples							
Design Specifications for Environmental Health Programs: Some Examples X = Aids in solving problems		Air Quality	Water Quality	Wastes	Ecological Dysfunction	Environmental Chemicals	Food Safety	Radiation	Noise Pollution
	Air Pollution Control	X	X	X	X	X		X	
	Food Protection	X	X	X		X	X	X	X
	Radiation Protection	X	X	X			X	X	
	Solid Waste Management	X	X	X	X	X	X		
	Hazardous Waste Management	X	X	X	X	X	X		
	Insect & Rodent Control			X	X	X	X		
	Water Supply		X	X		X	X	X	
	Noise Control								X
	Environmental Control of Recreation Areas	X	X	X	X	X	X		X
	Institutional Environment Control	X	X	X		X	X	X	X
	Occupational Health and Safety	X	X	X		X	X	X	X
	Water Pollution Control	X	X	X	X	X	X	X	

FIGURE 21.3

environmental problems, whether they involve food safety, wastes, air quality, water quality, radiation, noise pollution, or environmental chemicals.

It is imperative that problems be accurately defined as to cause, time of day or season, geographic area, nature, intensity, and health and environmental effects prior to designing the program. The program design must then stand the scrutiny of critical evaluation to assure that the design will in fact prevent or solve the problems in an economical and societally acceptable manner. The net health, environmental, social, and economic impacts of proposed requirements should be thoroughly understood prior to implementation. A seemingly effective measure may produce undesirable problems of a more serious nature than the problem for which the program was intended.

Most environmental health and protection programs have been developed to address a single problem.

This has led to unnecessary inefficiencies and ineffectiveness along with poor utilization of personnel and other resources. Improving program design for federally mandated and similarly legislated programs may be difficult, but other programs can be designed and administered in a more creative manner. When properly designed, a program can address components of several environmental problems. This practice is common in such programs as food protection, institutional environmental control, environmental control of recreational areas, and occupational safety and health.

Program Support

All organizations require such basic support elements as purchasing, budget, personnel, and audit. In addition, several other support functions are essential to the development and delivery of environmental health and protection services.

Laboratory Support

Comprehensive laboratory support must be available in quantity and quality to undertake epidemiological investigations, determine environmental trends and needs, develop standards and regulations, carry out enforcement, inform the public, and design programs. Such services are available through public health laboratories, environmental laboratories, pollution control laboratories, agriculture laboratories, or, in a few jurisdictions, comprehensive laboratories serving various governmental agencies. At the federal level, more specialized services may be requested from the Centers for Disease Control and Prevention, the Environmental Protection Agency, the Food and Drug Administration, and the Department of Energy.

Epidemiology Support

Environmental epidemiology is a specialized epidemiological function that deals with extrapolations and correlations as well as direct cause-and-effect investigations. Early environmental health practice was geared primarily to communicable disease problems. Now, it also embraces the impacts of increasing amounts, types, and combinations of nonliving contaminants and other stresses. Such impacts are more subtle and long range in their effects. There is greater difficulty in measuring the effects as well as in precisely isolating and understanding the causes.

Some state and local environmental health and protection agencies do not have in-house epidemiological support and must receive such services through another agency, usually a health department. Sound environmental surveillance data and epidemiology are essential to determine needs, trends, and priorities and to design effective programs.

Legal Support

Environmental health and protection programs are authorized by legislative bodies at various levels of government, and they provide legal remedies when other efforts do not lead to compliance with specified requirements. When enforcement remedies are pursued, the advice, support, and involvement of legal counsel are necessary.

Many environmental health and protection agencies have specialized environmental law attorneys. Others may request assistance through the office of a city or county attorney, a state attorney general, or the United States Department of Justice, depending on the type of requirement being violated. The involvement of a skilled legal draft person is also essential when legislation is being drafted or amended.

Public Information and Education Support

Environmental health and protection is the public's business, and it cannot be properly understood, supported, or attained in the absence of continuing public information and educational activities. While all environmental health and protection personnel should be involved in these activities, it is appropriate that the agency utilize staff specifically trained and experienced in assuring a free flow of information and the attainment of new skills by the public, including the news media, target groups, citizen groups, professional groups, elected officials, and other agencies involved in the field of environmental health and protection.

Research Support

Environmental health and protection programs cannot be properly justified, prioritized, budgeted, designed, or implemented without the benefits of peer-reviewed research. Research is essential to the development of new methodologies for preventing and controlling problems, environmental remediation, analyses, and the education of target groups.

Most operating agencies and practitioners are not well equipped to conduct research, but they should be vital participants in the process by identifying research needs and communicating these needs on a routine basis to research institutions and agencies. The knowledge and skills of practitioners will be enhanced through continuing communication and coalitions with academic programs and individuals involved in environmental health and protection education and research.

Environmental Health and Protection Planning Support

Environmental health and protection planning is another key support function that has not been widely understood, developed, or utilized. While the field of environmental health and protection focuses on prevention in many program areas, a preponderance of effort and funds is devoted to remediation of contamination and pollution created as a result of earlier actions taken by other interests in the public and private sectors.

Environmental health and protection practitioners must have the knowledge, skills, and authority to become effectively involved in prevention during the planning, design, and construction stages of a diverse range of activities, including energy development and production, land use, transportation methods and systems, facilities construction, resource development and utilization, and product design and development. Developing the capacity and authority to function effectively in environmental health and protection planning will be necessary as environmental health and protection agencies strive to function in a primary prevention mode, rather than secondary prevention or treatment

of the environment after the contamination or pollution has been produced and emitted.

Data Support

Data collected and published annually by the Public Health Foundation (PHF)[15] include only a very small portion of the total environmental health and protection programs and expenditures of state and local governments. Because these data are limited and other sources are inadequate and incomplete, a perception exists that environmental health and protection activities are not nearly as large and significant as other components of public health practice. Comprehensive annual reporting of environmental health and protection program information would reveal a manifold increase in environmental health and protection activities beyond that reported by the Public Health Foundation. Such accurate and comprehensive program information should be essential to educational institutions and public health policy leaders as they strive to plan, prioritize, and deliver services.

Additionally, surveillance and status data in the area of environmental health and protection are inadequate. These data should include environmentally related morbidity and mortality, specified environmental contaminant and pollution levels, and other environmental/ecological conditions.

State-of-the-art environmental health and protection information systems would enhance the level of informed decision making at all levels of government and industry.[16]

Fiscal Support

Historically, environmental health and protection programs were financed by general fund tax revenues. Currently, environmental health and protection agencies are finding it necessary to be creative in funding additional services or, in some areas, retaining existing levels of funding. Existing activities and proposed expansions must be evaluated and prioritized so as to address the higher priorities in any specific jurisdiction. Where additional general fund support is not available, agencies must consider reallocating budgets from lower priority activities or developing new sources of revenue, such as fees for service, pollution taxes, or other market–based incentives.

Prioritizing funding requests will require the best skills in epidemiology, toxicology, and risk assessment. Developing creative funding mechanisms will require that agency personnel have basic knowledge and skills in public financing and environmental economics. Marketing such budget requests will increasingly require competency in risk communication and public policy development.

Building and Travelling Bridges

Effective environmental health and protection programs depend on developing and utilizing constantly travelled communication bridges and network processes connecting a wide variety of groups and agencies involved in the struggle for a quality environment and enhanced public health. A few such agencies and interests include land use, energy production, transportation, resource development, the medical community, public works officials, agriculture, conservation, engineering, architecture, colleges and universities, product design and development, economic development, chambers of commerce, environmental groups, trade and industry groups, and elected officials. These relationships should be a matter of organizational policy, and they should be institutionalized rather than being left to chance or personalities.

PREVENTION

In addition to developing environmental health and protection planning, other approaches are necessary to assure more effective prevention methods. According to EPA's Science Advisory Board:

> . . . end-of-pipe controls and waste disposal should be the last line of environmental defense, not the front line. Preventing pollution at its source—through the redesign of production processes, the substitution of less toxic production materials, the screening of new chemicals and technologies before they are introduced into commerce,

energy and water conservation, the development of less-polluting transportation systems and farming practices, etc.—is usually a far cheaper, more effective way to reduce environmental risk, especially over the long term . . .

> Pollution prevention also minimizes environmental problems that are caused through a variety of exposures. For example, substituting a non-toxic for a toxic agent reduces exposures to workers producing and using the agent at the same time as it reduces exposures through surface water, groundwater, and the air.

> Pollution prevention also is preferable to end-of-pipe controls that often cause environmental problems of their own. Air pollutants captured in industrial smokestacks and deposited in landfills can contribute to groundwater pollution; stripping toxic chemicals out of groundwater, and combusting solid and hazardous wastes, can contribute to air pollution. Pollution prevention techniques are especially promising because they do not move pollutants from one environmental medium to another, as is often the case with end-of-pipe controls. Rather, the pollutants are not generated in the first place.[17]

PERSONNEL

The field of environmental health and protection requires the involvement of scores of disciplines as well as interdisciplinarily trained personnel. Additionally, personnel are needed in roles varying from routine inspection and surveillance through management, policy, education, and research. Depending on the type of agency and sophistication of programs, effective efforts demand an alliance of physical scientists, life scientists, social scientists, educators, physicians, environmental scientists, engineers, data specialists, planners, administrators, laboratory scientists, veterinarians, attorneys, economists, political scientists, and others in order to fully utilize the variety of environmental health and protection activities.

Environmental health and protection professionals are those who have been educated in the various environmental health and protection technical areas as well as in epidemiology, biostatistics, toxicology, management, public policy, risk assessment, risk communication, risk management, environmental law, social dynamics, and/or environmental economics.[18] For the most part, such professionals are graduates of environmental health science and protection programs accredited by the National Environmental Health Science and Protection Accreditation Council, or they are graduates of schools or programs accredited by the Council on Education for Public Health.

Other professionals in environmental health and protection include those educated in other essential professions and disciplines, such as epidemiologists, biostaticians, toxicologists, chemists, geohydrologists, biologists, physicians, health educators, attorneys, public administrators, economists, educators, engineers, meteorologists, and social scientists.[18]

Professional Shortage

A 1988 United States Public Health Service Bureau of Health Professions report indicated that only 11 percent of the environmental health and protection work force had formal education as environmental health and protection professionals. It also estimated a need for 120,000 more such professionals to address problems in several key areas.[18]

The 1990 EPA Science Advisory Board publication states that:

> The nation is facing a shortage of environmental scientists and engineers needed to cope with environmental problems today and in the future. Moreover, professionals today need continuing education and training to help them understand the complex control technologies and pollution prevention strategies needed to reduce environmental risks more effectively.

> Most environmental officials have been trained in a subset of environmental problems, such as air pollution, water pollution or waste disposal. But they have not been trained to assist and respond to environmental problems in an integrated and comprehensive way. Moreover, few have been taught to anticipate and prevent pollution from occurring or to utilize risk reduction tools beyond command-and-control regulations. This narrow focus is not very effective in the face of intermedia problems that have emerged over the past two decades and that are projected for the future.[17]

Other significant employers of environmental health and protection personnel, such as the Departments of Defense and Energy and the private sector, have also emphasized the unmet need for properly qualified professionals.

Training

Competencies for environmental health and protection professionals as practitioners should include:[3(pp42–45)]

- relevant environmental health and protection sciences, such as biology, chemistry, physics, geology, ecology, and toxicology
- environmental health and protection technical issues
- epidemiology
- biostatistics
- etiology of environmentally induced diseases
- risk assessment, communication, and management
- communications and marketing
- interest group interactions
- personnel and program management
- organizational behavior
- public policy development and implementation
- environmental health and protection planning
- cultural issues
- strategic planning
- financial planning and management
- environmental health and protection economics
- environmental health and protection law
- federal, state, and local environmental health and protection organizations
- federal, state, and local political processes

Few graduates of single discipline programs such as chemistry, engineering, or biology, are trained in the foregoing competency areas. Programs accredited by the National Environmental Health Science and Protection Accreditation Council assure that their graduates who are trained specifically in environmental health and protection professionals, have been trained in most of these competency areas. Schools and programs accredited by the Council on Education for Public Health require that their graduates be trained in many of these competencies.

Continuing Education

Formal education in environmental health and protection was once considered to be a vaccine that would prevent ignorance and ineffectiveness later in one's career. However, such formal education is inadequate by itself, and it does not provide personnel all the knowledge and skills needed for leadership and effective careers. Continuing education is an essential component of a career, not only to increase effectiveness, but also to meet ongoing specific needs as they are encountered. Such continuing environmental health and protection education should be budgeted, timely, relevant, economical, and convenient, as well as strongly supported by management.

Specific knowledge and skills that many environmental health and protection personnel have not acquired during formal education include organizational behavior, administrative skills, the political process, environmental health and protection law, financial impacts of programs, financial management, program planning and evaluation, developing and implementing public policy, epidemiology, toxicology, risk assessment, risk communication, and behavior modification.

ACCESS TO SERVICES

Access to comprehensive environmental health and protection services contributes more to protecting and enhancing the health status of the public than does access to health care services. Environmental health and protection services are vital to the health and well-being of our citizens. Everyone requires and expects the benefits of services that protect against toxic chemicals, polluted air and water, contaminated food, unsafe drinking water, noise pollution, unintentional injuries, dangerous radiation exposures, solid wastes, hazardous wastes, vector-borne diseases, inadequate shelter, and global environmental health and protection problems.

THE FUTURE

It is reasonable to assume that environmental health and protection will become an even higher priority issue in our society. It is likely that the public will expect and demand greater levels of protection from both the public and private sectors.

Population growth and shifts, resource development and consumption, product and materials manufacture and utilization, wastes, global environmental deterioration, technological development, changing patterns of land use, transportation methodologies, and energy development and utilization will create additional and unanticipated problems. The competencies of properly prepared environmental health and protection practitioners will be required if prevention and control efforts are to anticipate and keep pace with these changes.

The targeted education, involvement, and leadership of public health professionals will require significant changes in their current preparation and philosophy. As environmental health and protection issues assume a higher priority and demand greater visibility and emphasis, the tendency to diversify the programs into new agencies will increase. Retaining existing environmental health and protection services in traditional health departments will require significant changes in essential knowledge and skills of public health leaders, as well as changes in health department organization and priorities to keep pace with public and political expectations. Enactment of health care reform proposals might mandate the transfer of some health department responsibilities to other agencies, possibly resulting in environmental health and protection (and the other public health programs that are retained) being accorded greater emphasis within health departments.

CONCLUSION

Environmental health and protection are vital parts of public health, regardless of whether they are organizationally within the official public health agency. The environment and its protection requires the ability to do risk assessment and to communicate those risks. It requires skills and support services if efforts to protect human health and the environment are to be successful. The environment will remain high on the public health agenda.

REFERENCES

1. Gordon LJ. Who will manage the environment? *Am J Public Health.* August 1990;80:904–905.

2. Health Resources and Services Administration, Public Health Service. *Educating the Environmental Health Science and Protection Work Force: Problems, Challenges, and Recommendations.* Rockville, Md: US Dept of Health and Human Services, Bureau of Health Professions; 1991.

3. Committee on the Future of Environmental Health, National Environmental Health Association. The future of environmental health. *J Envir Health.* 1993;55(4):28–32.

4. Shattuck L, et al. Report of the Sanitary Commission of Massachusetts. Boston: Harvard University Press; 1850.

5. *Reducing Risk: Setting Priorities and Strategies for Environmental Protection.* Washington, DC: US Environmental Protection Agency, Science Advisory Board; 1990.

6. *The Health Scientist Survey: Identifying Consensus on Assessing Human Health Risk.* Washington, DC: Institute for Regulatory Policy; 1991.

7. *Healthy People 2000: National Health Promotion and Disease Prevention Objectives.* Washington, DC: US Dept of Health and Human Services; 1990. PHS publication no. 91-50212.

8. Hileman B. Expert intuition tops in test of carcinogenicity prediction. *Chem and Engineering News.* 1993;71(25):35–37.

9. *Regulatory Program of the United States Government.* Washington, DC: US Office of Management and Budget; 1990

10. Landy MK, Roberts MJ, Thomas SR. *The Environmental Protection Agency: Asking the Wrong Questions.* New York, NY: Oxford University Press; 1990.

11. Health Resources and Services Administration, Public Health Service. *Identifying State Environmental Health Services.* Rockville, Md: US Dept of Health and Human Services, Bureau of Health Professions; 1993.

12. Gordon LJ. The future of environmental health, and the need for public health leadership. *J Environ Health.* 1993;56(5):38–40.

13. *National Profile of Local Health Departments.* Washington, DC: National Association of County Health Officials; 1990.

14. Browner C. Public health—an EPA imperative. *EPA Insight Policy Paper;* November 1993. EPA-175-N-93-025

15. *Public Health Agencies 1991: An Inventory of Programs and Block Grant Expenditures.* Washington, DC: Public Health Foundation; 1991.

16. Roper WL, Baker EL, Dyal WW, Nicola RM. Strengthening the public health system. *Public Health Rep.* 1992;107(6):609–615.

17. *Reducing Risk: Setting Priorities and Strategies for Environmental Protection.* Washington, DC: US Environmental Protection Agency, Science Advisory Board; 1990.

18. Health Resources and Services Administration, Public Health Service. *Evaluating the Environmental Health Work Force.* Rockville, Md: US Dept of Health and Human Services, Bureau of Health Professions; 1988.

CHAPTER

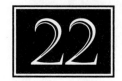

Primary Care and Public Health

Robert G. Harmon, M.D., M.P.H.

Primary care is a broad term with many definitions. It has also been the subject of a lengthy debate among public health leaders. Some authorities, such as Winslow, Terris, and Miller, claim that primary care and "personal health services," as they are often called in the public health literature, are an integral part of public health practice. Others, such as Emerson, Bellin, Hanlon, and Jonas, maintain that primary care should be the responsibility of another sector, leaving public health resources devoted to population–based prevention programs.[1]

The inclusion of a primary care chapter in a textbook of public health practice is likely to be a surprise for some. To omit it, however, would leave a large gap, especially in light of the major commitment to primary care and personal health services in the current United States public health system.

This chapter provides a definition of primary care and shows its relationship to preventive services. It then reviews the role of government at the federal, state, and local levels in the provision of primary care services, especially to medically underserved populations in the

United States. Finally, it highlights important areas for research required to support future policy decisions related to primary care.

INTRODUCTION

Public health agencies and programs have a long tradition of "filling the gaps" in the United States health care system. These gaps have been numerous in the absence of universal health insurance, especially among low-income and vulnerable populations such as women and children. While this gap-filling role has resulted in an expansion of the categorical, personal, public health services delivered, it has not necessarily resulted in the provision of comprehensive primary care.

Some states and communities have delegated primary care responsibilities for low-income populations to teaching hospitals or other providers, whereas others have implemented major governmental initiatives. Nonetheless, most public health officials agree that primary care is an important link between population-based prevention programs and the individual client, especially among underserved, often low-income, rural and inner-city high-risk populations. If primary care systems for these groups are well designed, public health status and services can benefit.

The chronic lack of primary care resources and access have been a major barrier to progress in public health. Scarce public health resources have often been used to fill the gaps in primary care programs, while worthy population-based prevention programs have been neglected. There was renewed expectation in early 1994 that health care reform in the United States would eventually bring universal access to primary care services, allowing public health efforts to focus on a clear prevention mission. Unfortunately, the demise of health care reform later in 1994 put public health back into the position of continuing to provide primary care services.

DEFINITIONS OF PRIMARY CARE

Primary care was defined by the Millis Commission in 1966 as:

> . . . the delivery of first contact medicine, the assumption of longitudinal responsibility for the patient regardless of the presence or absence of disease, and the integration of physical, psychological, and social aspects of health to the limits of the capability of the health personnel.[2]

This definition was refined by the Institute of Medicine in 1978 to read, "accessible, comprehensive, coordinated and continual care delivered by accountable providers of personal health services."[3]

Both the World Health Organization and the United Nations Children's Fund, at the Alma-Ata international conference in 1978, defined primary health care as "essential health care needs made universally accessible to individuals and families in the community by means acceptable to them, through their full participation and at a cost that the community and the country can afford."[4] The famous goal of *health for all by the year 2000* was also set at Alma-Ata.

Especially relevant to public health is the concept of **community-oriented primary care (COPC),** a term originated by Sidney Kark and Joseph Abramson and defined as "a strategy whereby elements of primary health care and of community medicine are systematically developed and brought together in a coordinated practice." They listed the fundamental features of COPC as the use of epidemiology and clinical skills, a defined population for which the program has assumed responsibility, defined programs to address the community's health problems, and community involvement and accessibility to the program's services.[5]

COPC has been characterized by Fitzhugh Mullan as "the reunion of the traditions of public health and personal clinical health services to facilitate community diagnosis, health surveillance, monitoring and evaluation."[6] This integration has made COPC attractive to public health agencies. COPC has been tried in a variety of settings in the United States, including the Denver Department of Health and Hospitals, the Maricopa County Department of Health Services, Dallas Parkland Hospital, and many community and migrant health centers. Success in achieving true COPC has been limited, however, due to a lack of reimbursement for nonclinical services such as epidemiology and outreach.

Philip Lee has pointed out the critical difference between primary *health* care and primary *medical* care.[7] The former refers to a comprehensive, prevention-oriented model, whereas the latter refers to a biomedical, cure-oriented model. Most public health professionals acknowledge the importance of primary medical care, but only as a component of a broader, comprehensive primary health care and public health system.

CLINICAL PREVENTIVE SERVICES

A key interface between primary care and public health involves the provision of clinical preventive services. These are personal interventions in the clinical setting devoted to screening, counseling, immunizing, and providing chemoprophylaxis for health promotion and disease prevention in asymptomatic individuals.

The publication of the *Guide to Clinical Preventive Services* in 1989 was a milestone in bridging the gap between primary care clinicians and public health professionals.[8] The guide rigorously reviewed 169 interventions to prevent 60 different illnesses and conditions. It rejected the concept of the "annual physical exam" and instead recommended a specific periodic health examination schedule by age, sex, and various risk factors. For example, anemia screening was recommended for pregnant women and infants, but not for other groups.

The guide's protocols provide a scientific basis for determining which interventions are effective and worthy of recommendation, which are not, and which are in need of more research. Many of the protocols are gradually being incorporated into health insurance and managed care benefit packages as well as into public health practice guidelines. A major revision and update of the guide has recently been completed and released.[9]

GOVERNMENTAL ROLES, RESPONSIBILITIES, AND PROGRAMS

Government at all levels has contributed significantly to primary care in this country. Legal mandates, provision of services, and professional training are just some of the government contributions to primary care that are summarized here.

Legal Mandates

Under the United States Constitution, unless the federal government has enacted special programs such as Medicare and Medicaid, the provision of medical care for those unable to pay (the medically indigent) is the responsibility of the states and/or their political subdivisions—the counties, cities, towns, and other local government entities. This includes primary care as well as hospital, long-term, mental health, and other types of care. Some states, for example, Hawaii, carry this responsibility out directly, whereas others, for example, California, delegate it to local entities.

The result is a significant indigent primary care role for public health agencies in the United States, especially when compared to other countries such as Canada and Western European nations, where national health insurance has been in effect for decades. In addition to Medicaid, hundreds of other federal, state,

and local government programs have been created to address the primary care needs of underserved populations. The public health sector has labored for decades to assure adequate personal as well as population–based services for all.

Federal Primary Care Activities

Federal primary care activities include Medicaid and Medicare programs, health centers, and maternal and child health grants. These are described next.

Medicaid and Medicare

Medicaid eligibility, coverage, and reimbursement for maternal and child health care have been expanding since the late 1980s. This has been a source of relief and new revenue for overburdened health departments. Medicaid managed care systems have also been expanding, and in light of the demise of health care reform, Medicaid block grants are likely to expand more rapidly. In 1993, 8 out of 33 million, or 24 percent, of Medicaid beneficiaries were enrolled in some form of managed care. This has provided some Medicaid populations with a better, regular source of primary care, but it has also resulted in disruption of services in some locations due to start-up problems.

The Rural Health Clinics Act (P.L. 95-210) was enacted by Congress in 1977. The purpose was to promote primary care practice in rural underserved areas by nurse-practitioners and physician's assistants by providing cost–based reimbursement for Medicare and Medicaid beneficiaries. By 1992, over 800 clinics were certified, and it appeared that barriers of inadequate reimbursement rates and state resistance to nurse-practitioner and physician's assistant practice were lessening.

The Federally Qualified Health Center (FQHC) Program was established by act of Congress in 1989. Its purpose was to assure reasonable Medicare and Medicaid cost-based reimbursement to primary care clinics serving medically underserved areas and populations. Eligible entities included community and migrant health centers, health-care-for-the-homeless projects (see below), and other public and private nonprofit clinics meeting similar criteria (called "look-alikes"). As of January 1993, more than 900 programs had been approved under Medicare, and over 630 community, migrant, and homeless programs and 98 look-alike programs (about one-third of which were public) had been included under Medicaid. In 1991, Medicaid payments to FQHCs increased by $115 million, or about 30 percent. The program is now viewed as an important new resource for building primary care systems for the underserved.[10]

Health Centers

Federal funding for Community and Migrant Health Centers (CMHCs) began in the 1960s as part of the Johnson administration's war on poverty. Initial support came from the Office of Economic Opportunity for neighborhood health centers. This authority was later replaced in the 1970s by Section 330 of the Public Health Service Act (P.L. 94-63) for community health centers and Section 329 for migrant health centers. Grantees agreed to provide a comprehensive package of primary care services to an inner-city or rural medically underserved area or population, regardless of ability to pay. This support helped to develop a nationwide network of community-based providers and boards with significant political influence.

By 1992, the program had grown to 571 grantees serving 6.9 million people in 1,500 sites with a federal grant budget of $594 million. These resources still fell far short of the overall need of over 37 million Americans living in medically underserved areas or populations. Utilization data revealed that 85 percent of CMHC patients had incomes below 200 percent of the federal poverty level, 36 percent were Euro-American, 31 percent were African-American, 28 percent were Hispanic, and 5 percent were Asian or other ethnic groups. Fiscal year 1992 data revealed 38 percent of CMHC revenue was from federal grants, 30 percent from Medicaid, 13 percent from state and local government and other grants, 7 percent from insurance payments, 7 percent from patient payments, and 5 percent from Medicare. This shows that CMHCs have de-

veloped diversified funding sources, although 40 percent of their clients continue to be uninsured.[11]

By law, no more than 5 percent of funds have gone to public grantees such as local health departments (LHDs). About 95 percent have been awarded to community-based, private, nonprofit corporations with consumer-majority boards of directors. Many public health leaders have long objected to this 5 percent limit on public participation, but advocates of community control have defended it as a key element in the success of the program. Both models have demonstrated success, and cost comparisons have shown few significant differences.

Public health officials have also criticized the lack of coordination between CMHCs and LHDs. A 1990 report by the National Association of County Health Officials revealed that among 130 pairs of responding CMHCs and LHDs with overlapping service areas, only 28 percent reported a high level of interaction. Thirty percent reported a moderate level of interaction, 41 percent reported a minimal level, and 2 percent reported none. Most of the interaction was around maternal and child health and adult primary care services. Chief enabling factors for interaction included identification of mutual interests, physical proximity, fiscal advantage, and social relationships. Chief hindering factors included lack of initiator, time constraints, lack of mutual goals, and political factors.[12] Based on these findings, follow-up projects have been funded to build more linkages between the two parties. This is logical because both are serving similar populations.

Two new federal primary care programs appeared after 1987. The Health Care for the Homeless Program was enacted in 1987 under Section 340 of the Public Health Service Act. By 1992 it had grown to 119 grantees with 495 sites serving 500,000 people and a federal budget of $55.8 million. The Health Services for Residents of Public Housing Program began in 1991 under Section 340A of the Public Health Service Act and has grown to 14 grantees with 40 sites serving 73,000 people and a federal budget of $6 million in fiscal year 1992. Neither program has a limit on public grantees. Both support innovative new approaches to outreach and service delivery to populations that are especially hard to reach.

Maternal and Child Health

Title V of the Social Security Act authorizes the Maternal and Child Health (MCH) Block Grant to the states and territories, which in turn must earmark at least 30 percent of their federal allotment for preventive and primary care services for children. In fiscal year 1992, at least $164 million was available for this primary care. Also available was a significant part of the remaining $383 million allocated for Children with Special Health Care Needs and other MCH programs. MCH Block Grant set-asides, including Special Projects of Regional and National Significance (SPRANS) and Community Integrated Service Systems (CISS), provided $92.5 million and $6.3 million, respectively, in 1992. Some of this money went to primary care demonstrations and training.

In addition, there are other categorical MCH programs supporting primary care and personal health services. Included are family planning grants of $149 million in 1992 to 85 grantees with over 4,000 clinics serving more than four million clients; perinatal grants to CMHCs of $45 million in 1992; and Healthy Start, an infant mortality reduction project, which provided $61 million to 13 cities and two rural areas in 1992.

Health Professions Training and Deployment

The government has also been involved in the training and deployment of health professionals. The aim has been to provide better, more accessible care to underserved populations and areas.

National Health Service Corps

The National Health Service Corps (NHSC) was created by Congress in 1970 (P.L. 91-623). Its purpose is to provide financial support to health professional students and practitioners in return for service in designated inner-city and rural Health Professional Shortage Areas (HPSAs). As of 1992 there were over 2,100 primary care HPSAs in the United States needing an estimated 4,400 primary care practitioners and 3,600 dentists, mental health, and other professionals to care for an estimated 35 million underserved Americans. The deployed field strength in 1992, however, was only about 1,200, down from a peak of about 3,000 in the mid-1980s.

The reason for the shortfall was budget cuts in the early 1980s, which cut the number of NHSC scholarships from a peak of about 1,700 in 1980 to 47 in 1989. It was presumed that a physician surplus would result in more providers for HPSAs, but this did not materialize. Instead the NHSC was revitalized in the early 1990s with budget increases, which by 1993 brought the total funding up to $120 million, approaching the peak of $150 million in 1980. In the late 1980s, federal and state loan repayment incentives were added to scholarships. By 1993, loan repayments, which can amount to over $35,000 per year per individual, accounted for about two-thirds of all NHSC awards.

The NHSC has been one of the most successful programs for bringing bright, young primary care health professionals to needy areas. Since the program started, over 16,000 have served, with a default rate of less than five percent. Still, the program is not without problems, including retention beyond mandatory service, which has averaged at best only about 30 percent for one extra year; unhappiness with assignments, which are often in remote rural areas; and collection of what is owed by defaulters, which can amount to three times the amount of the scholarship plus interest.

Federal Training Grants

Over $84 million in primary care health professions training grants was awarded to academic institutions in 1992. This included $42.6 million for family medicine, $17.2 million for general internal medicine and pediatrics, $14.5 million for nurse-practitioners and midwives, $4.9 million for physician's assistants, $3.8 million for general dentistry, and about $1 million for general podiatry and osteopathy. New requirements for these grants mandate training linkages to shortage and underserved areas.

Although relatively small sums compared to the $5.6 *billion* spent by Medicare on direct and indirect support of hospital residency training, these training grants are considered critical in reversing the recent trend of fewer than 20 percent of medical students seeking generalist training and practice instead of specialist careers. In the United States, only about one-third of practicing physicians are generalists. Of these, 42 percent are family and general practitioners, 39 percent are general internists, and 19 percent are general pediatricians. Canada has about 50 percent generalists, nearly all of whom are family and general practitioners, whereas in the United Kingdom the mix is 70 percent generalists and 30 percent specialists.[13]

To correct these deficiencies, the Federal Council on Graduate Medical Education has called for reforms, including a goal that 50 percent of residency positions and 50 percent of the physician workforce be in the generalist disciplines.[12] There is also widespread interest in greatly increasing the training and deployment of primary care nurse-practitioners, certified nurse-midwives, and physician's assistants. These professionals have become an especially valuable resource in public health agencies, CMHCs, and other facilities serving the disadvantaged. Several studies have shown that their quality of care is as good or better than that delivered by physicians alone.

Other Programs

There are, of course, many other federal programs that contribute significantly to primary care within the public health sector. In the Health Resources and Services Administration in 1992, there were 122 projects in the Rural Health Outreach Program funded at $21.2 million, and there were another $276 million in Ryan White comprehensive AIDS grants. In the Centers for Disease Control, with its budget of $1.6 billion, there were dozens of programs supporting injury, communicable disease, and chronic disease control.

In the Substance Abuse and Mental Health Services Administration, with its budget of $2.0 billion, two large block grants and many categorical prevention and treatment programs support primary care. The primary

care research contributions of the National Institutes of Health, with its $10.0 billion budget, and the Agency for Health Care Policy and Research, with its $123.0 million budget, are noteworthy. Finally, the Indian Health Service is also a major direct primary care provider to about 1.3 million Native Americans.

Three Circles of Cooperation

In 1991, HRSA proposed a model of three interlocking circles of primary care, public health, and health professions training.[14] This is shown in Figure 22.1. The purpose was to encourage HRSA grantees in these areas to cooperate in an effort to make services more user-friendly. Successful examples of such cooperation have been recognized in Miami, Tucson, and Beaufort, South Carolina, among other places. Evidence of such linkages has been increasingly required in grant applications.

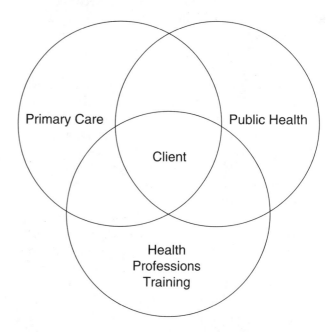

FIGURE 22.1 HRSA's Three Circles of Cooperation. SOURCE: Adapted from Harmon R, Carlson R. HRSA's role in primary care and public health in the 1990s. *Public Health Rep.* January-February 1991; 106(1): 6–10.

State Primary Care Activities

The states and territories play a critical role in assuring adequate primary care services, especially for the disadvantaged. Most, but not all, serve as a source of funding and coordination, while delegating the service delivery role to local health departments and/or private sector entities, such as community and migrant health centers or visiting nurse associations. Seven state and three territorial health agencies also serve as the Medicaid single state agency, with all of the primary care responsibilities and opportunities involved.[15]

Data on primary care spending by state and territorial health agencies are not readily available. A proxy measure is spending on *noninstitutional personal health services*. In fiscal year 1989, state health agencies reported spending $5.8 billion in this area, or 61 percent of their total expenditures. Over half of these expenditures were for MCH services, including the Women, Infant, and Children (WIC) Nutrition Program and the Children with Special Health Care Needs Program. Of this amount, $3.0 billion was from federal grants or contracts, $2.3 billion was from state appropriations, and the remainder was from other sources, including Medicaid, local government, and fees.

Coordinating these diverse personal health service programs is a difficult task for state and territorial health agencies. Many have chosen to establish, with federal grant support, state offices of primary care. As of October 1993, there were over 50 such offices. In addition, federal grants had also been awarded to 50 states for offices of rural health, many of which were colocated with primary care. These offices are responsible for such functions as needs assessments, planning, identification of shortage areas, operation of state primary care health professions scholarship and loan repayment programs, placement of health professionals in shortage areas, educating the public, and many other critical functions. They are also working closely with over 36 federally subsidized state primary care associations, which serve as a statewide or regional umbrella organization representing primary care providers to the underserved.

Many states, such as Florida, California, Alabama, Michigan, Virginia, and North Carolina, have developed ambitious plans to combine federal, state, and local government and private resources to build a better primary care infrastructure for the underserved. A critical factor in these plans is the approval of federal waivers to loosen requirements under Medicaid and Medicare block grants.

Local Primary Care Activities

A broad array of public and private entities provide primary care to the disadvantaged at the local level. The list includes, but is not limited to, local health departments, public and private teaching hospitals and their clinics, community/migrant/homeless/public housing health centers, private office-based practitioners, school–based clinics, free clinics, and managed care organizations.

Of special interest to readers of this textbook is the role of local health departments. The most recent study of this role was carried out by the National Association of County Health Officials (NACHO) with support from the CDC in 1991.[16] NACHO found that the majority of reporting local health departments provided *some* primary care services, such as immunization (88 percent) or well–child care (78 percent), but only 21 percent provided *comprehensive* primary care that met the United States Public Health Service definition. This low percentage was related to the fact that 77 percent of the respondents serve populations of less than 100,000. The percentage went up with size of population served.

Miller and Moos cite numerous impressive case studies of urban and rural primary care systems for the underserved. Recently there has been a trend in metropolitan areas such as Chicago and New York City towards merging large urban public health and hospital systems into comprehensive primary care models. These have proven successful in Denver, Cincinnati, Phoenix, and elsewhere.[1]

YEAR 2000 OBJECTIVES

Healthy People 2000[17] lists 32 objectives related to primary care services and providers. Of special note are the following:

- 21.3: increase to at least 95 percent the proportion of people who have a specific source of ongoing primary care for coordination of their preventive and episodic health care (1986 baseline was 82 percent for the general population, 80 percent for African-Americans and low-income populations, and 70 percent for Hispanics)
- 21.5: assure that at least 90 percent of people for whom primary care services are provided directly by publicly funded programs are offered, at a minimum, the screening, counseling, and immunization services recommended by the United States Preventive Services Task Force
- 21.7: increase to at least 90 percent the proportion of people who are served by a local health department that assesses and assures access to essential clinical preventive services

These ambitious objectives illustrate a continuing role for public health agencies in primary care, at least to assure that it is delivered appropriately.

CONCLUSION

There was a hope that health care reform would allow health departments to return to core public health functions and leave primary care services to the medical care system. Unfortunately, there has been an increase in the number of uninsured who require primary care services since health care reform collapsed. Thus, it appears that health departments must continue to provide "safety net" primary care services for the indigent.

Another issue of concern is the role of Medicaid. Health departments have relied on Medicaid payments to cross-subsidize the provision of services to the uninsured. As managed Medicaid efforts move medical patients out of public health agencies, public health will no longer be able to cross-subsidize the uninsured, creating additional difficulties for already financially strapped health departments.

There is an urgent need for more primary care health services research to determine conclusively which delivery models have the best quality of care and outcomes. Several questions require answers. For example,

should health departments abandon their primary care and personal health clinics in favor of strictly population-based programs? Studies in North Carolina and California suggest that birth outcomes for low-income pregnant women receiving prenatal care in public health clinics are better than in private practice settings, perhaps because of enhanced case management and social services. It might be premature to close these clinics if a better alternative is not available. As another example, should the public health specialty clinic model be abandoned in favor of a generalist model? It is conventional wisdom that comprehensive primary care is the best alternative, especially from the perspective of client convenience, but hard evidence is lacking. Finally, does capitated managed care, especially as delivered by staff or group model health maintenance organizations, have better primary care outcomes than traditional fee-for-service care? These and similar questions must be answered if future policy directions are to be based on scientific facts rather than opinions.

Public health professionals clearly must continue to at least be well informed about primary care and personal health services. To neglect this area would leave a serious gap in the core functions of public health.

REFERENCES

1. Miller CA, Moos MK. *Local Health Departments: Fifteen Case Studies*. Washington, DC: American Public Health Association; 1981.

2. Millis JS. *The Graduate Education of Physicians*. Report of the Citizens' Commission on Graduate Medical Education. Chicago, Il: American Medical Association; 1966.

3. Institute of Medicine. *A Manpower Policy for Primary Health Care*. Washington, DC: National Academy of Sciences; 1978.

4. *Alma-Ata 1978: Primary Health Care*. Report of the International Conference on Primary Health Care, Alma-Ata, USSR. Geneva, Switzerland: World Health Organization; September 6–12, 1978.

5. Institute of Medicine. *Community Oriented Primary Care: Conference Proceedings*. Washington, DC: National Academy Press; 1982.

6. Mullan F. Community-oriented primary care: an agenda for the 80's. *NEJM*. 1982;307:1076–1078.

7. Lee P. Assessing the primary care paradigm. In: *Proceedings of the National Primary Care Conference, I.* Washington, DC: Health Resources and Services Administration, US Public Health Service, Dept of Health and Human Services; 1993.

8. US Preventive Services Task Force. *Guide to Clinical Preventive Services: An Assessment of the Effectiveness of 169 Interventions.* Baltimore, Md: Williams & Wilkins; 1989.

9. US Preventive Services Task Force. *Guide to Clinical Preventive Services: Second Edition.* Baltimore, Md: Williams & Wilkins; 1996.

10. Fisher R, Jones J. *Access to Primary Care in Underserved Areas: Expanding Medicaid, Medicare, and Public Health Services Through the FQHC Program.* Washington, DC: The George Washington University; January 13, 1993. Issue Brief no. 613.

11. Bureau of Primary Health Care. *Assuring Access for the Underserved in Health Care Reform.* Rockville, Md: Health Resources and Services Administration, US Public Health Service, Dept of Health and Human Services; February 1993.

12. *Report on the Nature and Level of Linkages Between Local Health Departments and Community and Migrant Health Centers.* Washington, DC: National Association of County Health Officials; December 1990.

13. Council on Graduate Medical Education. *Third Report: Improving Access to Health Care Through Physician Workforce Reform: Direction for the 21st Century.* Rockville, Md: Health Resources and Services Administration, United States Public Health Service, Department of Health and Human Services; October 1992.

14. Harmon R, Carlson R. HRSA's role in primary care and public health in the 1990s. *Public Health Rep.* January-February 1991;106(1):6–10.

15. *Public Health Agencies 1991: An Inventory of Programs and Block Grant Expenditures.* Washington, DC: Public Health Foundation; December 1991.

16. *Primary Care Assessment: Local Health Departments' Role in Service Delivery.* Washington, DC: National Association of County Health Officials; October 1992.

17. *Healthy People 2000: National Health Promotion and Disease Prevention Objectives.* Washington, DC: US Dept of Health and Human Services; 1990. PHS publication no. 91-50212.

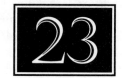

CHAPTER

23

Maternal and Child Health

Trude Bennett, Dr.P.H.
Alan Cross, M.D., M.P.H.

This chapter reviews the history and current status of public health involvement in the provision of maternal and child health services. Linkages between socioeconomic status and maternal and child health are emphasized. Programs that are community based and family centered and that provide integrated delivery of comprehensive services are advocated.

HISTORY

In the early years of the twentieth century, social reformers concerned about child labor and high infant mortality rates successfully lobbied for the creation of the Children's Bureau, whose mandate was to gather data and report on child welfare. The Children's Bureau involved local communities in studying the social and economic correlates of infant and maternal mortality, including income, housing, nutrition, sanitation, and access to medical care. The Bureau's findings demon-

strated a clear link between poverty and maternal health risks that created disadvantages for newborns.[1]

The Sheppard–Towner Act

Recognizing the need for public action, the Children's Bureau spearheaded passage in 1921 of the Maternity and Infancy Act (also called the Sheppard–Towner Act for its congressional sponsors). Federal matching funds were used to set up maternal and child health divisions in state health departments. These agencies coordinated child health programs and public maternity care services, including prenatal care, nutritional counseling, health education, and household assistance for poor and immigrant populations, particularly in the large northeastern cities. The Sheppard–Towner Act was controversial due to its assumption of public responsibility for health care, involvement in family life, and emphasis on prevention over cure. Although credited with saving many lives, the act was defeated in 1929, resulting in diminished public efforts just as the needs of women and children increased with the Great Depression.

The Social Security Act

The Sheppard–Towner Act served as the model for Title V of the Social Security Act of 1935, the purpose of which was to address the needs of vulnerable children and families affected by the depression. Title V provided rural and economically disadvantaged women and children with maternal and child health services, comprehensive services for "crippled" children, and child welfare and protective services. Through a separate administration, the Social Security Act provided income assistance for indigent families in a program that served as the forerunner of Aid to Families with Dependent Children (AFDC).[1] Despite the understanding that poverty and poor health are closely related, health and social welfare programs have continued to be funded and administered separately.

The 1960s

In the early 1960s, the emerging civil rights movement shifted the paradigm from a charitable obligation to a political commitment to achieving equality and compensating for racial injustices of the past. New programs emerged in the 1960s and 1970s that focused attention on economic and racial disparities in health outcomes and health services utilization. Medicaid (Title XIX) became the primary government funding mechanism for indigent health care. Neighborhood health centers reached out to communities with wide-ranging projects to improve nutrition, reduce lead exposure, and expand employment opportunities, in addition to providing primary care. New programs included maternal and infant care projects, family planning services, children and youth projects, the Head Start early childhood education program, the Special Supplemental Food Program for Women, Infants, and Children (WIC), school lunch programs, Title I educational assistance, and implementation of legislation guaranteeing the right to education of the handicapped

(PL 94-142).[1] This diversity of programs aimed at poverty, education, nutrition, and health acknowledged the complex interaction between socioeconomic circumstances and health outcomes.

Most of these programs were federally initiated but financed and administered through partnerships between the federal and state governments. Programs targeted specific populations defined by strict eligibility requirements. They were operated by different state government units responsible for education, welfare, nutrition, and health and thus delivered in communities by several different agencies. This approach divided the needs of high-risk women and children into categorical programs at the local level. Despite the fragmentation and limited funding, multiple evaluations have documented the effectiveness of these programs in improving the health and well-being of women and children.

The 1980s

In the early 1980s, the Reagan administration's new federalism gave states greater autonomy to determine program priorities, but it also provided less money for program implementation. Advocates succeeded in maintaining a specific block grant to states that was dedicated to MCH needs. However, total MCH block grant funds in 1983 were 18 percent lower than the amount made available for maternal and child health programs in the previous year.

The categorical programs consolidated into the MCH block grant were those for "crippled children," maternal and child health, lead-based paint poisoning prevention, sudden infant death syndrome, adolescent pregnancy prevention, genetic disease testing and counseling, hemophilia diagnostic and treatment centers, and services to disabled children eligible for Supplemental Security Income. The earlier federal mandates for uniform enactment of these programs for poor and minority populations had been seen by many as a form of protection against politically motivated disparities among states. Under the block grant strategy, some states have reported greater efficiency and a heightened ability to respond to local needs. However, the impact of uneven availability of various programs due to the states' greater discretionary power has not been fully determined.[2]

In the late 1980s, attention turned to the United States' poor international ranking in infant mortality (twentieth among the nations) and the large racial gap in infant health outcomes (African–American infant mortality was twice that of Euro-Americans). In recognition of inadequate access to prenatal care for many women lacking private insurance coverage, Medicaid benefits were extended to the near poor and enhanced to allow reimbursement for a wider array of services, including nutrition, health education, psychosocial services, and care coordination. However, expanded eligibility for Medicaid maternity care without parallel growth in the pool of prenatal care providers may have added to the stress of overloaded public clinics in need of additional resources.

The 1990s

The 1990s offer tremendous challenges and opportunities for public health workers in the field of maternal and child health. More than ever, studies confirm the strong relationship between poverty and health for the MCH population. Some problems have persisted and intensified, and new problems have emerged. In 1989, 12.6 million children under the age of 18 were living below the federal poverty level. Conditions are worse for children in racial and ethnic minority families: in 1990, poverty rates for children under 6 years of age were 50 percent for African-Americans and 40 percent for Latinos, compared with 14 percent for Euro-Americans.[3]

The large increase in female-headed households, combined with limited educational and employment opportunities for women, makes individual responsibility for children's social and economic needs unattainable for many families. AFDC benefit levels average less than 50 percent of the poverty level in most states. On a given day, 100,000 children are homeless throughout the United States. In 1989, 2.4 million children were reported to be abused or neglected. A growing number of children are known to be infected with HIV or affected by the use of harmful substances.

The emotional toll of societal violence on the nation's children is unknown. The number of children dropping out of school each year is at least 446,000. In 1990, approximately 25,000 cases of measles, 5,000 cases of mumps, and 4,000 cases of whooping cough were reported, with the nation's record of early immunization lagging behind most countries in the developing world.[4]

Emerging in the 1990s is a model of community–based comprehensive services coordinated and integrated at the local level. Rather than categorical programs administered with a separate set of rules and regulations aimed at a highly targeted population, efforts are now underway to pool the resources at the local level, eliminate the bureaucratic barriers among programs, and offer combinations of services to women and children based upon individual needs and available resources in the community. Client participation, agency collaboration, and the use of private and charity dollars to enhance local programs are all part of this new paradigm. New mandates for family-centered, community-based care should be compatible with creative approaches initiated through community mobilization and organization.

MAJOR FEDERAL MCH PROGRAMS

MCH programs in local health departments are largely determined by major federal programs that are funded and administered through various combinations of federal, state, and local collaboration. To assist in understanding these programs, key elements of federal legislation and regulations are described in this section. Each state and local health agency carries out these programs in different ways as allowed by federal law, so it is impossible to describe all the variations. However, each health agency has a manual for the operation of each of these programs. It should be consulted for local details that cannot be provided here.

Title V

Title V continues to play a key role in funding and shaping public health programs for women, children, and families at the state level.[5] The federal Title V program is currently administered by the Maternal and Child Health Bureau of the Health Resources and Services Administration (HRSA). HRSA is an agency of the United States Public Health Service within the Department of Health and Human Services.

Maternal and Child Health Block Grants

In fiscal year 1994, Congress allocated a total of $687,034,000 for Title V funding to the states for a combination of mandated and discretionary purposes. States received 85 percent of this amount as maternal and child health block grant funds, for which the states must match every four dollars of federal money with three dollars of their own contribution. In their block grant applications, states must demonstrate that they will use the funds to achieve objectives consistent with the Public Health Service's objectives for the year 2000. These objectives include reduction of adolescent and unintended pregnancy, substance use during pregnancy, severe complications of pregnancy, low birthweight and infant mortality, and unintentional childhood injury; and promotion of breastfeeding, immunization, genetic screening, and primary care for infants.[6] At least 30 percent of block grant funds must be used for children's preventive and primary care and at least 30 percent for services for children with special health care needs.

Utilizing maternal and child health block grant funds, states are expected by the federal government to:

- provide and assure mothers and children (especially those with low income or limited availability to services) access to quality MCH services
- reduce infant mortality and the incidence of preventable diseases and handicapping conditions among children
- reduce the need for inpatient and long-term care services
- increase the number of children appropriately immunized against disease and the number of low-income children receiving health assessments and follow-up diagnostic and treatment services

- otherwise promote the health of mothers and infants by providing prenatal, delivery, and postpartum care for low-income, at-risk pregnant women
- provide rehabilitation services for blind and disabled individuals under the age of 16 years
- provide and promote family-centered, community-based coordinated care for children and adolescents with special health care needs (those with or at risk for chronic or disabling conditions) and facilitate the development of community–based systems of services for such children and their families
- assure provision of services in areas of special concern, including: mental retardation, SIDS, pediatric AIDS, adolescent pregnancy, STDs, childhood injury prevention, substance abuse, lead poisoning, homelessness, and violence
- conduct needs assessments every five years and meet expanded requirements for planning, data collection, and reporting

The remaining 15 percent of the MCH block grant money is allocated for Special Projects of Regional and National Significance (SPRANS) grants. These are demonstration projects that are fully funded (that is, no matching funds are required) from competitive applications for MCH research and training; genetic disease testing, counseling, and information dissemination; hemophilia diagnostic and treatment centers; and other special projects.

MCH block grants and Title V have been undergoing severe scrutiny in Congress. Cuts originally proposed by Congress have been largely restored. However, it remains difficult, given the current federal legislative climate, to predict the eventual shape, state, or amount of MCH block grants. Given the precarious status of the nation's most vulnerable populations, mothers and infants, the developments surrounding Title V funding deserve careful attention.

Other New Programs

When appropriations for Title V exceed $600 million (as they did for the first time in 1992), 12.75 percent of the funds over that level are designated for the new Community Integrated Service System (CISS)

Program. Preference will then be given to the following projects in local areas with high rates of infant mortality: maternal and infant health home–visiting programs; projects to increase participation of obstetricians and pediatricians; integrated MCH service delivery systems; MCH centers providing pregnancy services for women and preventive and primary care services for infants under the direction of a not-for-profit hospital; MCH projects to serve rural populations; and outpatient and community-based service programs for children with special health care needs.

Two new programs authorized under the Public Health Service Act are also to be administered by the MCH Bureau of the HRSA: Emergency Medical Services for Children (EMSC), in which states work in partnership with medical schools, and the Pediatric/Family HIV Demonstration Grant Program, which provides comprehensive services to pediatric and adolescent AIDS patients and their families. The bureau also administers the Healthy Start infant mortality reduction initiative, whose projects in predominantly urban areas were spearheaded by coalitions involving public, private, religious, and other community-based organizations.

WIC

The Supplemental Food Program For Women, Infants, and Children, or WIC, is funded and administered by the Department of Agriculture in partnership with the states. Eligibility criteria include poverty and risk of poor nutrition for pregnant and postpartum women, nursing mothers and their infants, and children up to five years of age. Program benefits include vouchers for nutritious foods and infant formula, nutrition education, and referrals to comprehensive maternal and child health services.

Early Periodic Screening, Diagnosis, and Treatment

Early Periodic Screening, Diagnosis, and Treatment, or EPSDT, is part of the federal Medicaid program. It provides support for physicians, nurse–practitioners, and other qualified midlevel practitioners to perform well-child screening exams on Medicaid-enrolled children from birth to age 21 years. Each state is required to develop an appropriate schedule for these examinations, provide outreach to inform eligible families of this service, and assist with transportation and follow-up as needed. Although EPSDT is the largest federal-state program of child preventive services in the country, it continues to be vastly underutilized, with less than a third of the eligible examinations actually occurring.

Family Planning

Most family planning services provided through health departments are funded through Medicaid as funding has waned for Title X of the Public Health Service Act. Thus, eligibility for family planning services tends to be restricted to women who qualify for Medicaid. The expansion of non-AFDC Medicaid eligibility for pregnant women usually ends 60 days postpartum, so those mothers who lose Medicaid coverage can be started on birth control, but they generally cannot continue such services. Some states have recently sought federal Medicaid waivers to extend the period of eligibility for family planning coverage. Many health departments have special family planning programs for teenagers, sometimes located at or adjacent to high schools in order to increase access.

Other Programs

Numerous programs related to maternal and child health fall outside the realm of the MCH Bureau. For example, child welfare services are administered by the Administration on Children and Families, and the WIC nutritional supplementation program is housed within the Department of Agriculture. Many other federal agencies work with the bureau to serve the needs of women and children, for example, the Substance Abuse and Mental Health Services Administration (SAMHSA) which works in the area of perinatal substance abuse.

OBRA 89

The Omnibus Budget Reconciliation Act of 1989, or OBRA 89, uses several mechanisms to facilitate collaboration among agencies serving the MCH population:

- Requirements for coordination between Title V programs, WIC, and Medicaid were strengthened.
- Services provided by Title V agencies to Medicaid-eligible persons must be reimbursed by Medicaid.
- Interagency agreements are required to eliminate duplication of services.
- Standards must be set for EPSDT.
- Adequate outreach services need to be developed.
- Other programmatic cooperation must be facilitated, confidentiality assured, and billing procedures established.

State interagency agreements include such provisions as toll-free telephone hotlines and referral services, media campaigns about the importance of prenatal care, and door-to-door canvassing for recruitment of pregnant women. Some states train "resource mothers" to support and assist women in enrolling in Medicaid, WIC, and early prenatal care. Provider recruitment efforts and tracking systems to assure continuity of care for high-risk infants are aspects of other states' incentives. OBRA 89 also required the development of a joint application for enrollment in Title V programs, Medicaid, Head Start, community/migrant health centers, health care for the homeless, and WIC, thus reducing bureaucratic complexity.[7]

The Nature of State Public Health Systems and MCH Services

One of the national health promotion and disease prevention objectives for the year 2000 is to "increase to at least 90 percent the proportion of people who are served by a local health department that is effectively carrying out the core functions of public health."[6] Efforts to achieve this aim will be designed according to states' organization of public health systems. Every state and territory, as well as the District of Columbia, has a state health agency. The majority function as independent agencies, but about a third are part of consolidated superagencies within state government. The Institute of Medicine, in its 1988 report *The Future of Public Health,* recommended that state health departments serve as lead agencies for a wide range of health-related activities.[8] Currently, Medicaid, mental health, environmental services, and other programs are often administered under other agencies, and maternal and child health functions are divided up under different authorities.

Each state is characterized by one of three patterns of organization: (1) a highly centralized system in which the state has administrative authority, sets uniform statewide standards, and hires personnel as state employees; (2) a decentralized system in which local health programs are responsible to mayors or county commissioners; and (3) a system in which the state agency contracts with and monitors the performance of local providers, such as community health centers and visiting nurses' agencies, but does not sponsor local health departments. In some states, local governments share authority for their health departments with the states. In others, state authority applies to health departments and local authority to other agencies (verbal communication with C. A. Miller, Professor Emeritus, University of North Carolina, Chapel Hill, School of Public Health).

Prioritization and implementation of maternal and child health services varies among states according to organizational and other factors. In highly centralized states, MCH programs developed by the state may be mandated at the local level. In other states, there may be great diversity in county MCH services. In a survey of local public health agencies conducted in 1990, the two most commonly reported services provided were immunizations (92 percent) and child health services (84 percent). Other maternal and child health programs were WIC (69 percent), family planning (59 percent), prenatal care (59 percent), services for handicapped children (47 percent), and obstetrical care (20 percent).[9] States vary in the extent to which personal health care services are provided at local health department sites, based largely on funding sources and availability of alternative providers for Medicaid–eligible and uninsured populations. With major Medicaid eligibility expansions mandated for pregnant women and young children, public programs have seen a dramatic increase in the demand for services in areas lacking private providers who are willing to treat Medicaid clients.

HEALTH SERVICES FOR MCH POPULATIONS

MCH populations include women of childbearing age, pregnant women, infants and toddlers, school-age children, and adolescents. Special needs and programs for these vulnerable groups are addressed next.

Women of Childbearing Age

The public health services offered to women of childbearing age have traditionally focused on reproductive needs and have not always provided comprehensive health care for women. Family planning clinics that target young and multiparous women for the prevention and spacing of pregnancies often provide the major source of primary care for low-income women. Some providers advocate expanding the range of medical services in family planning settings for that reason. Family planning approaches have utilized school-based clinics and postpartum follow-up, seeking to disseminate educational materials regarding available forms of birth control. Screening for sexually transmitted diseases has also become an important component of family planning services.

Contraception and family planning services were significantly restrained by the Reagan and Bush administrations, but the Clinton administration has begun to reverse many of these regulations in spite of strong congressional reaction. FDA approval of Norplant and Depo-Provera could significantly alter family planning programs by providing long-term reversible contraception, but it also raises concerns about acceptability, costs, service delivery, and possible ethical concerns related to these new contraceptives. Greater understanding of cultural differences in fertility decision making will be required to promote the use of family planning services and contraceptive technology while respecting women's reproductive autonomy.

Abortion

Abortions are rarely provided through health departments, but referrals frequently were made to abortion clinics until such actions were forbidden by the Reagan administration. Now that this rule has been reversed, health departments can again play a role in assisting women who choose to terminate pregnancies. The introduction of noninvasive abortion procedures could greatly simplify the early termination of pregnancy and potentially make early abortion more readily available and less costly.

Infertility

Infertility remains a large problem with a wide range of causes. Advanced forms of assisted reproductive technology generally are not available to those of low income and are often not covered by standard insurance policies. However, some basic infertility services, such as the enhancement of ovulation, are available to most women. The prevention and early treatment of venereal disease is an important component of the prevention of infertility.

HIV and STDs

HIV infection and other sexually transmitted diseases represent a rapidly growing risk to women of reproductive age, particularly those in lower socioeconomic groups. Public education and condom use are the major prevention strategies available at this time. HIV testing has been recommended for pregnant women now that studies have shown that treatment with AZT early in pregnancy can significantly reduce HIV transmission from mother to baby. This recommendation runs counter to the current tradition of the need for informed consent in HIV testing. All pregnant women should be offered information about HIV disease, modes of transmission, behavioral risks, and risk reduction strategies. As with any form of screening, HIV screening must be contingent upon availability of services for ongoing evaluation, monitoring, and treatment.

Preconceptional Health Promotion

Preconceptional health promotion is a newly emerging and promising field. Many of the important events in fetal development occur in the first few weeks of pregnancy, before the woman even knows of her condition. To prevent fetal damage in those vulnerable early weeks, it is critical for the prospective mother to reduce the hazards of the uterine environment by avoiding alcohol and drug use and optimizing her health status with good nutrition, vitamin supplements, rest, and exercise. Preconceptional health promotion programs provide education and encouragement to women before pregnancy to modify their behavior and reduce early risks to fetal development.

Breast and cervical cancer screening and detection of other chronic diseases are also important functions for health departments. These services can be provided to women of childbearing age in conjunction with preconceptional health promotion.

Pregnant Women

The use of prenatal care early and regularly throughout pregnancy has been demonstrated repeatedly to be associated with improved pregnancy outcomes. Traditional prenatal care services were designed to detect early signs of medical problems, such as preeclampsia, that are known to complicate the latter months of pregnancy and increase maternal and infant morbidity and mortality. The Institute of Medicine and the American College of Obstetrics and Gynecology have recently advocated modifications of prenatal visit schedules to screen women early in pregnancy for risk of preterm delivery and to monitor closely those women found to be at high risk. Additional efforts have focused on using home visitation, social support services, and educational materials to reduce stress and modify maternal behavior in order to achieve optimal birth outcomes.

The malpractice crisis in obstetrics has caused many family physicians and some obstetricians to stop delivering babies with the result that delivery services and even prenatal care are less available, particularly for the poor and those living in rural areas. This trend has intensified the demand on public clinics as sites for prenatal care. In efforts to control hospital costs, women are being discharged routinely one or two days postpartum after uncomplicated deliveries. Early discharge of mothers and newborns results in the need for more careful follow-up for early identification of postpartum complications and infant health problems.

Women in the workforce often face additional challenges in meeting their health needs. Pregnant women often work at jobs that do not permit time off for prenatal care visits. The physical stresses of work, the need for day care services, and the lack of adequate health insurance for pregnancy-related services further undermine the provision of prenatal and delivery care for many women.

Infant and Toddler Health

Many health departments have the capacity to provide only well-child care, leaving families to find other means for dealing with acute and chronic illness. This division of health care services does not serve the population well, and it impedes the development of trusting and consistent relationships between patients and providers. Well-child care lays the basis for prevention and early intervention, but it needs to function in the context of comprehensive care.

Well-child care consists of assessment, counseling, and some medical interventions tailored to the stage of development and the needs and resources of the family. The assessment of growth and development provides a sensitive measure of child health, nutrition, and family functioning. Screening for anemia, deficits in hearing and vision, and abnormal blood pressure are recommended in early childhood. Under special circumstances, additional screening might be warranted for tuberculosis, lead poisoning, and hemoglobinopathies. By age four, children should have received a screening dental examination. Assessments also should be made of the child's risk status for illness and injuries as well as exposure to tobacco smoke and other environmental hazards. Additionally, it is important to identify potential problem areas in the family's critical role of nurturing and providing essential resources for the child.

Counseling

Counseling is tailored to the developmental level of the child and the resources and capacities of the family. Counseling should focus on the three or four most pertinent issues that emerge from the assessment. Both counseling and assessment processes should be sensitive to the diversity of families' cultures and values. Counseling will be most successful when it is provided in a supportive environment with appropriate referral and follow-up. Because future developmental events are predictable, it is also possible to offer anticipatory guidance for problems likely to arise before the next scheduled visit.

Immunizations

Immunizations remain one of the most effective means of preventing disease. The schedule for immunizations is constantly being revised as new vaccines become available. The current immunization schedule requires at least six visits between birth and school entry, with as many as four immunizations given at some of those visits. Because of state regulations, virtually all children are fully immunized before school entry. However, there is far less success at immunizing young children adequately prior to their second birthday. Current estimates indicate that 40 to 50 percent of two–year-old children have not received all the recommended immunizations by 18 months of age. The United States now ranks among the worst of the nations of the Western Hemisphere in achieving full immunization of children under two years of age.

Day Care Sites for Service Delivery

Child day care centers become logical sites for the provision of health services to preschool children as more women join the workforce. Day care offers the opportunity to combine health care with services to enhance physical and cognitive development and social skills. Parents can benefit from health education and child development programs in the day care setting. There is also growing evidence that high-risk families benefit by home visitation that provides one-on-one assistance in parenting skills, enhancing child development and providing social support to mothers living under stressful circumstances.

School-Age Children and Adolescents

Health department staff often work closely with schools to provide important health services to the school-age population. On-site school nursing services have moved beyond the traditional screening programs for hearing, vision, and scoliosis to include health assessments of individual children at risk, counseling services, and even medical services such as illness care, family planning, and the treatment of chronic medical problems. In addition to providing specific health services, health department personnel often work in partnership with teachers to provide health education to students in the classroom setting as well as one-on-one.

School-based or school-linked clinics are emerging as a way of getting needed health services to the adolescent population. Services are often linked to the curriculum so that students who are learning about topics such as sexually transmitted diseases can have access to related services in or adjacent to the school building. Such linkages have also led to controversial programs such as condom distribution and family planning services. Substance abuse prevention, AIDS education, and violence prevention are the major issues dominating school health programs at this time.

MCH Services In the Future

Moving beyond health care reform, maternal and child health advocates are eager to assure that the historical lessons of federal MCH policy guide future steps. Some lessons learned include the advantage of comprehensive service models for low-income populations and the need to streamline and coordinate a full array of services to make them accessible and efficient. The importance of basing programs in community settings has been recognized as a means of assuring their acceptance and cultural competence. Orienting services to involve and meet the needs of entire families recognizes the impact of health problems on all family members and the therapeutic potential of family systems.

Another lesson from federal MCH policy is the need to make public systems more user-friendly for providers as well as patients, eliminating unnecessary bureaucratic hassles and providing adequate support for the care of traditionally underserved groups. Acceptability of services for both providers and patients requires elimination of the inequities and stigmatization traditionally attached to programs for low–income women and children. Thus, the trend in public health services for the MCH population has been and should continue to be towards community-based, family-centered, integrated delivery systems of comprehensive services with increased incentives for provider participation.

There is a major effort now underway to move Medicaid patients, many of them AFDC recipients, into managed care plans. Advocates suggest that these women and children will welcome better–coordinated mainstream medical care in the private sector over the care they currently receive in the public sector. However, private sector health care has not traditionally been organized to coordinate the range of care needed by low-income pregnant women, including outreach, nutritional, health education, psychosocial, care coordination, and follow-up services. The successful approaches of public providers in offering appropriate, comprehensive services for low-income families will need to be incorporated into new service delivery systems.

With the spotlight on the future of health care, maternal and child health providers will need to join with families and advocates to provide oversight to the change process, to build upon the lessons learned in this important realm of public health, and to assure governmental accountability for achieving the objectives of health reform for all of the nation's mothers and children.

CONCLUSION

Mothers and infants are our most vulnerable populations. Efforts have been expended since the early 1900s to assure services to mothers and children. We have developed, over the years, a network of programs designed to benefit maternal and child health. As forces develop that may threaten this range of services, public health must remain vigilant to assure services to these populations.

REFERENCES

1. Lesser AJ. The origin and development of maternal and child health programs in the United States. *Am J Public Health.* 1985;75(6):590–598.

2. Rosenbaum S. The Maternal and Child Health Block Grant Act of 1981: teaching an old program new tricks. *Clearinghouse Review.* August/September 1983:400–414.

3. National Center for Children in Poverty. *Five Million Children: 1992 Update.* New York, NY: Columbia University School of Public Health; 1992.

4. Brauerman P, Bennett T. Information for action: An advocate's guide to using maternal and child health data. Washington, DC: Children's Defense Fund; 1993.

5. US Dept of Health and Human Services. *Understanding Title V of the Social Security Act.* Washington, DC: Public Health Service, Health Resources and Services Administration, Maternal and Child Health Bureau; undated.

6. *Healthy People 2000: National Health Promotion and Disease Prevention Objectives for the Nation.* Washington, DC: US Dept of Health and Human Services; 1991. PHS publication no. 91-50212.

7. *Dedicated to Care for Children: a Report on States Use of OBRA 1986 Earmarked Title V Funds.* Washington, DC: Association of Maternal and Child Health Programs; 1990.

8. Institute of Medicine, Committee for the Study of the Future of Public Health. *The Future of Public Health.* Washington, DC: National Academy Press; 1988.

9. National Association of County and City Health Officers. National profile of local health departments. Washington, DC: 1992.

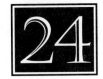

CHAPTER

24

Injury Control

David A. Sleet, Ph.D.

Mark L. Rosenberg, M.D., M.P.P.

Injury is the third leading cause of death in the United States and the leading cause of death for children and young adults.[1] Each year, about 149,000 injury-related deaths result in 3.7 million potential years of life lost prematurely before age 65.[2] This compares with less than 3.0 million potential years of life lost for cancer or heart disease alone and 400,000 for AIDS or stroke alone.

INJURY AS A PUBLIC HEALTH PROBLEM

Nonfatal injuries result in 114 million physician contacts every year, and more than one-quarter of all emergency room visits are for the treatment of injuries. Injuries are also the leading cause of hospital admissions for people under age 45 and the leading cause of medical spending for children ages 5–14.[3] One in four Americans will suffer a potentially preventable injury serious enough to require medical attention this year.

Using a new method of measuring disease burden, called Disability-Adjusted Life Years (DALYs), which combines the impact of both death and disability from a variety of causes worldwide,[4] the injury burden is even more impressive. Violence alone, including homicide, suicide, and war, account for about 50.1 million DALYs lost, causing more suffering than AIDS, malaria, tuberculosis, or ischemic heart disease.[5] Unintentional injuries account for 50.6 million DALYs.[4]

In 1993, motor vehicle crashes were the leading cause of death from injury, as shown in Table 24.1. Firearms were the second leading cause of death from injury, and they were third, after falls and motor vehicle crashes, as a cause of hospitalization. Although motor vehicles, firearms, falls, poisoning, fires and burns, and drownings account for 80 percent of deaths from injury, they represent only 36 percent of treated injuries not requiring hospitalization.

TABLE 24.1   Number of Deaths Caused by Injury and Rates Per 100,000 Population by Sex and Age, 1993, United States

| | (INCLUDES UNKNOWN AGES) | | | | | | |
| | MALES | | FEMALES | | TOTAL | | |
Cause of Death	No.	Rate	No.	Rate	No.	Crude Rate	Age Adj. Rate*
Motor Vehicle E810–825	28,531	22.68	13,362	10.12	41,893	16.25	15.97
Falls E880–E888	6,620	5.26	6,521	4.94	13,141	5.10	2.47
Drownings E830 E832 E910	3,569	2.84	821	0.62	4,390	1.70	1.72
Fires/Flames E890–E899	2,326	1.85	1,574	1.19	3,900	1.51	1.30
Poisonings E850–E869	6,476	5.15	2,061	1.56	8,537	3.31	3.07
Homicide/Legal Intervention							
E960–E978	20,290	16.13	5,719	4.33	26,009	10.09	10.71
Suicide E950–E999	25,007	19.88	6,095	4.62	31,102	12.06	11.23
Other	15,116	12.01	6,973	5.28	22,089	8.57	6.93
TOTAL E800–E999	107,935	85.79	43,126	32.67	146,715	58.60	53.40

*The age–adjusted rate excludes those of unknown age. The standard population used to calculate age-adjusted rates is the 1940 United States population, all races and both sexes.
SOURCES: National Center for Injury Prevention and Control; National Center for Health Statistics, Centers for Disease Control and Prevention (CDC), 1996
Note: NCHS Mortality Data Tapes are used for number of deaths; Demo-Detail postcensal estimates are used for population numbers.

Most severe and fatal injuries are the result of interactions between humans and technological developments and devices. Motor vehicles and guns account for the largest burden of injuries. Cigarettes, which ignite more house fires than any other ignition source, and home swimming pools, which drown more children than any other bodies of water, provide examples of human inventions that are major sources of preventable injuries.

Injuries not only harm individuals, they also place a tremendous burden on the United States economy. The aggregate lifetime cost for persons injured in 1988 was $180 billion. Unintentional injuries accounted for approximately two-thirds of those costs.[2]

PUBLIC HEALTH APPROACHES TO INJURY CONTROL

Applying a host-agent-environment approach to the injury problem has demonstrated that injury control programs can work to reduce the incidence and severity of injuries.[6] These programs have in common the application of a public health model and a scientific approach to injury prevention that includes surveillance of the magnitude of the problem, risk factor identification, intervention development, and program implementation. This approach is shown in Figure 24.1.

Injury prevention has not traditionally been embraced as a public health issue. One obstacle to addressing the injury burden in this manner has been the belief that injuries are "accidents" that occur by chance. This implies that injury patterns cannot be understood and that injuries cannot be prevented. In fact, most injuries, like many diseases, can be attributed to behavioral and environmental factors that can be modified to prevent injuries.[7] Injury control aims to prevent the medical, social, and economic consequence of events that are predictable and often preventable.

The term **injury** (or the specific type of injury, such as a broken arm, a burn, or a gunshot wound to the chest) describes the harm done. When referring to attempts to reduce harm, the term **injury control** is used because it includes injury prevention as well as reduction in the severity of injury through medical care and

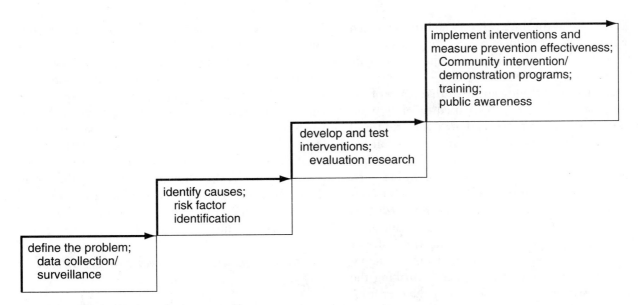

FIGURE 24.1 Public Health Model of a Scientific Approach to Prevention. SOURCE: National Center for Injury Prevention and Control, Centers for Disease Control and Prevention.

rehabilitation. Injury control thus encompasses all three of these phases: prevention, acute medical care, and rehabilitation.

The Epidemiologic Model

Epidemiology is the study of the occurrence, causes, and prevention of disease. Disease occurrence is measured and related to different characteristics of individuals and their environment. *Injury epidemiology* has developed in acknowledgement of the fact that injuries, like diseases, display long-term trends and geographic, socioeconomic, and seasonal variations. They also vary according to characteristics among individuals (including age, sex, and income) and their environments (such as neighborhood, workplace, or home). Epidemiologists ask the question, "Which characteristics explain differences in disease patterns or outcomes?" For epidemiologists working in the area of transportation-related injuries, the question might be phrased, "What predisposes the occurrence of a crash (for example, alcohol, bad weather, or other factors), and what influences the risk of an injury or other adverse health

outcome (for example, seat belt use, side impact protection, or other factors)?"

Conceptually, the epidemiologic model developed for disease can be applied to injury. This model includes a consideration of the contribution of and interaction between the *host* (the person injured), the *agent* (energy), the *vector* (the vehicle that may convey energy), and the *environment* (including physical and sociocultural factors).

The specific cause of an injury is the transfer of energy to a person at rates and in amounts above the tolerance level of human tissue. The amount of the energy concentration above the tolerance level of tissue determines the severity of the injury. Injury may be either *unintentional* (accidental) as in a fall or drowning, or *intentional* (deliberate) as in homicide, battering, murder, or suicide.

The epidemiological study of injury is relatively new. The twentieth century was almost two-thirds past before the agents of injury were accurately identified as various forms of energy (mechanical, thermal, chemical, electrical, or radiological ionization) or lack of essentials (such as oxygen in the case of asphyxiation and heat in the case of frostbite.)[8] Injury control is a much newer field than the epidemiologic study of diseases, and many fundamental problems of injury control are just beginning to be addressed.

Nonetheless, it is already apparent that many of the same approaches that have been used to understand and control disease can be used to understand and control injury. Injury results from the interaction between injury-producing agents, such as kinetic energy and playground equipment; and a susceptible host, such as a young and curious child. Injury can be controlled by preventing its occurrence or minimizing its severity. In the case of motor vehicle injury, damage to the host is brought about through a rapid transfer of kinetic energy when the car stops suddenly. Changing this pattern of energy transfer, either by making the host more resistant to it or by separating the host from the energy exchange, is part of the science of injury control.[9]

Factors and Phases of Injury

An important contribution to the epidemiology of injuries and the potential for prevention was made by Haddon.[9] Haddon perceived three phases of injury—preinjury, injury, and postinjury—for which human, vehicle, and environmental factors play an important role. Table 24.2 gives examples of Haddon's phases and factors.

In the preinjury phase of a car crash, human factors (such as intoxication), vehicle factors (such as faulty brakes), and environmental factors (such as poor visibility) can all contribute to the cause of the crash. During energy exchange in the injury phase, host factors (such as susceptibility to tissue damage), vehicle factors (such as energy absorbing automobile interiors), and environmental factors (such as pavement surface or combustible material) affect injury severity. In the postinjury phase, the condition of the host, the potential for further exposure to energy, and access to treatment and rehabilitation can substantially affect survival and the ensuing quality of life.

Countermeasures to Prevent and Control Injury

Haddon also devised a systematic classification scheme for preventing injury or controlling its severity by altering the damaging effects of energy exchange.[9] Robertson[10] points out that the interventions are applicable to environmental hazards generally, but they have relevance for many other injury control interventions. These interventions, with examples of each, include:

- *Prevent the creation of a hazard.* Ban the manufacture of flammable children's sleepware.
- *Reduce the amount of hazard produced.* Require that passenger vehicles, particularly utility vehicles, have low centers of gravity.

TABLE 24.2 The Haddon Matrix, with Examples of Influencing Factors and Phases in Injury

Phases	Factors		
	Human	Vehicle	Environment
Preinjury	alcohol intoxication	braking capacity of motor vehicles	visibility of hazards
Injury	resistance to energy	sharp or pointed edges and surfaces	flammable material
Postinjury	hemorrhage	rapidity of energy reduction	emergency medical response

SOURCE: Haddon W Jr. On the escape of tigers: an ecologic note. *Tech. Rev.* 1970;72:44.

- *Prevent the release of an existing hazard.* Require all cigarette lighters to be child-proof.
- *Modify the rate at which a hazard is released.* Limit the speeds that can be attained by automobiles and motorcycles.
- *Separate, in time or space, the hazard from the people at risk.* Separate pedestrian and bicycle paths from vehicle roads.
- *Place a barrier between the hazard and the people at risk.* Build four-sided fences around home swimming pools, with self-closing, self-latching gates that children cannot open.
- *Modify the hazard.* Use energy-absorbing materials on playground surfaces.
- *Make people at risk more resistant to damage from the hazard.* Provide sufficient warm-up and training programs to reduce or prevent sports-related injuries.
- *Begin to counter damage from environmental hazards.* Use smoke detectors and carbon monoxide detectors in the home.
- *Stabilize, repair, and rehabilitate people who are injured.* Provide prosthetic devices, wheelchairs, and special equipment to those injured.[8,10]

These countermeasures can be useful in conceptualizing how one might approach the prevention and control of injuries. Some have tried to integrate Haddon's approach with more modern health promotion approaches, whereas others have proposed a new behavioral science conceptual framework for intervention development.[11,12]

Injury Surveillance and Data

Public health practitioners agree that effective injury control requires collection and appropriate use of injury surveillance data. The fundamental elements of injury surveillance are described briefly here, with most of the major discussion points derived from Robertson's text.[8]

Several United States government and private agencies as well as many foreign governments maintain complex data systems that routinely or periodically collect injury data as part of public health practice. These data aid prevention planning by allowing researchers to measure trends, detect clusters, and identify factors related to injury. The systems are sometimes used to identify new injury risks, such as injuries associated with the use of snowmobiles,[13] or to identify the benefits of specific injury prevention interventions, such as the use of air bags in motor vehicles.[14]

Use of E-Codes

Although *The International Classification of Diseases*[15] specifies both N-codes, which indicate the nature of the injury, and E-codes, which indicate the external cause of the injury, E-codes are often missing or incomplete from injury reports, even in hospitals and health departments where injury coding is done systematically. These deficiencies severely limit injury control data-gathering efforts. In many cases, the medical history and chart notes are not detailed enough to allow classification by E-code.

Universal E-coding would provide much better information on trends and clusters of injuries by type and demographic characteristics. It would also allow injury control efforts to be better targeted. Additionally it would allow linkage of injury cause data with crash data, hospital treatment, and cost data, enabling better–targeted intervention planning and evaluation. Universal E-coding of hospital discharge records has been advocated by the Council of State and Territorial Epidemiologists, and several states now require it.

Steps in Injury Surveillance

Robertson outlined four steps to successful efforts in control based on injury surveillance that may be usefully applied to public health practice:[8]

1. conduct surveillance to identify injury types and contributing factors
2. identify one or more approaches to eliminating or reducing the hazard
3. implement prevention or intervention approaches among the populations at risk
4. monitor changes in the pattern of injuries over time[8]

An illustration of this approach is found in a program to reduce fatal falls among children in New York City. Epidemiologists from the New York City Health Department devised a surveillance system to monitor fatal falls of children and found that 66 percent of the children under five years of age who fell had crawled out of windows in high-rise buildings. The research also identified the geographical areas of the city where these deaths most frequently occurred.

To combat the problem, the health department promoted the installation of window bars to prevent children from crawling out. A campaign was launched in high-risk neighborhoods to persuade the parents or landlords to install the barriers, and eventually the health department required landlords to install such barriers when requested by tenants. As a result, the number of children who died from falling out of windows declined from 30 to 50 per year in the 1960s to 4 in 1980. Total reported falls also declined proportionately during the same period. In July 1986, the city changed the regulation to require barriers in buildings where children under age 11 lived.

Use of Surveillance Data

This experience shows the usefulness of injury surveillance to injury control and the importance of obtaining location-specific data to identify local injury problems. A campaign to install window guards in *all* homes in New York City, for example, might have been unnecessary.

Another example of the effective use of surveillance data comes from the health department of the State of Missouri. In that state, health and traffic safety databases have been merged into a statewide data linkage program to monitor the impact of not using safety belts, child safety seats, and motorcycle helmets on injury type and severity, care and treatment, and health care costs. These data provide important information to insurers, government-funded programs, and health care professionals, particularly when modifications in injury control programs or policies are being considered.

Detailed surveillance of the circumstances, frequency, and locations of serious injuries can guide recommendations for action by other agencies or organizations that may be in a position to implement preventive measures. For example, if a traffic intersection is the site of repeated crashes and injuries, this information can be used by the appropriate transportation agency in charge of traffic planning to reduce the problem. Knowing the geographic distributions of injuries can also be important in developing programs such as an emergency medical service or trauma care system.[16]

Example of a Good Surveillance System

A good surveillance system includes sufficient detail to identify types of injuries by cause and geographic location, and it helps identify environmental or behavioral modifications that could reduce the incidence and severity of injuries.[17] The Indian Health Service (IHS) provides a good example. IHS designed a supplemental data system, the IHS Severe Injury Surveillance System, that captures data on injury causes and contributing factors. The data are gathered on separate forms for each injury cause. The forms include not only the circumstances of the injury, but also a list of actions that might have prevented the injury or reduced its severity. The form for motor vehicle injury surveillance is presented in Table 24.3 as an example. Other data entry forms and further information about the IHS surveillance system are found in Robertson.[8]

IHS also developed a pilot computer software program that simplified data entry into the surveillance system. Later, IHS switched to use of the Centers for Disease Control and Prevention's database management system called Epi-Info, which, together with the IHS data entry forms, allowed for more efficient data entry and analysis and permitted uncomplicated modification for use in most communities.

As Robertson points out, this surveillance system can be used to target specific interventions.[8] For example, injury control specialists in White River, Arizona, found a cluster of 37 severe pedestrian injuries that occurred at night on a two-mile stretch of road during a two-year period. The tribal government, the State of Arizona, and IHS collaborated in installing lights that illuminated the road section at night.

TABLE 24.3 Sample of the IHS Motor Vehicle Injury Report Form

Community_____ Census tract _____ Location of the incident (specify road, street, or intersection and distance to an identifiable reference point, such as an intersection, business, or milepost number)

_____

_____

_____

Severity: __ fatal __ hospitalized __ ambulatory (fracture, loss consciousness only—exclude others)

Age __   Gender: M __   F __

Single vehicle occupant __
Fixed object __   If fixed object:
Tree__   Utility pole __
Rollover __   Bridge abutment __
Light __ Both   Pole __   Sign pole __   Other __

Animal on the road __   (What? _____)

Multiple vehicle occupant: Frontal __   Side __   Rear __

Motorcyclist __   Single Vehicle __   Multiple vehicle __

Pedestrian __   Crossing intersection __   Crossing elsewhere __

Walking along road __   Vehicle came off road __

Laying in road __   Other (What? _____)

Bicyclist __   Crossing intersection __   Crossing elsewhere __
On road parallel to traffic __   On road __
Against traffic __   Motor veh. came off road __   Other (What? _____)

Lighting: Daylight __   Dark __   Dark but lighted __   Dawn or dusk __

Signals: None __   Flashing warnings __   Red-yellow-green __
Stop sign __   Yield sign __
Other (What? _____)

Crash protection: __ Seat belt   __ Child restraint   __ Crash helmet

Roadway jurisdiction: __ City or town   __ County   __ State   __ Fed.

Modification that might have prevented the injury or reduced severity (check all that apply):

__ No pass stripe   __ Roadside hazard removal
__ Rumble strips   __ Signal or sign at intersection
__ Lengthen yellow phase at signalized intersection
__ Install or lengthen pedestrian walk signal
__ Median barrier   __ Reflectors on curve
__ Snow removal   __ Improve road skid resistance
__ Separate pedestrian walkway from road
__ Reflectors on vehicles or clothing
__ Lighted roadway   __ Curb to limit road access

__ Other (What? _____)

—Additional observations _____

SOURCE: Robertson LS. *Injury Epidemiology.* New York, NY: Oxford University Press; 1992:63–64

During the next two years, only two pedestrians were struck on the modified stretch of road. The Arizona Department of Transportation was so impressed by the success of the initial pedestrian lighting project that they have since widened roadways and pedestrian paths and added improved lighting set back from the road shoulder.

Summary

Every community stands to benefit from an injury surveillance system. Even if the numbers of injuries in a given community are too small to provide useful statistics, communities in adjacent areas can pool their data to detect county, state, or regional patterns. Until a national injury surveillance system is implemented, local communities may benefit from collecting their own surveillance information. Although many medical examiners, coroners, and hospitals collect injury data routinely, uniform mechanisms for assuring data quality are not yet in place. Issues of data quality will continue to be a formidable challenge for injury surveillance in the future.

PREVENTION

Prevention deserves special attention in considerations of injury control. Policies and programs that help reduce the occurrence of injuries also help reduce the economic costs and human suffering that accompany serious injuries.

Axioms to Guide Injury Prevention

Several axioms for injury prevention can help guide efforts in controlling injuries. These are explained and illustrated in the sections that follow.

Injury Results From Interactions Between People and the Environment

Both human and environmental determinants cause injury. The agent of injury will cause relatively little damage if the amount of energy reaching tissues is be-

low human tolerance levels. A tap water temperature of less than 40 to 44 degrees centigrade is not likely to acutely damage human tissue, although higher temperatures may. Approaches that control the environment by reducing hot water temperatures at the tap and that simultaneously target the elderly and parents of small children for education about hot water scald risks, including the need for reduced tap water temperatures, recognize the importance of this interaction.

Injury-Producing Interactions Can Be Modified Through Changing Behavior, Products, or Environments

Injuries can be reduced by modifying the weakest or most adaptable link in the chain of causation. Unsanctioned swimming in a home swimming pool is more easily reduced by placing an isolation fence or barrier between the child and the pool than by supervising the child's behavior at all times. During sanctioned swimming, supervision is the most important strategy. Changing the environment, the laws, the person, or the product can each lead to reductions in injuries.

Environmental Changes Have the Potential to Protect the Greatest Number of People

Changes to the environment that automatically provide protection to every person have the potential to prevent the most injuries. Automatic protections include barriers built into roads, fire sprinklers in buildings, air bags in automobiles, fuses in homes, and child-resistant packaging on consumer products. Such passive interventions have even more success when the public is informed and convinced of their need and benefit.

Effective Injury Prevention Requires a Mixture of Strategies and Methods

Three primary strategies, education/behavior change, technology/engineering, and legislation/enforcement, are widely recognized as effective in preventing injuries.[6] Individual behavior change, product engineering, public education, legal requirements, law enforcement, and changes in the physical and social environment work together to reduce injuries. The challenge in intervention planning is to select the most effective combination of strategies to produce the desired result.

Public Participation Is Essential for Community Action

Effective public policy requires the support and participation of community members. Local conditions and resource availability often determine the direction of injury prevention programs. Injury prevention is most successful when there is public participation, support for, and understanding of injury prevention methods. Without public support, laws that are designed to protect the public, such as laws requiring the use of bicycle helmets, may be ignored and/or repealed.

Cross-Sector Collaboration Is Necessary

Injury prevention requires coordinated action by many groups. Participation by community leaders, in addition to health department and public health officials, is necessary in planning and implementing injury prevention programs. There are a number of ways that other community members can contribute to a program's success, ranging from identifying problems to mobilizing community action and evaluating intervention effectiveness.

Violence Prevention

Violence is a public health problem that affects all segments of American society. The recent public health focus on violence has helped to define the problem in measurable terms. Violence includes suicide, attempted suicide, and acts of interpersonal violence, such as assault, rape, and partner, child, and elder abuse. These types of violence are shown in Figure 24.2.

Young people are disproportionately represented among the victims and perpetrators of violence. The average age of both violent offenders and victims has become younger and younger. Homicide is now the second leading cause of death for young African-American males and females.[18]

Firearms play a critical role in the escalating violence in our communities and in our schools. Between 1985 and 1991, homicide rates increased by 88 percent in the 15 to 24 age group, with almost one-fourth of all firearm fatalities in the United States occurring among this group. More than 60 percent of all suicides are committed with a firearm,[19] and 77 percent of the 105 confirmed cases of school-associated violent deaths in the United States between 1992 and 1994 involved a firearm, most often a handgun.[20]

Women are frequent targets of both physical and sexual assault by partners and acquaintances. Many of these assaults are fatal. In 1991, 5,475 women died as a result of homicide. Six out of ten female homicide

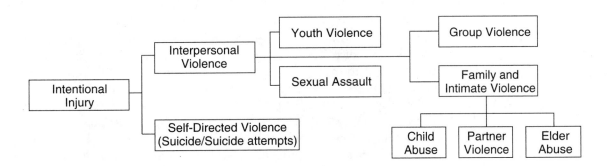

FIGURE 24.2 Types and Categories of Intentional Injury.

victims are murdered by someone they know; about half of these women are murdered by a spouse or intimate acquaintance. Over 99 percent of assaults on women, however, do not result in death, but result instead in long-term physical and psychological injury.

Victims of family and intimate violence represent tens of thousands of emergency room and physician visits. Seventy-five percent of battered women who are seen medically continue to experience physical abuse. In many instances, health care providers are unaware of the extent of the violence, are unsure how to communicate with the victim, and do not know how to refer the victim for additional help.

Guidelines

Although current knowledge about specific strategies to prevent violence is imprecise, some general guidelines can be followed at the individual and community level. These guidelines are equally useful in approaching the violence problem from either the criminal justice or the public health perspective.

Emphasize Primary Prevention. Primary prevention aims to prevent violence from occurring in the first place, rather than trying to identify people who have already perpetrated violence or people who have already been victimized. This means that the target audience for primary prevention programs is much broader than just the group of already–victimized individuals. Primary prevention efforts will probably have an impact on preventing and will help to generate a larger benefit than programs merely aiming to deliver services to victims.

Expect Complex Problems to Require Complex Solutions and Look for Synergy. The types and causes of violence are multiple and complex, and different forms of violence have different causes. Psychological, social, economic, and environmental factors play a very strong role. It follows that the solutions must be multiple and complex as well. Effective prevention programs require combinations of interventions aimed at many different factors and delivered through many channels simultaneously.

New solutions may require new approaches. The large–scale social factors that contribute to violence include poverty, discrimination, lack of opportunity for education and employment, alcohol and other drugs, lack of adequate housing, and easy access to firearms by youth. Thus, an effective prevention program might include interventions to reduce discrimination; enhance opportunities for education, training, and employment; reduce alcohol and drug use; enforce existing regulations; prevent access by youth to firearms; and provide adequate health and social services. These efforts, while requiring complex and broad–ranging actions, may result in a combined effect that is greater than would be normally expected.

Intervene Early and Focus on Children and Those Who Influence Children. The most effective interventions in the long run may well be those that shape attitudes, knowledge, and behaviors in children who are very young and still open to positive influences. The impact of early intervention may be felt over the course of a lifetime and passed on to successive generations. However, results of programs aimed at children are often difficult to measure, and evaluation will require a sustained commitment over time. Because children grow and develop under the influence of parents, teachers, peers, and media, programs aimed at children should include components focused on these groups as well as on the children themselves.

Work with the Community. St. Francis of Assisi urged, "seek first to understand and then to be understood."[21] Public health practitioners must listen to the communities that are affected and understand what they consider the best approaches to preventing violence among their residents, given their resources and the patterns of violence that occur. Those living with violence often have an excellent intuitive sense of what would be an effective intervention. Community participation must begin at the earliest point so the people who will be affected most are involved in designing the programs. New partnerships involving community-based organizations working with health departments, police, courts, schools, labor, academic institutions, social service agencies, and public housing authorities hold great promise for success.

To develop the most effective prevention programs for a given community, the characteristics of its violence problem must be assessed. In some areas, gangs may be the primary problem; in others, ethnic rivalry. In still others, violence against women may be the most prevalent problem. Surveillance and data analysis are also critical to monitor progress and evaluate the impact of interventions. Problems vary from one community to the next, and solutions must be culturally appropriate, specific, and sensitive.

Recognize that Safe Schools and Safe Communities Go Together. Schools must be safe if teachers are to teach and children are to learn, but schools must be more than just safe havens in a sea of violence. They must be part of a community-wide effort to prevent violence.

To be most effective, violence prevention education should be integrated into a comprehensive school health education curriculum. This means including violence prevention in the kindergarten through grade 12 curriculum, including it in teacher in-service training, and developing strategies to create safe school environments. Some of the interventions best suited to schools involve teaching skills in nonviolent conflict resolution. Another approach is to teach violence prevention through noncurricular methods, such as mentoring programs, peer mediation, and modeling by teachers. Schools must also develop strong policies that discourage violence and crime at school and provide sure and swift penalties for violators.

There is no greater threat to effective teaching and learning than an armed and violent student body. In order to achieve the year 2000 national health objective of every school in America being free of violence as well as offering a disciplined environment conducive to learning, there must be close cooperation between schools and their communities.

Evaluate Programs Scientifically and Use Epidemiologic and Behavioral Research to Learn What Works. Violence prevention programs must ultimately be evaluated. Unlike many other public health problem areas, little is known about what works in violence pre-

vention. There is a tension between doing something now and knowing what works, between analysis and action, between science and community. The importance of proceeding scientifically must be underscored so that program effectiveness can be determined while immediate and timely actions are taken to address urgent problems.

The temptation to attempt enormous, all–encompassing programs must be avoided, however. Slow, steady progress with small measured steps is necessary if feedback from experience is to guide program development. At the beginning, a program must be limited in scope: limited in the number of sites, problems addressed, and measurable outcomes.

Use a Scientific Approach to Help Evaluate a Wide Array of Strategies and Interventions to Prevent Firearm Injuries. Firearm homicides and firearm suicides have been responsible for almost all of the recent increases in youth violence. This presents a rare opportunity for substantial improvement in community well–being through the amelioration of a single risk factor. Better information on firearm injuries, especially nonfatal injuries, must be assessed to establish the risks and benefits of firearm ownership and access. Recent studies have shown that:

- The risk of suicide in a household member increases almost five-fold when a firearm is kept in the home.
- When a couple fights, the risk that one will die is 12 times higher when a gun is used than when some other weapon is involved.[19]

The ways conflicts are resolved and the ways firearms are used must be examined. The National Academy of Sciences has suggested that interventions should be targeted on modifying the availability of, access to, use of, storage of, and lethality of firearms.[22] Many of the interventions being advocated today, including gun buybacks, metal detectors, and waiting periods, have not yet been fully evaluated.

Finally, there must be a shift in the public discussion about firearm injuries, from a political or philosophical debate on gun control as an all-or-nothing intervention, to a discussion based on scientifically documented risks and benefits of firearm access and rigorously evaluated policy options. People must be informed that there are many ways to prevent injuries from firearms apart from banning guns—just as deaths from motor vehicle crashes were reduced not by banning automobiles but by building safer cars and safer roads, getting drunk drivers off the roads, and modifying driver licensing requirements.

Address the Problems of Alcohol and Other Drugs as They Contribute to Violence. Too little attention has been given to the role of alcohol and other drugs as factors that contribute to violence. The variety of ways that illegitimate drug use can be associated with violence have been examined, from a direct physiologic effect to violence associated with the business of drug-dealing or obtaining money to buy drugs. However, the ways that alcohol can lead to violence have been much less studied. Control of alcohol and other drugs can help control violence, and violence prevention components can also be built into alcohol and drug abuse prevention programs.

Use all the Strengths of the Criminal Justice Community. There is much to be gained from active enforcement of existing laws that are not strongly enforced. Community policing may be an effective way to enhance enforcement. Judges and judicial system personnel could also receive training that may help them recognize high-risk young people and perhaps lead to the modification of sentencing that would provide constructive alternatives for dealing with such youths. Incarcerated youths also need special attention and treatment in programs such as graduated aftercare. These young people are clearly at risk for perpetuating violence in the future. Out-of-school youths need special opportunities. They could be referred to opportunities for job training, parenting skills, and nonviolent recreation.

Speak to the Heart and Reflect a Clear Vision. Dr. William Foege, a former director of CDC, has said, "behind everything we do, behind everything we say, as the basis for every program decision, we must be willing to see faces."[23] These are the faces of children, children who see their friends, their brothers and sisters, and their parents abused, beaten, and shot down; faces of children and teachers who live and work and play in an atmosphere of constant fear. The victims of violence are clearly not just criminals, drug addicts, and delinquents.

Both media and educational resources must be used proactively to communicate the most important messages and findings clearly and convincingly. At the same time, the exposure of young children to violence in the media must be limited. Both science and the community must be listened to and understood and what is said must be communicated with respect and creativity.

CONCLUSION

Injury control is more readily accomplished when an epidemiologic perspective is employed. A focus on behavioral, environmental, and technological solutions can help prevent injuries by reducing or eliminating hazardous energy exchange.

Injuries are seldom randomly distributed. They are concentrated in physical space, in time, and usually among certain at-risk populations. Collection of data on when, where, how, and which people are injured can lead to the development of specific interventions to reduce injuries.

Further reductions in both unintentional and violence-related injuries and their associated medical care costs will require continued efforts by the public health community in surveillance and research, in building partnerships with public and private organizations, and in the development of state and local health department strategies and injury control programs. Injuries affect people's lives in dramatic ways, and the practice of public health in this area can do much to prevent tragedies and alleviate suffering.

ACKNOWLEDGMENT

Many people from the National Center for Injury Prevention and Control contributed significantly to the material in this chapter, and we wish to thank them collectively for their work both on this chapter and in advancing the field of injury control. In particular, Jim Mercy, Mary Ann Fenley, and Mark Moore (the Kennedy School of Government) helped develop the principles for violence prevention programs. Lee Annest assisted in injury data retrieval, and Garry Egger (Sydney, Australia) helped develop axioms to guide injury prevention. We appreciate the contribution of Chris Branche-Dorsey, Julie Russell, Mary Lynn Harris, Patricia A. Skousen, and Gwen Ingraham in processing and editing this manuscript.

REFERENCES

1. *Vital Statistics Data Tapes.* Hyattsville, Md: National Center for Health Statistics; 1991.

2. Rice DP, MacKenzie EJ, et al. *Cost of Injury in the United States: A Report to Congress, 1989.* San Francisco, Ca: Institute for Health and Aging, University of California and Injury Prevention Center, Johns Hopkins University, Baltimore, Md; 1989.

3. Graves EJ. *1991 Summary: National Hospital Discharge Survey.* Hyattsville, Md: National Center for Health Statistics; 1993. Advance Data from Vital Health Statistics, #227.

4. The World Bank. *World Development Report 1993; Investing in Health: World Development Indicators.* New York, NY: Oxford University Press; 1993.

5. Foege WH, Rosenberg ML, Mercy JA. Public health and violence prevention. *Curr Issues Public Health.* 1995;1:2–9.

6. National Committee for Injury Prevention and Control. *Injury Prevention: Meeting the Challenge.* New York, NY: Oxford University Press; 1989. *Am J Prev Med (Suppl).*

7. Sleet DA. Injury prevention. In: Cortese P, Middleton C, eds. *The Comprehensive School Health Challenge.* Santa Cruz, Ca: ETR Associates; 1994:443–489.

8. Robertson LS. *Injury Epidemiology.* New York, NY: Oxford University Press; 1992.

9. Haddon W Jr. On the escape of tigers: an ecologic note. *Tech Rev.* 1970;72:44.

10. Robertson LS. *Injuries: Causes, Control Strategies and Public Policy.* Lexington, Ma: DC Heath; 1983.

11. Gielen AC. Health education and injury control: integrating approaches. *Health Educ Q.* 1992;19(2):203–218.

12. Geller E, Berry TD, Ludwig TD, Evans RE, Gilmore MR, Clarke SW. A conceptual framework for developing and evaluating behavior change interventions for injury control. *Health Educ Res.* 1990;5(2):125–138.

13. Centers for Disease Control. Injuries associated with the use of snowmobiles—New Hampshire, 1989–1992. *MMWR.* January 13, 1995;44(1):1–3.

14. Sleet DA, Kallberg VP. Airbags and their potential in Finnish motor crashes. *J Traffic Med.* 1992;21(1)(suppl):1873.

15. *International Classification of Diseases.* 9th rev. Geneva, Switzerland: World Health Organization 1977.

16. Pepe PE, Mattox KL, Fischer RP, Matsumoto CM. Geographic pattern of urban trauma according to mechanism and severity of injury. *J Trauma.* 1990;30:1125–1132.

17. Baker SP, O'Neill B, Ginsberg M. *The Injury Fact Book.* 2nd ed. New York, NY: Oxford University Press; 1992.

18. Rosenberg ML, Fenley MA, eds. *Violence in America.* New York, NY: Oxford University Press; 1991.

19. Mercy JA, Rosenberg ML, Powell KE, Broome CV, Roper WL. Public health policy for preventing violence. *Health Aff.* Winter 1993:7–29.

20. Kachur SP, Stennies GM, Powell KE, et. al. School-associated violent deaths in the United States, 1992 to 1994. *JAMA.* 1996; 275(22):1729–1733.

21. Bartlett J, Kaplan J, eds. *Bartlett's Familiar Quotations.* Boston: Little, Brown and Company; 1992.

22. Reiss AJ Jr., Roth JA eds. *Understanding and Preventing Violence.* National Academy of Sciences, Washington, DC: National Academy Press; 1993.

23. Foege WH. Quoted by Sleet DA. In: The Joseph Mountain Lecture. Atlanta, GA: Centers for Disease Control; 1984.

CHAPTER

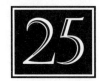

The Public Health Laboratory

K. Michael Peddecord, Dr.P.H.
Ronald L. Cada, Dr.P.H.

Public health laboratories contribute significantly to the capacity of health departments to carry out their core functions of assessment, policy development, and assurance. They were initially developed out of a need to monitor the presence of infectious diseases. Over time, as nonmicrobial contamination of the environment became more of a concern, laboratories developed the capacity to monitor many of these threats as well. In addition to providing surveillance testing, public health laboratories have often been required to provide high-quality, low-cost diagnostic testing for patients enrolled in public health programs and hospitals. Many state laboratories have also assumed a significant role in the assurance of laboratory testing quality in community clinical laboratories through inspection and education services.

Resources have seldom met demands for services. Many laboratories are poorly positioned to meet the current challenges of public health reform. This chapter provides an overview of core laboratory responsibil-

ities and offers a vision for the future. It is anticipated that new technology and changes in the health care system will result in a significant reduction of the routine screening and testing now done in public health laboratories. A growing need for effective surveillance of the quality of community laboratory services will require the effective public health laboratory to increase its capacity to operate in this arena. Enhanced communication, information management, and analytic skills will be necessary if public health laboratories are to continue to be viable and effective entities.

ROLE OF THE PUBLIC HEALTH LABORATORY

In many situations, laboratory testing provides the objective data that underpin public health decision making. Decisions to treat individual patients, provide access to a program for HIV/AIDS patients, prosecute a company found to be polluting a water supply, incarcerate a drunk driver, shut down a public water supply, or condemn a shipload of dried milk powder, among other possible examples—all are based on laboratory information. Laboratory results are as important as other, often subjective, observations of disease and health in the search for solutions to public health problems.

Beginnings

Public health laboratory services were identified as a core function of community health during the 1890s. Laboratories were charged with tracking the distribution of the enteric and respiratory infections that periodically exploded among populations crowding into urban centers at that time. The unique responsibility of public health laboratories was to assist with the task of community health assessment through the scientific identification and measurement of disease incidence and prevalence in susceptible populations. As the relationship between host, agent, and environment was identified for specific disease agents, public health laboratories contributed to disease prevention by using environmental monitoring to estimate disease risk. The need for more adequate characterization and quantification of environmental hazards will continue to challenge the capabilities of public health laboratories.[1]

Shift in Emphasis to Personal Health Care

More recently, since the passage of Medicare and Medicaid legislation, public health departments have become increasingly involved in the delivery of personal health care services. In many local public health agencies, laboratories were merged or integrated with publicly owned hospital labs. The unique community assessment role of public health laboratories often disappeared as the tests they performed became indistinguishable from those of hospital and private clinical laboratories. As increasing resources were needed to support growing public health clinic and hospital workloads, priorities were adjusted, often resulting in a change in emphasis from epidemic surveillance and sanitation efforts to clinical testing services for individual patients supported by health insurance reimbursements.

For those patients who are poor and whose costs are not covered by third party payers, the public health laboratory is often the only viable alternative for needed clinical testing because of the tax-based financial subsidy inherent in most public health laboratory operations. In addition, costs for clinical testing are usually lower in public health laboratories than in the private sector. This increasing attention to patient–based clinical testing has clearly detracted from the ongoing missions of infectious disease surveillance, epidemic investigations, and environmental risk factor analysis.

Public health laboratories, especially at the state and local level, often find themselves in the position of providing services in areas considered unprofitable by commercial testing facilities. For example, testing for the potential of rabies transmission by examination of animal tissue has always remained in the community health laboratory, both because it is a form of environmental disease monitoring and because this labor-intensive analysis has not been automated and would not be profitable in commercial systems. Another example is the use of enteric pathogen serotyping as a surveillance mechanism for tracking disease outbreaks. This activity is essential for understanding the distribution of these organisms in population groups, but it is not particularly helpful in individual patient interventions. As a result, these and similar tests are ignored by the clinician's commercial testing facilities.

Impact of New Technologies

A growing number of laboratory tests are now available for use by the general public. Rapidly developing technologies promise an ever increasing list of procedures intended to be performed by nonlaboratorians in locations where clients live and work, rather than by individuals specifically trained in laboratory processes working in closely controlled institutional environments. More and more laboratory tests can now be done at the patient's bedside, at nursing stations, in shopping malls, in physician's offices, or at remote clinics and environmental sites. Patient self-testing or home testing for blood glucose and pregnancy are examples of over-the-counter test kit technologies readily available with or without a physician's order. The list of home-use tests is expected to grow dramatically over the next decade as individuals request more control over their personal health and manufacturers respond to this market demand. The extent to which these testing methodologies can be safely and effectively used and interpreted by personnel without extensive laboratory training is a current topic of considerable debate.[2]

Especially germane here is the impact this trend will have on the current activities of public health laboratories. The additional options created by generally available test kits increases the complexity of decisions about how and where to provide needed testing services and how to provide clients with the information they need to correctly use home test kits and appropriately interpret and respond to test results.

The Reference Laboratory and Improvement Activities

Since their inception, public health laboratories have collected specimens for testing when an issue of public health importance was at stake.[3] These specimens come from a variety of sources, including other laboratories.[4] Over time, public health laboratories have become *reference laboratories* for a number of procedures that have implications for community health.

As their expertise improved, some public laboratories developed strategies beyond the passive reference role and began activities to systematically improve the quality of testing in other laboratories. These activities were buttressed by early surveys of medical testing laboratories, which indicated that test results were often below minimally acceptable levels.[5,6] Concerns were raised that poor results were so widespread as to constitute a serious threat to the public health. Comprehensive efforts to externally monitor laboratory quality were first introduced in military hospitals during World War II.[7] They were followed by similar efforts in private hospital laboratories in the late 1940s.[6] This external quality control activity run by many state health departments is now a major component of laboratory accreditation and regulatory programs.[8]

REGULATION OF PUBLIC HEALTH LABORATORIES

Despite the lack of credible empirical evidence that modern laboratory services constituted a threat to public health,[9] a federal law requiring licensing of all clinical laboratories was enacted in 1988. Primarily intended to bring clinical laboratory testing in physicians' offices under regulatory oversight, the Clinical Laboratories Improvement Amendments Act of 1988 (CLIA' 88) brought an estimated 135,000 previously unregulated testing sites under a complex system of federal licensure.[10] This highly contentious law classifies tests based upon their technical complexity as well as the risk to patients of incorrect results.

A major reason that federal regulations have prompted concern by public health officials and their laboratories is because personnel standards under CLIA' 88 are based, to a great extent, on previous federal requirements designed for clinical laboratories in hospitals and independent commercial settings.[11] Some public health laboratory leaders believe it is essential to develop standards that recognize the unique nature of public health laboratory testing.[12]

Practice Standards and Guidelines

The use of practice standards and guidelines to improve the accuracy of laboratory testing is well established in laboratory practice and continues to be an area of emphasis of regulatory agencies, public health laboratorians, and their professional associations.

Government Contributions

The recent evolution of practice guidelines for HIV/AIDS testing services provides an example of how federal agencies, such as the Centers for Disease Control and Prevention (CDC), and public health laboratories have worked to standardize and improve testing services for HIV antibody and T lymphocyte immunophenotyping. Public health laboratory officials at CDC and at state and local public health laboratories as well as test kit manufacturers recognized the need to evaluate performance, develop a consensus, and establish guidelines for HIV testing. After a number of ad hoc meetings of experts, the Association of State and Territorial Public Health Laboratory Directors (ASTPHLD) formed a human retrovirus testing committee to oversee this process.[13] Manufacturers, laboratory scientists, and pathologists from commercial and hospital laboratories contributed to the formulation of practice guidelines. CDC provided "official" sanction to many of the practice recommendations by publishing them in supplements to the *Morbidity and Mortality Weekly Report* (*MMWR*).[14]

In the mid-1980s, as the testing requirements to support response to the HIV epidemic exploded onto the public health scene, CDC reorganized its efforts in laboratory training and other improvement activities such as proficiency testing. Most of these new efforts were focused on HIV/AIDS and related testing. The existing centralized, government-run training model was replaced by programs run through a National Laboratory Training Network (NLTN).[15] Seven regional Area Laboratory Training Alliances (ALTAs) were developed to serve as clearinghouses to assess, facilitate, and evaluate training activities. These centers work through training coordinators in state government laboratories.

Voluntary Guidelines to Improve Quality

While some standardization is clearly accomplished by regulation at both the state and federal levels, it is also achieved through the use of voluntary or consensus guidelines. The National Committee on Clinical Laboratory Standards (NCCLS), for example, is a consortium of representatives of laboratorian professional organizations, government, and industry that has a well-defined process to identify procedures in need of standardization and then to draft, review, and promulgate voluntary practice standards.[16]

PUBLIC HEALTH LABORATORIES TODAY AND TOMORROW

In 1988, The Institute of Medicine delineated assessment, policy development, and assurance as the core functions of public health.[17] As the profession fur-ther refines the characteristics of these core functions, it is increasingly clear that public health laboratories have much to contribute to the accomplishment of each. Information obtained from laboratories is important in assessing risks to community health, establishing priorities for public policy making, and assuring the availability and reliability of laboratory tests for decisions related to individual patient diagnosis and treatment.

Current Status

Not surprisingly, the roles, responsibilities, and priorities of a given public health laboratory today correlate closely with the mission of its parent agency. The public health agency that is a leader in disease control and environmental protection, for example, will likely support a laboratory program that provides leadership in information services for those areas of interest. However, if the parent public health agency is heavily involved in providing direct medical services, its laboratory will likely have as its priority the provision of clinical laboratory testing. Community health programs would no doubt be enhanced by the separation of clinical laboratory responsibilities from those more traditionally associated with public health agencies, but such a separation would likely be impractical and unrealistic as well as inefficient in some jurisdictions within the present system.

The fragmentation of the public health system over the past several decades is mirrored in public health laboratories today. A number of traditional public health laboratory functions have been transferred from public health agencies to other agencies and institutions. For example, while the study of the distribution of salmonella infections in the United States population is the responsibility of the CDC, the monitoring of water supplies, one of the vehicles of transmission for these organisms, is the purview of the Environmental Protection Agency. Similarly, the monitoring of food supplies, the most common vehicle for salmonella outbreaks, is the responsibility of the Food and Drug Administration. At the state level, these responsibilities are often distributed widely to such entities as state departments of agriculture, consumer protection, and/or natural resources. Until these activities are unified or coordinated effectively, efficiency and effectiveness will not be maximized. As a lead agency for public health policy development in the United States, the CDC will have among its most important tasks the provision of leadership and assistance to states and selected local laboratories in assuring a public health laboratory system that is truly functional.

Public Health Laboratories of the Future

The existence and future direction of laboratory testing in support of public health is not just a challenge for public health laboratorians. As described previously, laboratory information is essential to the existence of a scientific base for public health services. In a recent review of public health laboratories, Walter Dowdle, deputy director of CDC, expressed concern over a lack of resources in public health and concluded that public health laboratories have generally not fared well during recent cutbacks. However, he also observed that a number of state laboratories had continued to thrive even in this environment.[18]

In order to thrive in changing times, public health agencies need to make an honest evaluation of their capabilities and be willing to adjust to new realities, including adjusting their laboratory services. A public/private planning venture[19] involving public health laboratory directors, public health leaders, and laboratorians from the private sector assessed present public health laboratory structure and services and recommended changes to respond to national trends. Sadly, many of the needed capabilities envisioned in this planning document and espoused as core functions of public health are currently not available or are poorly developed in many public health agencies. These include monitoring of nutritional status and systematic assessment of environmental contaminants, among other capabilities.

The Impact of Health Care Reform

Under current conditions and under most health care reform scenarios, significant clinical and epidemiological laboratory roles would remain the purview of state and local health departments. In an improved system, laboratory services should be universally available in a timely manner to the client, either the individual patient or the community. The experience of private sector commercial laboratories may provide excellent models in this respect. These laboratories have connected networks of local, regional, and national testing facilities linked by electronic and courier networks. A rational system of public health laboratory services would share many characteristics of these private sector systems.

Given the demand for high-quality, cost-effective services, it is clear that many smaller local agencies may not choose to maintain full-service laboratories. Even very large local departments may find it more effective to pool their resources with the state or other local health agencies. In some instances, sharing services with public or private hospital laboratories may be reasonable, as long as the information is available to public decision makers for assessment. The test of the utility of such mergers and reorganizations should be the continued ability to provide information in support of health programs, not short-term cost savings and political correctness.

It was the expectation of some that an evolving system of health care delivery would free public health departments from the responsibility for personal health care services. Under such a scenario, the public health laboratory could have returned to its primary purpose of protecting and promoting the public health through population-based programs.[20] The American Public Health Association (APHA) developed a vision of public health services in a reformed United States health care system.[21] Unfortunately, the envisioned health care reform did not occur. Thus, it appears that the average public health laboratory will retain significant responsibility for providing clinical laboratory services to a large, medically underserved population.

A Vision of the Future Public Health Laboratory

What should the "typical" public health agency laboratory look like in the future? Although there will never be an archetypal laboratory, it is anticipated that future public health laboratories will be different from public health laboratories supported today. It is likely that they will have the characteristics discussed next.

Highly Integrated

The future public health laboratory will be integrated with intrastate and interstate public health laboratory testing. Information technologies and transportation systems will allow efficient integration.

Connected to Personal Health Care Information Systems

The electronic information highways envisioned under health care reform will funnel selected laboratory test results to the local, state, and federal health agency. Public health laboratorians/epidemiologists will monitor communicable disease in the community, converting data into useful assessment information. On a routine basis, supplemental data will be collected from personal health care providers or special studies and integrated with routine, organized community surveys.

Involved in Health-Related Environmental Testing

Food and water testing as well as other environmental testing will be expanded and directed more to health risk measurement. Testing will often depend on remote sensing systems with information passing to the health and environmental authorities for analysis and interpretation. Food monitoring will obtain real-time input from laboratories in food processing facilities in order to monitor changes in the endemic distribution of organisms and the emergence of potential community pathogens or toxins.

Committed to Quality Assessment

Local, state, and federal laboratories will be positioned to assist personal health care providers and various professional organizations in monitoring and improving laboratory performance. Reference specimens of interest will be processed as needed for disease monitoring by the public health testing system. Feedback to personal health care laboratories will provide an opportunity to assure the quality of testing services in the private sector.

Devoted to Laboratory Improvement

Most regulation of personal health care and environmental laboratories will have been replaced by a system of practice guidelines and peer review through professional accreditation agencies. Local or regional public health laboratories will monitor proficiency and patient–testing outcomes with an emphasis on feedback and focused interventions, using practice sanctions as a last resort. Information on testing problems will be used to design training and other intervention strategies. Local or regional organizations will coordinate delivery of training through traditional and innovative distance-based learning methods. Affiliations with local community colleges, universities, laboratory training programs, and schools of public health will enhance available public and private sector resources.

Dedicated to Providing a Safety Net of Bottom-Line Assurance Testing

Some orphan tests that are too specialized for managed-care plans will find a home in the public health system if there is a consensus on public benefits and cost-effectiveness of such testing. In some instances, local health agencies, because of their expertise in managing selected diseases (for example, HIV, TB), will contract with the managed-care plans to provide personal health care services. Laboratories will provide or arrange for needed support services for diagnosis and treatment as well as monitoring of these diseases and conditions.

Committed to a Rapid Response and Research

In some jurisdictions, resources will be allocated to improve assessment methods. Research and development sections will seek improvements in operations as well as basic and applied assessment testing. These centers may be affiliated with universities or research institutes.

CONCLUSION

There is little opportunity for transformation of the public health laboratory until public health and laboratory leaders develop a consensus vision of the future. As communication and testing technology continue to evolve, they present additional management challenges. Laboratory directors and managers were historically judged on their scientific knowledge and their ability to perform skilled analyses. As technology and competition change the laboratory industry, laboratory directors and managers must increasingly become system and information managers.

The challenge is to participate in the development of effective reporting systems that produce standardized information for disease reporting. The ability to understand the decision-making needs of clients and the programs they serve, the menu of available tests, and the test procurement options available from the industry is now an essential skill for laboratory services managers. This transition to "testing–and–information" managers will require a radical shift of thinking for many laboratory directors. Laboratory directors who view their role as one of only providing a service rather than providing information for public health decision making will continue to play a minor role in their organizations. The capacity to balance and manage issues of turnaround time, cost of testing, analytic quality, and legal issues will be the benchmark of the effective laboratory information manager and director of the future.

ACKNOWLEDGMENT

Ongoing funding of the Laboratory Assurance Program is provided by the Centers for Disease Control and Prevention provided under a cooperative agreement with the Association of Schools of Public Health. This funding has provided Professor Peddecord an op-

portunity to continue learning about public health laboratory testing at local, state, and federal levels.

REFERENCES

1. Burke TA. Understanding environmental risk: the role of the laboratory in epidemiology and policy setting. *Clin Chem.* 1992;38:1519-1522.

2. Ferris DG, Fischer PM. Elementary school students' performance with two ELISA test systems. *JAMA.* 1992;268:766–770.

3. Inhorn SL, ed. *Quality Assurance Practices for Health Laboratories.* Washington, DC: American Public Health Association; 1978.

4. Valdiserri RO. Temples of the future: an historical overview of the laboratory's role in public health practice. *Annu Rev Public Health.* 1993;14:635–648.

5. Schaeffer M, ed. *Federal Legislation and the Clinical Laboratory.* Boston, Ma: GK Hall Medical Publishers; 1981.

6. Belk WP, Sunderman FW. A survey of the accuracy of chemical analysis in clinical laboratories. *Am J Clin Pathol.* 1947;17:853–861.

7. Shuey HE, Cabel J. Standards of performance in clinical laboratory diagnosis. *Bull US Army Medical Dept.* 1949;9:799–815.

8. *Clinical Laboratory Improvement Amendments of 1988; Final Rule.* Washington, DC: Dept of Health and Human Services, Health Care Financing Administration; February 28, 1992. Federal Register 57;40:7002–7288.

9. Kenney ML. Quality assurance in changing times: proposals for reform and research in the clinical laboratory field. *Clin Chem.* 1987;33:728-736.

10. Clinical Laboratories Improvement Act of 1967. Washington, DC: US Dept of Health, Education, and Welfare; 1967. Code of Federal Regulations Title 42, Part 74.

11. Sweet CE. Effect of CLIA-88 on public health laboratories. *Clin Microbiol Newsletter.* 1993;15:60–62.

12. Hausler WJ. Commentary by a state public health laboratory director. Paper presented at Session 1090 of the 121st Annual Meeting of the American Public Health Association: San Francisco, Ca; October 25, 1993.

13. *Committee on Retrovirus Testing: Second Consensus Conference on Human Retrovirus Testing.* Washington, DC: Association of State and Territorial Public Health Laboratory Directors; 1987.

14. Centers for Disease Control. Interpretation and use of the Western blot assay for serodiagnosis of human immunodeficiency virus type 1 infections. *MMWR.* 1989;38:1–7.

15. Gore MJ. Keeping up with changing times: how the National Laboratory Training Network helps. *Clin Lab Sci.* 1993; 6:268–271.

16. National Committee on Clinical Laboratory Standards. *NCCLS Handbook.* Wayna, PA: National committe on Clinical Laboratory Standards; 1989.

17. Institute of Medicine, Committee for the Study of the Future of Public Health. *The Future of Public Health.* Washington, DC: National Academy Press; 1988.

18. Dowdle WR. The future of the public health laboratory. *Annu Rev Public Health.* 1993;14:649–664.

19. Counts JM. LIFT 2000: laboratory initiatives for the year 2000. *Clin Chem.* 1992;38:1517–1518.

20. Lee PR, Toomey KE. Epidemiology in public health in the era of health care reform. *Public Health Rep.* 1994; 109:1–3.

21. American Public Health Association. APHA's vision: public health and a reformed health care system. *Nation's Health.* July, 1993:9,11.

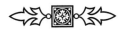

PART FIVE

THE FUTURE OF PUBLIC HEALTH PRACTICE

CHAPTER

The Future of Public Health

C. William Keck, M.D., M.P.H.
F. Douglas Scutchfield, M.D.

Significant gains in health status and life expectancy have occurred over the past two hundred years in the United States as well as in most other industrialized nations. Many attribute those gains to advances in clinical medicine that tend to be dramatically and impressively chronicled in the electronic and print media. Indeed, our capacity to diagnose and treat illness has advanced rapidly during this century. The reality remains, however, that most of the improvements in quality and length of life have come from measures aimed at protecting populations from environmental hazards and pursuing behaviors and activities that are known to be health promoting. Health departments and other community agencies are responsible for developing the programs and relationships with individuals and neighborhoods that will continue to improve the health of citizens of this country.

BACKGROUND

From 1993 through 1994, the Clinton administration stirred a great professional and political debate

through its proposal to significantly change the health care system in the United States in a manner that would provide universal access to health care while controlling the costs of that care. The public health system and its functions were only a minor portion of that discussion. Public health leaders around the country were aware that their discipline was at risk of being ignored while debate focused on illness care, and they were galvanized to define better the role of public health and acquire the resources necessary to carry out effective health promotion and disease prevention activities. The combination of well-documented public health system problems and the need to convince policy makers of the importance of public health in society resulted in clear descriptions of both the core functions of public health and the resources that would be required to assure their existence in each community.

Federal efforts to reform the system came to naught and were largely abandoned by the end of 1994. The pressure created by the high cost of illness care, however, began to drive efforts of cost control across the country, and a dramatic shift to large-scale experimentation with managed care began in many communities. At the same time, a new Congress bent on budget reduction is proposing significant financial cuts and restructuring of many federally supported public health programs. These realities are producing a substantially changed environment for public health agencies. A clear understanding of role, significant community support, substantial flexibility, and real leadership will be required for public health agencies to survive and thrive and make continuing contributions to health status.

THE CONTRIBUTIONS OF PUBLIC HEALTH

Public health policies and actions have significantly improved the health status of the population of this country. Their contribution is summarized in this section.

Public Health Measures and Previous Health Status Gains

Significant gains in population health status during the nineteenth and early twentieth centuries were based on activities assuring the availability and safety of food and clean water, the adequate disposal of sewage, the provision of adequate and safe shelter with minimal crowding, and the adoption of personal behaviors that were health promoting. Due to these measures, substantial control of many communicable diseases was accomplished before the advent of vaccines and antibiotics. For example, tuberculosis deaths declined as a result of improved physical environments and better nutrition; the impact of fecally/orally transmitted pathogens declined with the separation of sewage and drinking water; and vectorborne conditions improved with vector habitat control.[1] These changes, combined with the discovery of vaccines and antibiotics, modified the major causes of death from infectious diseases at the turn of the century to chronic diseases (including heart disease, cancer, and stroke) currently. There has been a concomitant rapid gain of life expectancy from less than 50 years in 1900 to more than 75 years in 1990.

During the past 20 years or so, there has been a growing emphasis on population-based prevention programs aimed at reducing risks for chronic disease. Programs aimed at reducing tobacco use, controlling blood pressure, diminishing obesity and dietary fat, reducing risks for occupational and home injury, and promoting use of seat belts and automobile air bags have contributed to a decline of 50 percent in stroke deaths, 40 percent in coronary heart disease deaths, and 25 percent in death rates for children.[2]

Potential for Further Gains in Health Status

The Centers for Disease Control and Prevention reviewed the major causes of premature death in United States citizens.[3] Their findings confirm that 50 percent of premature mortality in this country is directly related to individual lifestyle and behavior, 20 percent is related to environmental factors, an additional 20 percent is directly related to one's inherited genetic profile, and only 10 percent is related to inadequate access to medical care. This means that fully 70 percent of the premature mortality suffered by the United States population will require population-wide strategies for effective control.

Traditional discussions of health status include a list of the major causes of death for the population of interest. That information is listed in Table 26.1 for the United States.

From a public health/preventive perspective, however, the real question is what underlying risk factors caused the fatal conditions listed in Table 26.1. The underlying causes of many of the premature deaths occurring in our population are listed in Table 26.2.

These factors, which are closely linked to the determinants of health discussed in Chapter 3, are at the root of the finding that 50 percent of premature mortality in the United States is due to factors related to lifestyle. These factors are at the root of preventable conditions that carry a high cost in terms of morbidity and mortality. They also carry a high economic cost. For example, it has been estimated that costs of more than $110 billion can be attributed to alcohol and drug abuse and

TABLE 26.1 Ten Leading Causes of Death in the United States, 1990

Cause of Death	No. of Deaths
All Causes	2,148,463
Heart Diseases	720,058
Cancer	505,322
Stroke	144,088
Accidents	91,983
Chronic Obstructive Lung Diseases	86,679
Pneumonia/Influenza	79,513
Diabetes	47,664
Suicide	30,906
Cirrhosis of Liver	25,815
HIV Infection	25,188

SOURCE: *Healthy People: The Surgeon General's Report on Health Promotion and Disease Prevention*. Washington, DC: US Dept of Health and Human Services, Public Health Service, 1979.

TABLE 26.2 Leading Underlying Causes of Death in the United States, 1990

Cause of Death	No. of Deaths
Tobacco	400,000
Diet/Inactivity	300,000
Alcohol	100,000
Certain Infections	90,000
Toxic Agents	60,000
Firearms	35,000
Sexual Behavior	30,000
Motor Vehicles	25,000
Drug Use	20,000

SOURCE: McGinnis JM, Foege WH. Actual causes of death in the United States. *JAMA*. 1993; 270:2207–2212.

of $65 billion to smoking. Health care costs created by specific preventable problems include $100 billion annually from injuries, $70 billion from cancer, and $135 billion from cardiovascular diseases.[2] Improving access to medical care will have little impact on diminishing the death and disability reflected in the disease and economic figures just cited. AIDS will not be controlled by actions taken in doctor's offices, low-birth weight babies will not be prevented solely by the work of obstetricians, and heart disease will not continue to decline without extensive community outreach and education.

Human health is also directly related to the quality of the environment. Factors such as air pollution, food and water contaminants, radiation, toxic chemicals, wastes, disease vectors, safety hazards, and habitat alterations are at the root of the 20 percent excess mortality related to environmental issues in the United States. Long-term human health is dependent upon achieving ecological balance and maintaining health-promoting home, work, and leisure environments.

PUBLIC HEALTH IN AN EVOLVING SYSTEM

The United States is currently discussing significant changes in the mechanisms utilized to pay for and deliver illness care. It is certain that there is an ongoing major evolution of the health care delivery system, but it is not at all certain what the exact nature of the evolved system will be, including how much attention will be paid to the issues of environment, health promotion, and disease prevention.

In many ways the debate about health care reform is miscast. For the most part, the wrong question is being addressed. Attempts are made to seek better ways of providing and paying for illness care rather than to determine what should be done to create the healthiest population possible. With the courage and the foresight to frame the debate in these terms, it is readily apparent that improved health status depends on illness care reform *and* on public health reform.

For too long, those professionals who concentrate on the diagnosis and treatment of illness have been separated from those who concentrate on health promotion, disease prevention, and control of the environment. Instead of a seamless web of integrated services and activities focusing first on minimizing risks and then on early diagnosis and treatment of emerging disease, two separate systems have developed and evolved into two distinct cultures that are often at odds with one another. It is the responsibility of public health practitioners to help society understand the value of each approach and the need to integrate them into a quest for improving health status.

Obtaining medical care is very important for that segment of the population for whom access is denied or inappropriately restricted. The approximately 10 percent of excess mortality in citizens of the United States that is related to inadequate access to medical care occurs principally in that group for whom access to care is limited. No illness is "deserved," and every member of society should have access to those interventions that have been developed to diagnose and treat disease and minimize suffering. It is also worth noting that significant contributions to disease prevention can be made in the context of a single patient's interaction with a physician or other health care provider. The activities described in the *Guide to Clinical Preventive Services*[4] are particularly recommended for their proven capacity to improve health and prevent disease and injury. Nonetheless, it is population-based services that have the greatest potential to contribute to overall gains in health status.

THE CORE FUNCTIONS OF PUBLIC HEALTH

Population-based services are provided from a variety of sources in most communities. These sources include state and local health departments, community health agencies (for example, family planning agencies, heart associations, kidney associations, cancer societies, mental health agencies, and drug abuse agencies, among others), hospitals, and schools, to name several. However, this chapter focuses on the local health department because it is only the local health department that has statutory responsibility for the health status of its constituent population. It is the health department, in most locations, that is ultimately responsible for the assurance that all citizens have access to the services they need in the community, no matter which groups or organizations ultimately deliver those services. This focus on the health needs of the entire community by an agency ultimately responsible to that community for its performance emphasizes the importance for health of "a governmental presence at the local level (AGPALL)."[5]

Institute of Medicine Report

There exists wide variation in the size, sophistication, capacity, and roles of local health departments in the United States. In their report, *The Future of Public Health,* the Institute of Medicine's Committee for the Study of the Future of Public Health described widespread agreement across the country that "public health does things that benefit everybody," and that "public health prevents illness and educates the population."[6(p3)] However, they found little consensus on how those broad statements should be translated into action. Indeed, there is such great variability in resources, available services, and organizational arrangements " . . . that contemporary public health is defined less by what public health professionals know how to do than by what the political system in a given area decides is appropriate or feasible."[6(p4)] The committee concluded that "effective public health activities are essential to the health and well–being of the American people, now and in the future," but the variability across the country is so great that this essential system is currently in "disarray."[6(p6)]

In an effort to provide a set of directions for the discipline of public health that could attract the support of the whole society, the committee proposed a public health mission statement and a set of core functions. The committee defined the mission of public health as "fulfilling society's interest in assuring conditions in which people can be healthy."[6(p7)] The committee further found that "The core functions of public health agencies at all levels of government are assessment, policy development, and assurance."[6(p7)]

The committee's definitions of these core functions are as follows:

- *Assessment.* Every public health agency should " . . . regularly and systematically collect, assemble, analyze, and make available information on the health of the community, including statistics on health status, community health needs, and epidemiologic and other studies of health problems."[6(p7)]
- *Policy Development.* Every public health agency should " . . . exercise its responsibility to serve the public interest in the development of comprehensive public health policies by promoting use of the scien-

tific knowledge base in decision-making about public health and by leading in developing public health policy. Agencies must take a strategic approach, developed on the basis of a positive appreciation for the democratic political process."[6(p8)]

• *Assurance.* Every public health agency should " . . . assure their constituents that services necessary to achieve agreed upon goals are provided, either by encouraging actions by other entities (private or public sector), by requiring such action through regulation, or by providing services directly." Each public health agency should also " . . . involve key policymakers and the general public in determining a set of high-priority personal and community-wide health services that governments will guarantee to every member of the community. This guarantee should include subsidization or direct provision of high-priority personal health services for those unable to afford them."[6(p8)]

Response to the Report

This report, *The Future of Public Health*, was completed in 1988. Since its appearance it has generated considerable discussion and action. Many in the public health community were (and many still are) uncomfortable with the characterization of public health as a system in "disarray," particularly when looking at the capacity and work of their own agencies. Dissenters note that public health workers have accomplished much in an atmosphere of diminishing resources and devalued public health skills. However, few argue with the committee's suggested mission statement and core functions or with its recommendations for change in order that the mission can be addressed more adequately.

One illustrative response to the Institute of Medicine report has come from the state of Washington. Building on the base established by the institute, the Washington State Department of Health and its Core Governmental Public Health Functions Task Force sought to prepare for public health reform efforts in that state by developing a common definition of the institute's core functions and the role they play in improving a community's health. This effort presaged the work of that state's Public Health Improvement Plan Steering Committee, which sent to its legislature at the end of 1994 a *Public Health Improvement Plan* intended as a blueprint for improving health status in Washington through prevention and improved capacity for public health services delivery.[7] This plan is worthy of careful review by all other states as an excellent example of how public health issues can be understandably described and public health services effectively delivered.

The National Association of County Health Officials (NACHO) responded to a need voiced by many local health officials for a guide to assist local health departments in developing their roles and services in light of the findings of the Institute of Medicine and the changing structure of the health care delivery system. In July 1994, the association published its *Blueprint for a Healthy Community: A Guide for Local Health Departments,* in which it examined the core public health functions in the context of what services are required to create and maintain a healthy community.[8]

NACHO identified 10 *essential elements* that must be present in any community striving for the highest level of health possible. Health departments are responsible for assuring that all the essential elements are provided, and provided well, by some community-based entity. The 10 essential elements identified by NACHO are

1. *Conduct a community diagnosis.* Collect, manage, and analyze health-related data for the purpose of information-based decision making.
2. *Prevent and control epidemics.* Investigate and contain diseases and injuries.
3. *Provide a safe and healthy environment.* Maintain clean and safe air, water, food, and facilities.
4. *Measure performance, effectiveness, and outcomes of health services.* Monitor health care providers and the health care system.
5. *Promote healthy lifestyles.* Provide health education to individuals and communities.
6. *Provide laboratory testing.* Identify disease agents.
7. *Provide targeted outreach and form partnerships.* Assure access to services for all vulnerable populations and the development of culturally appropriate care.
8. *Provide personal health care services.* Treat illness, injury, disabling conditions, and dysfunction (ranging

from primary and preventive care to specialty and tertiary treatment).

9. *Promote research and innovation.* Discover and apply improved health care delivery mechanisms and clinical interventions.

10. *Mobilize the community for action.* Provide leadership and initiate collaboration.

The *Blueprint* correctly notes that some of these elements are directly provided by health departments and that health departments should assure that those provided by others are provided effectively. The *Blueprint* also notes that certain capacities must exist in a local health department in order for it to carry out this combined role of service provision and oversight. These capacities are health assessment, policy development, administration, health promotion, health protection, quality assurance, training and education, and community empowerment.

Although stated somewhat differently, the Institute of Medicine's list of core functions for public health, augmented and expanded by the work of the state of Washington and the National Association of County Health Officials, is quite similar to the list that appears in the public health section of the Clinton administration's unsuccessful health care legislative proposal. The descriptions and examples of population-based services in the latter document defined the basic activities in which effective state and local health departments should be engaged.[9] A reformed health care delivery system should recognize the importance of these services for maintaining and improving health and assure that the agencies providing these services are integrated into the reformed delivery system in an effective manner.

Enhancing the Federal Capacity to Support Local Public Health

The federal government has some responsibility to assure a stable funding base for the delivery of the core public health functions. Effective implementation of the core functions and some other activities of state and local health departments will require the improvement of federal capacities in several areas. An effective and efficient national capacity in surveillance and health statistics, laboratories, and epidemiological services will be essential. Consolidating currently fragmented public health data systems and integrating them into a new regional and national data network would provide timely information to support the development of public policy, the development of budgets, and the efficient administration of programs.

In addition to funding and information, the federal government must also accept some responsibility for providing technical support to health departments struggling with complex problems and the means to carry out responsible research on health risks and the effectiveness of intervention efforts. It would be very helpful to eventually have a guide to effective public health interventions that parallels the existing *Guide to Clinical Preventive Services.*[4]

Public Health Functions in Addition to Core Functions

Most health departments will have responsibilities that go beyond the variously defined core functions of public health. The nature of the additional responsibilities will depend upon the needs of the community served by a particular department. Although many assume that health departments would no longer have a need to provide medical care in a revamped health care system, it could very well be that some departments would have a very active health care role. In some areas the health department is the major or sole source of primary care for a community, and a revamped health care delivery system may recognize those strengths and allow departments to build on them, particularly if the appropriate mix of other medical providers does not move to provide services to some of the country's currently medically underserved areas. Some health departments may very well become health maintenance organizations, or managed-care providers, themselves.

Those localities where significant portions of the population receive medical care from non-health department managed-care providers may offer new opportunities for collaboration between local health departments and managed-care entities. This is especially likely in those states where Medicaid waivers have been granted to move Medicaid recipients into managed-care systems. Health departments will negotiate with managed-care companies to become providers of such services as clinical preventive services, community outreach, case finding, client tracking, and transportation, among others.

Local and state health departments are also very important for the advancement of knowledge about population-based services. Wherever possible, these departments should form links with academic centers for health and provide support for community-based research, including demonstration projects and program evaluation efforts.

CAPACITY OF HEALTH DEPARTMENTS TO FULFILL CORE AND OTHER FUNCTIONS

Since the publication of the Institute of Medicine report on *The Future of Public Health* in 1988, there has been growing agreement in the public health community that the core functions of public health make sense. The profession has been busy defining the particulars of those functions in the interim, as described earlier. The growing unity of thought about public health's core functions, however, begs the question of whether or not local and state health departments actually have the capacity to fulfill the core functions and the other tasks that may be required of them by their own communities. Indeed, available evidence suggests that there is great variability in capacity among the diverse agencies found at local and state levels.

Organizational Diversity

Chapter 7 in this book reviews the structure, governance, financing, and capacities of local health departments. The diversity that characterizes health departments is perhaps an indication of just how problematic it can be to provide public sector services in a democracy. Competition for attention and resources among many interests in a system with multiple decision makers and policy makers makes it difficult to at-

tain and sustain coherence and consistency of function.[6(p123)] In addition to the organizational variability of local public health agencies, there is also a great deal of programmatic variability that results from the deliberate delegation out of public health departments of a number of responsibilities previously considered to be in the purview of public health.

The Institute of Medicine report noted that the coherence of public health activities is damaged by the administration of environmental health, mental health, and indigent care programs by separate agencies.[6(pp108–112)] This separation of responsibilities encourages the development of separate programs and fragmented data systems that impede integrated problem analysis and risk assessment. The result is diminished coherency in the efforts of government to provide service, and a division of constituencies that might otherwise coalesce around a broad vision of the mission of public health.[6(pp123–124)]

Funding

In addition to the problems noted above, most local health departments must cope with inconsistent funding sources. Some local departments are comparatively well funded, but many face severe financial constraints and must rely heavily on sources of revenue that may very well result in inadequate and unstable funding.

Public Health Training in the Workforce

Most public health workers, including some public health leaders, have not had formal training in public health. The Institute of Medicine report noted the need for well-trained public health professionals with " . . . appropriate technical expertise, management and political skills, and a firm grounding in the commitment to the public good and social justice that gives public health its coherence as a professional calling."[6(p127)] The report further noted that public health leadership requires an appreciation of the role and nature of government. It also requires the capacity to continue to learn in order to stay current with the evolution of the discipline.

The Public Health Faculty/Agency Forum was constituted with support from the Centers for Disease Control and Prevention shortly after the Institute of Medicine report was published. This was done in an effort to respond to a recommendation of the report that "firm practice links" should be established between schools of public health and public health agencies as a way of improving health department staffing.[10] An initial step of the forum was to delineate those competencies that, in the forum's view, should be universal in public health professionals if the core functions were to be adequately accomplished. The forum recognized four major public health disciplines, behavioral sciences, environmental public health, epidemiology/ biostatistics, and public health administration, each with its own set of unique competencies. The forum agreed, however, that many competencies, including analytic skills, communication skills, policy development/program planning skills, cultural skills, basic public health sciences skills, and financial planning and management skills, transcended the boundaries of those four disciplines. It recommended that more public health students and workers receive training in these areas by requiring practicum experiences in local health agencies for students; improving communication and collaboration among agencies and schools through such efforts as joint programs, research, and technical assistance, among others; making education and training programs more relevant to practice; and increasing the resources devoted to linking academia with practice.[10]

Despite these recommendations, however, too few of those currently employed in public health come to their jobs with the requisite values and skills, implying that significant on-the-job training is an integral part of the job experience for most. There are, of course, no formal standards for this kind of learning experience, so the presence of the values and skills required is inconstant at best in those who receive their training in public health in this manner. Moreover, there are no licensing or credentialling agencies for public health workers, as there are for physicians and nurses, for example, so it is difficult to obtain data on the public health workforce and to ascertain skill levels.

Staff Size

An important indicator of the capacity of an agency's staff to fulfill the core functions of public health is the size of its staff. The large majority of health departments are small. NACHO's *National Profile of Local Health Departments*[11] reveals that 26 percent of local health departments in the United States have four or fewer employees and an additional 20 percent have between five and nine employees. Twenty-two percent employ ten to twenty-four people, and only 10 percent have one hundred or more employees. Not surprisingly, the report also indicates that larger health departments are most likely already to be carrying out the core public health functions. It is the larger departments that are most likely to have significant numbers of staff with the public health or related training and resultant capacity to pursue assessment, policy development, and assurance functions.

Technical Capacity

Technical capacity is closely linked to the issue of staffing, although it also includes the availability of equipment that might be required to provide for preventive health services, analysis of environmental health problems, laboratory services, and health education activities, among others. Few data exist regarding the distribution of equipment and facilities, but it is probably reasonable to assume that it follows the same distribution characteristics as the staff required to utilize it.

Accomplishment of the core functions relies heavily on the capacity of local health departments to collect, analyze, and use information. There are no data available on the quantity and quality of computer hardware or software or of the technical expertise currently available in local health departments, although the increasing capacity and diminishing cost of computers brings data processing and electronic communication capabilities within the theoretical reach of most agencies. The current perception of public health leaders is that the larger, more sophisticated agencies are becoming part of the "information superhighway," that the smallest agencies largely are not involved with much data processing or information sharing, and that medium–sized agencies are beginning to improve their capacity to process information.

Leadership

The importance of leadership in public health is emphasized in Chapter 9. There is no objective scale by which leadership can be measured, although most people seem to have a good notion of whether it is present or absent. Certainly, there are no formal efforts to measure the effectiveness of leadership in the public health world. There have been discussions of the nature of that leadership, however, with some praise mixed in with an apparent consensus that public health leadership is generally lacking.[6] That consensus has fueled efforts to provide leadership training opportunities at the national level (the Public Health Leadership Institute, a program of the Western Consortium for Public Health, funded by the Centers for Disease Control and Prevention in 1991) and, in some states, for those in public health leadership positions.

Harlan Cleveland suggests that successful public health leaders will be those who understand that from now on the public's health will depend on the art of making creative interconnections. All problems in the real world are interdisciplinary, interprofessional, and international. Because all problems increasingly require a combination of contributions from a variety of disciplines for solution, the successful leader must begin with the aptitudes and attitudes of the generalist.[12] The generalist leader, according to Dr. Cleveland, must be skeptical of inherited assumptions, curious about science-based technology, broad in perspective, eager to pull people and their ideas together, interested in issues of fairness, and self-confident enough to work in the open in an increasingly open society.[13]

Attitudes may be as important as skills in this regard. Dr. Cleveland calls leadership the "get-it-all-together" profession and notes that the following attitudes are indispensable to the management of complexity:[13]

- an acceptance that crises are normal, tensions can be promising, and complexity is fun
- a realization that paranoia and self-pity are reserved for people who do not want to be executives
- a conviction that there must be some more upbeat outcome than would result from adding together the available expert advice

- a sense of personal responsibility for the situation as a whole

Although leadership is difficult to measure objectively, there are several questions one can ask to assess whether a local health department is well led. For example, is the department respected in its community by both community leaders and citizens? Is the opinion of department leaders actively sought when the community faces public health problems? Does the department seek and maintain collaborative working arrangements with other community groups and agencies in such a manner that services to the public are provided efficiently and effectively? Is the department successful working within the political system? Are interactions with the medical community (physicians and hospitals) strong and productive? Is the department considered a source of innovative problem solving? Does the department exhibit a history of adequate and stable funding? Is the department involved in teaching and research? There are many other questions that could be listed here as well. It is the sum total of impressions garnered from pursuing questions such as these that leads to a judgment of the quality of leadership present in a particular local health department.

The quality and nature of public health leadership will be increasingly critical as practitioners struggle to bring some focus to the activities of all the disciplines and professions that impact the public's health. Health is the arena where social forces come together, and the growing awareness of the interrelationship of factors that influence health will continue to expand areas of involvement for health departments. Flexible and innovative public health leadership is essential for society increasingly to make decisions in all areas of human endeavor that are health promoting rather than health destroying.

PUBLIC HEALTH AND MANAGED CARE

The number of individuals receiving medical care through managed-care organizations has been growing steadily. All indications are that this trend will continue because managed care is showing some success in decreasing the costs of medical care, and cost consciousness is expected to remain a dominating concern of those who pay for health services. A basic precept of managed care is the importance of achieving optimal health status in enrollees in order to minimize the occurrence of costly illness and injury. Given this concern for the health status of subscribers, formal relationships should increase between managed-care companies and other organizations working to improve population health status. The organization traditionally responsible for the health status of populations is the local public health department, so it is logical to hope that the coming years will see substantially more cooperation, coordination, and collaboration than currently exists between local public health departments and managed-care companies.

This synergy of interests is most apparent in "maturing" managed-care markets where a significant portion of the population is enrolled in managed care. The growth of Medicaid managed care includes, as subscribers, population groups with less-than-average health status, often in a capitated rather than a discounted fee-for-service plan. This should make managed-care organizations even more concerned with maintaining and improving the overall health status of enrollees. Managed-care organizations actually face a severe downside risk by accepting responsibility for individuals who need more social and health services than the average enrollee of several years ago.

It is public health departments and other community agencies that have the experience, skills, and services to meet the special needs of socioeconomically disadvantaged people. If the pundits are correct in predicting that almost all communities are moving toward managed care, then the imperative for collaboration between health departments and managed-care organizations is even more powerful. Without collaboration, it is likely that Medicaid reimbursements to health departments will diminish as current health department Medicaid clients are forced to enroll in managed care, with a resultant decrease in the capacity of health departments to cross-subsidize health services for the growing number of uninsured. Without collaboration, it is also likely that managed-care organizations will either fail to meet the

needs of many of their enrollees or be forced to duplicate services currently based in health departments.

One can hope that the logical approach of developing local collaborative networks of health departments, managed-care organizations, hospitals, academic institutions, and others to assess community health needs and develop a coordinated response focused on improving community health status would become the norm across the nation. Managed-care organizations have the resources to support efforts to develop community partnerships such as these, and they stand to benefit if amelioration of community health problems improves the health status of their enrollees. Enlightened self-interest has the potential to improve both the health of subscribers and the organization's financial picture.

THE EFFECTIVE HEALTH DEPARTMENT OF THE FUTURE

The public health system in the United States is in a state of significant flux. Some of the characteristics of this evolving system include shifts towards the provision of services based on demonstrated need and potential impact, modelled after the year 2000 objectives for the nation; multidisciplinary team-based approaches to problem solving; growing community involvement; closer linkages between prevention and treatment services; and closer linkages between practice and academia.

To be effective, public health agencies of the future must be aware of these continuing waves of change and exhibit the understanding and flexibility required to adapt activities to their environment so that public health services will be appropriately designed and effectively delivered. Also to be effective, public health departments must be positioned as the health intelligence centers of their respective communities; that is, they must be the source of epidemiologically based thinking and analysis of their community's approach to dealing with health matters. They must be facilitators of strong and meaningful community participation in the assessment and prioritization of community health problems and issues. They must be major participants in public policy decision making, and they must both deliver and broker the delivery of services needed by their constituent populations. Finally, they must be focused on health outcomes as measures of the impact of interventions.

Accomplishing these tasks will require that health departments work from the strongest organizational base possible and that they hone and expand the capacities that are necessary to accomplish the core functions of public health and the other services assigned to them by their respective communities.

Many local health departments are too small and too resource-poor even to attempt to play the role now expected of them, let alone to be taken seriously as players by community decision makers. The findings of the Institute of Medicine described in *The Future of Public Health* and the description of local health departments contained in Chapter 7 demonstrate clearly that the old penchant for home rule has outlived its usefulness. To be effective, health departments must represent a constituency large enough that geographic boundaries of authority make sense to the citizenry, that funding is stable, and that the tax base is adequate to provide the local share of resources needed to assure that at least the core functions of public health are accomplished.

Effective health departments will require a governance structure that clearly delineates policy and administrative functions between the board of health (or other governing body) and the director of the department. Additionally, the primary concern of governance must be the description and solution of public health problems in the constituent community rather than the political correctness of the department's actions.

Those of today's public health leaders, who are reluctant to embrace community participation and adopt new ways of thinking and acting, may actually be significant barriers to the change that is required if every citizen is to be served by a strong and effective public health agency. Effective health departments will have leaders who exhibit commitment, charisma, and drive, and who embrace collective action, community empowerment, consumer advocacy, and egalitarianism.[14]

New technology is moving the nation into an information-rich future. Dealing appropriately with this reality will require computer equipment and analytical skills that provide access to the information available and allow for the correct interpretation of its meaning. Health departments must be able to analyze

information about the world they find themselves in and determine the appropriate response to it. This means they must be connected to the "information superhighway" and be capable of recognizing information and trends that are relevant to the health of their constituents. Every department should subscribe to a large electronic network, such as *Compuserve* or *Internet*, and be connected with the Centers for Disease Control and Prevention through *PCWonder* and the developing *Information Network for Public Health Officials (INPHO)*. Departments must be able to collect and analyze information from their own communities, as well. At a minimum, agencies should be proficient in the use of the computer software package *Epi-Info*, but they should also be thinking imaginatively about the potential use of home computers and interactive television in assessing community perceptions of health needs and priorities. These capacities are basic to future policy and program development and evaluation.

The effective health department will enable individual citizens to take responsibility for decision making related to the community's health as well as their own. Citizens will be involved both in setting the community's priorities for public health issue study and action and in assessing the impact of programs and services designed to improve community health.

It is doubtful that any health department has available the resources needed to carry out the community's full public health agenda. Thus, assuring that all citizens receive the services they require for good health will require that public health departments build strong collaborative and cooperative linkages with other community health agencies and with the illness care system in the community. These collaborative arrangements will be with other health departments, other departments of local government, community health centers, school systems, and community agencies such as Planned Parenthood, the American Lung Association, the American Cancer Society, neighborhood block clubs, and environmental groups, to name just a few. Such collaboration is necessary for effective health promotion and disease prevention efforts to occur. Joint programming and service and referral arrangements with hospitals, managed-care companies, group medical practices, individual physicians, and other providers of illness services are necessary to assure that each citizen has access to a seamless web of services that promote health, prevent illness, diagnose disease early, and provide disease treatment that is efficient and effective.

Improvements in those activities and services intended to advance the public's health are strongly dependent upon increasing knowledge of the effectiveness of current or planned actions. They also depend upon the ability to bring well-trained professionals into the field of public health. The practice of and the academic base for public health have been allowed to become relatively isolated from one another. This reality has been recognized, and work is underway to link the two settings in a manner that will improve the level of training of local public health workers and increasingly focus research efforts on public health administration and service delivery concerns. If at all possible, the effective local health department will welcome students and faculty from academic settings who have the potential to contribute to the understanding of local public health issues and strengthen the capacities of the local public health workforce. The health department should also be supportive of its current employees who wish to pursue additional public health training and/or become adjunct or part-time faculty members. The Public Health Training Network under development by the Public Health Practice Program Office of the Centers for Disease Control and Prevention is an important example of low-cost, high-quality professional training made possible by the use of distance-learning techniques.

CONCLUSION

This is an extraordinary time, and change is in the air. It is a time when no one is clearly in charge of the public health world. Consequently, there are remarkable opportunities for entrepreneurial efforts to reshape the public health system. It is a time for public health leaders to take responsibility for shaping the profession's collective destiny. If that leadership can be exerted so that the public health system can break out of old molds that are no longer functional, there is every reason to believe that public health workers will provide a valuable service to their communities, and that it will be recognized as

such. The most important element of that recognition, of course, will be steady, measurable gains in community health status.

REFERENCES

1. McKeown T. *Medicine in Modern Society—Medical Planning Based on Evaluation of Medical Achievement.* London, England: Allen & Vawin; 1966.

2. *Health Care Reform and Public Health.* Washington, DC: Office of Disease Prevention and Health Promotion, US Public Health Service; 1993.

3. *Healthy People: The Surgeon General's Report on Health Promotion and Disease Prevention.* Washington, DC: US Dept of Health and Human Services, Public Health Service; 1979.

4. *Guide to Clinical Preventive Services.* 2nd ed. Baltimore, Md: Williams & Wilkins; 1996.

5. American Public Health Association, et al. *Model Standards: A Guide for Community Preventive Health Services.* 2nd ed. Washington, DC: American Public Health Association; 1985:4.

6. Institute of Medicine, Committee for the Study of the Future of Public Health. *The Future of Public Health.* Washington, DC: National Academy Press; 1988.

7. Washington State Department of Health. *Public Health Improvement Plan.* Olympia, Wa: Washington State Department of Health; 1994.

8. *Blueprint for a Healthy Community: A Guide for Local Health Departments.* Washington, DC: National Association of County Health Officials; 1994.

9. *Health Security Act, Title III—Public Health Initiatives, HR3600.* Washington, DC: 103rd Congress; 1993.

10. Sorensen AA, Bialek RG. *The Public Health Faculty Agency Forum: Linking Graduate Education and Practice, Final Report.* Gainesville, Fl: University Press of Florida; 1993.

11. *National Profile of Local Health Departments.* Washington, DC: National Association of County Health Officials; 1990.

12. Cleveland H. Leadership in the new world disorder. Presented at the Public Health Leadership Institute; November 8, 1992; Washington, DC.

13. Cleveland H. *The Knowledge Executive: Leadership in an Information Society.* New York, NY: E.P. Dutton; 1985.

14. Lloyd P. Management competencies in health for all/new public settings. *J Health Admin Ed.* Spring, 1994;12(2):187–207.

INDEX